Thanks for
neighborliness,

Sprawl Kills

How blandburbs steal your
time, health and money.

Joel S. Hirschhorn, Ph.D.

PUBLISHERS

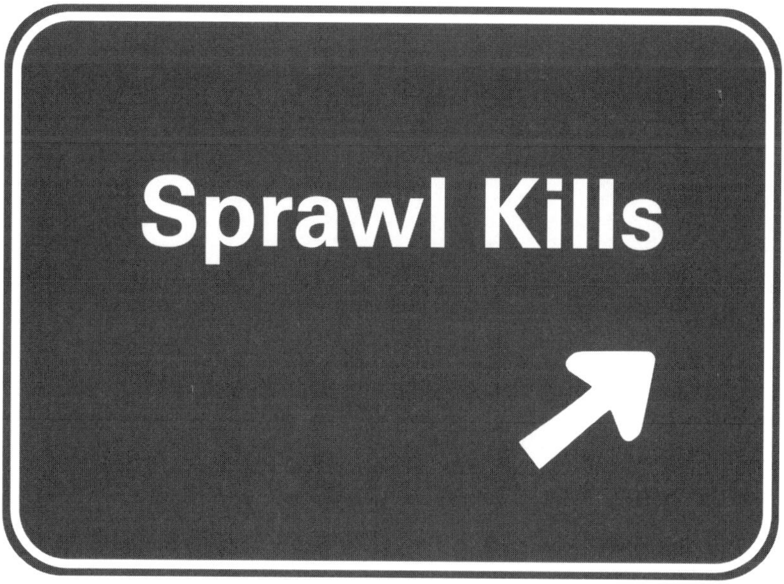
Sprawl Kills

FOR YOU,

READER, CITIZEN,
AND CONSUMER

COME JOIN ME
ON A MIND-WALK
TO A BETTER PLACE

CONTENTS

Printed in the United States of America.

Published by Sterling & Ross Publishers
115 W. 29th St. New York, NY 10001

www.sterlingandross.com

Cover Design by Ben Peterson

Page composition/typography by Ben Peterson

ISBN: 0-9766372-0-0

FIRST EDITION

10 9 8 7 6 5 4 3 2 1

LIST OF FIGURES

ACKNOWLEDGMENTS

I owe my introduction to smart growth, land use, urban revitalization and related subjects to my former position as Director of Environment, Energy and Natural Resources at the National Governors Association, where I was allowed to design and obtain funding for a number of projects and publications. I had the good fortune to be at NGA when then Maryland Governor Parris Glendening was Chairman and I directed his special initiative "Where Do We Grow From Here?" As part of this initiative, the Growth and Quality of Life Tool Kit was developed and made available to governors and the public. Through directing many projects and organizing various meetings related to smart growth I gained a deep understanding of the complexities of the subject; these were enabled by funding from the Robert Wood Johnson Foundation, the David and Lucile Packard Foundation, the U.S. Environmental Protection Agency, the U.S. Department of Transportation, the U.S. Department of Housing and Urban Development, the Centers for Disease Control and Prevention, and others.

Several of my associates at NGA provided helpful comments on early drafts of this book, especially Tracey Westfield and Ethan Brown.

Many of the ideas in *Sprawl Kills* were developed and tested in many public talks I gave over the past several years and in a number of articles. I thank the audiences who provided feedback and the many readers who sent me their thoughts and comments. Many colleagues and strangers provided the encouragement needed to write a hard-hitting book. In particular, Elizabeth Revelise provided support and comments when times were difficult.

Over several years my wife, Jacqueline Rams, put up with my obsessive search for perfection in content and writing, and the stress of getting a book published.

FOREWORD

Sprawl Kills is a wake-up call for America. This country has managed to engineer an everyday world that has contributed to an enormous public health burden. Dr. Hirschhorn's book helps to identify the fact that our health is under siege from forces within the built environment and that our communities are not as safe and healthy as we are led to believe.

Sprawl Kills highlights the recent widespread attention given to the relationships between where we live, how we travel, and our health, and makes a convincing argument that our communities may deter or entirely prevent people from choosing healthy behaviors and living well.

Sprawl Kills considers various possibilities for the way we have been developing our communities and how that pattern of development has upset the balance of human behavior. For example, over the past several decades, we have found innovative ways to engineer routine forms of physical activity out of our daily lives. Few people are using active approaches to complete simple tasks such as climbing the stairs, mowing the lawn, or even walking or bicycling to nearby destinations. This is complicated by the notion that most Americans seek the most convenient way of doing things, often translating into less physical activity. With the rising percentage of children and adults who are overweight and obese we need to consider more carefully how community design supports healthy behavior.

This book highlights how our neighborhoods were once valued for the presence of people who walked and biked along their sidewalks and streets. Now opportunities for walking and biking have been socially and physically engineered out of our daily routines. This is especially damaging to children for whom physical activity is a vital part of their overall development and understanding of what is good about the neighborhoods in which they are being raised.

In public health we often use indicator species to determine the state of the environment. The appearance of these species and the status of their health usually express the viability of their habitat. This basic scientific method can be used to illustrate the state of our communities and their inhabitants, especially the children. Children are an ideal indicator of a healthy community, but regrettably if we use children as our indicator of analysis it would reveal an environment poorly designed to support important behaviors of childhood such as physical activity, even very basic forms of activity such as walking and bicycling. And this is easily reflected in the precipitous decline in the number of children who walk or bicycle to school – now only 13% manage to do so regularly.

A possible factor influencing this is our current development patterns and sprawl. Sprawl has influenced how children seek out active play, and now the unfortunate reality is that most children spend more time watching television or playing computer games than being physically active. This may explain why nearly half of young people today are not vigorously active on a daily basis, and why the percentage of children who are overweight has almost tripled in the last 30 years. These data bring to light a trend that affects our social and cultural capacity to build healthy communities, and sadly this trend has gone largely unnoticed, and most of America has accepted sprawl as the norm without realizing the detrimental impacts on their health.

Sprawl Kills brings to light the reasons why we should be concerned about this nation's development trends and why we need to support efforts to create healthier communities. Dr. Hirschhorn does an extraordinary job of identifying the impacts of the built environment and transportation and how they shape our choices and opportunities to engage in healthy lifestyles.

Sprawl Kills makes a persuasive connection that the auto-dominant design of most communities has contributed to thousands of pedestrian injuries and fatalities annually, and its ability to provide clean air and water, mitigate noise and land pollution, and minimize the impacts of urban heat islands. All of these issues not only disturb healthy human functioning, but also damage a sensitive eco-system that is struggling to cope with increasing encroachment on Mother Nature. The result is often avoidable disability, premature loss of life, and extraordinarily high economic consequences.

It is a common belief that people don't appreciate their health until they get sick, their freedom until they are restricted, or their prosperity until it is threatened. The primary argument of *Sprawl Kills* is that all three of these values are under siege because of the disconnect that has occurred between how we design our communities and how they support a healthy lifestyle. Dr. Hirschhorn provides an excellent overview of the dilemma we are in and a powerful call to action. *Sprawl Kills* helps us to recognize our role in the scheme of this crisis and how we can make a difference in shaping our communities so they can provide choices to be healthy. We have a great challenge before us that requires better collaboration in how we build our cities. We must commit ourselves to develop a viable strategy that supports healthier community design. Dr. Hirschhorn challenges our current thinking and provides an influential discussion with innovative solutions to reclaim our communities and create healthy places for everyone to have the choices to live well and prosper.

A resounding message from *Sprawl Kills* is that we are all accountable to leaving a legacy for future generations to thrive and grow. The challenge lies in leaving a legacy for our children, our neighborhoods, our cities, and this nation that is built upon creating and supporting a built environment that offers choices to be healthier. Leaving a legacy of this magnitude will result in many other beneficial outcomes; most importantly it will advance the value of our cities, improve the quality of life and help develop better health outcomes. This book is a must read for anyone recognizing their accountability to do something to improve their community and leave something of significance for future generations to respect, cherish and grow.

RICHARD E. KILLINGSWORTH
Director & Associate Research Professor
School of Public Health
The University of North Carolina

PREFACE

I know that millions of Americans like living in today's suburbia. They believe they have achieved the American dream. They have a large house on a large lot in the middle of what was previously known as 'nowhere'. They merrily drive to just about every event in their lives. But there are also millions of Americans (and increasingly those who used to belong to the first group) who think the dream has turned to nightmare, and pejoratively call it "sprawl." There are two basic ways of framing the suburbs-sprawl debate, each having strong believers and advocates:

CONVENTIONAL THINKING: Suburban life is good; it is your American dream. The term sprawl is a negative view of suburbia and disrespects the majority of Americans who live in and like suburbia. People who condemn sprawl criticize the American dream and want to deprive you of reaching or keeping it— particularly spacious homes. Suburbia is your right, the right to own private land and a home. Some traffic congestion is just the reasonable price you pay for affordable housing, a high quality suburban life, and many shopping opportunities. Sprawl is a sign of American prosperity and success that people in other nations envy. There is more than enough land to provide this American dream for a growing population.

ALTERNATIVE THINKING: Suburbia is geography, places outside cities. For 50 years suburbs have been designed on the sprawl model alone, with all key parts of daily life widely separated on land, requiring constant motor vehicle use. Public space is mostly for cars and shopping, not social interaction. Suburbs can be designed compactly, however, so you can get to most things by walking or short vehicle trips, and live in a close-knit, neighborly community with great public spaces. But the land development and home building industries, with government help, produce sprawl. You are deprived of housing and transportation choice and quality of life benefits. Uncontrolled sprawl development is eating up our natural world, paving it over, and reducing cherished greenspaces.

I expect that by the time you finish this book you will vigorously support the alternative framework. Americans will choose alternatives to sprawl once they are armed with the right information. *Sprawl Kills* provides the most compelling case ever presented for rejecting sprawl and choosing its beneficial alternative by providing a broader scope of evidence and information than ever before available. Do not equate sprawl with suburbia. Suburbia is not the enemy, sprawl is. Suburbia was not always dominated by sprawl and it does not have to remain so.

I have read about, studied, and lived in sprawl. I have listened to all the arguments made by sprawl's defenders. I was born and raised in New York City where walking was my passion and everyday mode of transport, and my family did not have a car until I started college. I was and remain a walkaholic. I have also lived in Meriden, Connecticut; Troy, New York; Madison, Wisconsin; Houston, Texas; Washington, D.C.; and some foreign places, not as a tourist, but because of work, including Cairo, Egypt; Amsterdam, the Netherlands; Paris, France; and Jakarta, Indonesia.

America has settled for a lowered quality of life by surrendering to sprawl. After fifty years of sprawl dominance, few Americans appreciate what preceded sprawl and what can and should replace new sprawl. So many business interests, what I call the "sprawl industry," have prospered while destroying our natural environment, social fabric, and personal health. Housing is needed. But we know how to build communities that offer incredible benefits over sprawl. Sprawl should no longer be successful. But it is.

People who like sprawl have plenty to choose from in the marketplace. Sprawl subdivisions are everywhere. In high growth areas trying to accommodate substantial increases in population, sprawl is almost the only housing choice. True, consumers may have to settle for sprawl housing at greater distances from their jobs to get a house they can afford, but they see that as a rational tradeoff. With better information, it doesn't have to be that way.

Sprawl Kills is primarily for consumers and explains how they can use their power in the housing market — for the people who like sprawl, the people who hate it, and those who are ambivalent about it. But I know that urban designers and planners, architects, real estate professionals, developers, home builders, social scientists, and health professionals will benefit from this new treatment of familiar subjects.

After fifty years of American housing and culture being dominated by sprawl, many people do not know any other style of living. They have had no other choice, assuming they ruled out living in a city or old town. Can those who like sprawl see their world differently? Only if they better understand how sprawl harms them. And only if they believe there is a practical alternative to sprawl. As you read, you will understand and you will believe that we can do better than sprawl.

Others see sprawl as evil and the cause of just about every ill of American society. As you read, such feelings will turn from anger to a pragmatic strategy of embracing a true alternative form of housing and community.

What if sprawl is not an issue for you? If you are willing to consider new information, what I present will allow you to better appreciate your current non-sprawl form of living. The challenge for sprawl residents is to see beyond the choices already made. You will experience what I call "data of the absurd." So much unbelievable information about sprawl and its consequences that you will end up questioning how the nation ever allowed it to spread across the land.

In seeking the alternative to sprawl, however, consumers face housing that masquerades as something different than run-of-the-mill sprawl. Why do developers and builders play such games? Because they know that many consumers desire something other than sprawl. Yet they do not offer authentic alternatives because building sprawl housing is so much easier and less expensive for them.

I call true alternatives to sprawl "HEALTHY PLACES." More than 200 of them have been built in many states and the rate is accelerating. People seeking HEALTHY PLACES have different perspectives. Some want a solution to the mounting traffic congestion plaguing so many areas of the country and yet others seek a higher quality environmental setting. Still others think in terms of a higher quality of life associated with old-fashioned, walkable neighborhoods. Oddly, few people realize that perhaps the best reason to seek an alternative to sprawl is protecting and improving their health through active living, which is not the same thing as exercise.

For some years, many books, newspaper stories, magazine articles, and television programs have strongly attacked sprawl. The attacks focus on automobile dependence, traffic congestions, ugly surroundings, rapid consumption of land, and loss of environmental quality. Much of this activity is part of the national "smart growth" movement. Unlike other works, the focus in *Sprawl Kills* is on helping consumers make better housing decisions, and not on abstract public policy or lofty social and environmental goals.

The housing and real estate market can be made to work better, if consumer demand for HEALTHY PLACES asserts itself. Rather than selling smart growth on the basis of idealistic principles, such as protecting the natural environment or saving cities, *Sprawl Kills* uses a market-based approach. Market forces can displace sprawl through the informed decisions of consumers to choose a better housing product that gives them greater benefits. Consumer demand can also pressure government to remove the regulatory distortions of the housing market that now favor sprawl. Let sprawl compete in a fair market against HEALTHY PLACES. Blaming the government does not work. Citizens must take responsibility and seek a solution within *their* control.

Just like appreciating peace requires knowing something about the horrors of war, consumers must know about the harm of sprawl to appreciate its alternative. Presenting material about the negative aspects of sprawl is necessary for understanding the benefits of the alternative to sprawl. Make no mistake; this is not so much a book about sprawl as it is about housing, community, and health.

"Sprawl kills" is not a cute metaphor. It is a fact. *Sprawl really does kill people.* Sprawl makes people fat, tired, depressed, stressed, more likely to die in auto accidents, and succumb to very serious disease. "Sprawl kills" is also an idea that needs to spread like a virus. These two simple, powerful words convey the key motivational message. They define the problem for which HEALTHY PLACES are the solution.

Scientific evidence reveals that about 70 percent of a person's health and longevity can be controlled and only about 30 percent is genetically programmed. Much of that 70 percent can be associated with the built-environment that surrounds people in their everyday lives. Readers will learn that sprawl creates a set of conditions and behaviors that indisputably harm health. Americans need to take sprawl personally, not as some abstraction, nor unalterable feature of American society. Sprawl may be ugly, but that is a matter of taste. That sprawl is unhealthy is far more important. In fact, sprawl kills more than just people.

Sprawl Kills will show you that it is best to see overweight and obesity as *a cause* of disease rather than as a disease itself, sedentariness as *a cause* of overweight and obesity, and a poorly designed built environment as *a cause* of sedentariness.

Some analogies are useful. For most of us, the case against cigarette smoking is compelling. Yet about a quarter of Americans still smoke, which means some 75 million people. Using seat belts in automobiles and not driving while intoxicated are also agreed to be in the interest of drivers. Yet millions of drivers do not practice these safety measures.

No case made against sprawl will entirely remove the desire for it or get rid of what already exists. No laws will be passed to outlaw sprawl. But the 'big picture' is not the number one issue. What matters most are the individual decisions that are made about where to live. More of those decisions can and should be made for true alternatives to sprawl – HEALTHY PLACES. But this requires more determination and work. Sprawl is for lazy consumers.

One thing is clear. Consumers deserve more choice in the housing marketplace. If sprawl is about the only option, then it is an illusion to believe that consumers really prefer sprawl, as the sprawl industry will have us believe.

When more people choose HEALTHY PLACES over sprawl to selfishly improve their own lives, the world will change for the better, one consumer at a time. Automobiles did not become safer and more reliable, and cigarette smoking did not drop dramatically just because of what companies or the government did. Consumers changed and those changes dictated an industry change. The population sent clear messages about what they believed served their own interest. American industry resisted. In the case of automobiles, competition came to the rescue from foreign automakers. In the case of cigarettes, information came to the rescue, about preventable disease and death. Consumers must act.

Consumers *can* change the American housing industry – the sprawl industry that has succeeded for 50 years. Innovative developers are already overcoming obstacles and building HEALTHY PLACES to meet consumers' needs. The goal of *Sprawl Kills* is to spread information about HEALTHY PLACES to help loosen sprawl's grip on the nation. Throughout the book I provide information about actual HEALTHY PLACES to illustrate the concepts discussed. I have selected these places to show geographical diversity, and communities built from scratch on greenfield sites as well as smaller neighborhoods built or improved within existing cities and suburbs. There is real progress providing HEALTHY PLACES throughout the nation. Yet statistically, sprawl dominates the housing market despite its shortcomings.

This is what must be learned. The design of the built environment affects everything people do. But most people have not recognized the impacts of the built environment on the quality of their lives. That helps explain why sprawl has remained so successful long after it served some critical needs after World War II. And why more consumers have not yet become a force for change in the marketplace.

For the first time *Sprawl Kills* exposes the sprawl industry's political power, particularly of land developers and home builders. This story is ripped not from the headlines but from the shadows of sprawl. Consumers need to understand how – *and by whom* – they and the housing market are manipulated. But illuminating the sprawl industry lacks the pizzazz of divulging the truth about the automobile and fast-food industries, for example. The reason is simple. Everyone buys housing, yet pretty much no one is familiar with specific companies, except perhaps the one that built their home. Unlike companies such as McDonald's and General Motors, that millions of consumers immediately recognize, sprawl industry companies are largely invisible.

The paradox is that even though sprawl surrounds everyone, it is also "un-branded." Success and profit in the sprawl industry do not require name recognition. If you are a consumer and can name the largest home builders in the nation, you are unique – for examplePulte and D.R. Horton. You will see why not being in the public's awareness has helped the sprawl industry maintain its monopolistic control of the real estate market. You will learn about the politics of sprawl that until now have been hidden from public view, and you will probably become angry and outraged. You will learn who makes up the small army of sprawl apologists and supporters. Consumers continue to be betrayed and deceived. It is time for truth about the sprawl lobby and its corruption of the housing market by spending and dirty tricks.

Fortunately, no market domination is perfect. The long overdue replacement of sprawl with HEALTHY PLACES is emerging. But more than technical changes in planning, building and street design are at stake. Think in terms of a cultural revolution that reshapes lives and society for the better. To succeed, the politics of sprawl must be confronted and overcome, which is why the first chapter is about the power and corrupting influences of the sprawl industry.

Great books change the world, like Rachel Carson's *Silent Spring* and

Ralph Nader's *Unsafe At Any Speed*; they did what Albert Einstein said was needed: "We cannot solve the problems we have created with the same thinking that created them." We need new thinking about sprawl, housing, community and American culture. With your help this book will spark a housing revolution and shake up the debilitating sprawl culture that harms all of us.

Imagine you are house hunting. First you visit a typical sprawl subdivision and examine a wonderful large estate house on a one-acre lot on a quiet cul-de-sac street with no sidewalks. Your commute to work in another suburb will be at least 90 minutes one-way and that of your spouse 60 minutes to get downtown. The congested commute roads have big box stores, a major mall and many strip malls. Later, you inspect a much smaller home on a small lot in a new HEALTHY PLACE, close to other small houses, all with front porches. A ten-minute walk takes you to the town center that has all the stores you normally use plus several eateries or to a great park and a system of scenic trails for walking or biking. You would save 2 hours a day commuting. Your spouse could walk to a light rail station for a 20-minute trip downtown and a short walk to the office. But the house is only 2,000 square feet compared to 3,100 square feet for the sprawl house, and it has just a small patio in back and a tiny front yard. Financially, the 55 percent larger sprawl house with two extra rooms and a large deck is *$55,000 less.*

Psychologically, the conspicuous consumption of the sprawl house is valued more, because its physical attributes are visible and immediately available. The HEALTHY PLACE house is disadvantaged. You are buying *imagined experiences* that you hope will happen: use of the trails, more free time because of less car use, better relationships with close-by neighbors, and more use of downtown theaters, museums and restaurants. You can only estimate how the lower car, lawn maintenance and utility costs may offset the higher monthly mortgage cost. You might even get rid of one car. Further, you can theorize whether adaptation to the larger sprawl house might mean *less* satisfaction over time (typical with conspicuous consumption), and whether your use of the outdoor amenities and the extra time you get in the HEALTHY PLACE might provide *more* pleasure over time (typical with inconspicuous consumption) and advance better health.

Such difficult housing decisions will be easier with the information and ways of thinking *Sprawl Kills* provides.

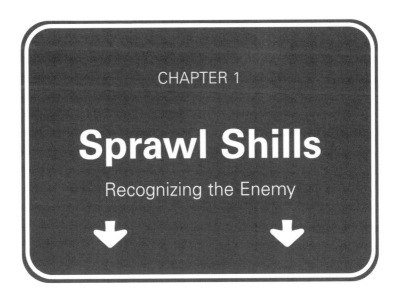

CHAPTER 1

Sprawl Shills

Recognizing the Enemy

Sprawl deceives.

A war rages in the United States; the people vs. the tyranny of relentless, runaway suburban sprawl. Residents trying to retain rural character, quality of life, farmland or greenspace fight business interests primed to profit from more land development. Local governments usually select sprawl over smart growth. But sprawl puppet-masters are beginning to lose control.

Throughout the nation the drama plays out daily, but the sprawl land war does not end. With so much money at stake sprawl battles are fought again and again. The Portland, Oregon metropolitan area is renowned for controlling sprawl. Yet in the spring of 2004 Bill Kenny with the "Coalition to Save the Valley," one of hundreds of grassroots groups trying to limit sprawl, was under attack, and wrote in *The Oregonian*: "Urban sprawl is not inevitable. It is a choice we make, in this case driven by the greed of speculators and an indifferent shrug by complicit public officials who lack the courage and vision to preserve what is unique and productive about the land we love."

Kenny's group was backing a courageous attempt by Councilor Carl Hosticka, of the Metro regional government, to define the Willamette River as the southern limit to the Portland urban growth area. Most local officials in the Willamette Valley backed the proposed ordinance, particularly Wilsonville Mayor Charlotte Lehan, living on land her ancestors bought in 1880. She and others believed it critical to save the agricultural and rural valley and its unique natural resources for eternity. She said, "I don't think we did Oregon land-use planning in the 1970s to be for 30 years and then it would (turn into) strip development." Rural lifestyle was in jeopardy. And Lake Oswego Mayor Judie Hammerstad said what so many Americans felt: "They're not making land like this anymore." Certainly not like this Oregon land treasure.

On the other side were Chris and Tom Maletis, who bought the 173-acre Langdon Farms Golf Club in 2002 in anticipation of getting inside the urban growth boundary. Land values could jump 1,000 percent. They hired expensive lawyers and a politically connected consultant, a partner in former Governor Neil Goldschmidt's firm and a board member of the Port of Portland who had to resign from an advisory committee to the Metro government because of his conflict of interest. Across the highway Wayne Russell operated a 72-acre nursery on land his family worked for four generations. His son agreed that expanding Portland's boundary across the river would end the valley's agriculture industry. Wayne Russell surrendered to development: "We think it's going to come across the river, so we might as well move on." Sell out, take the money and move on, like thousands of other large land owners across the nation. Supporting the boundary expansion was the Port of Portland and Beaverton Mayor Rob Drake who had worked at a company of the Meletis brothers and accused mayors on the other side of backing "the feel-good thing to do." Preserving the valley's character *would* feel good and was something to be proud of.

In March 2004, by a vote of 17 to 4 the Hostika ordinance to preserve the current growth boundary was supported by the Metro Policy Advisory Committee. But would the seven-member Metro Council, with power over land use in 24 cities and three counties, ultimately pass the measure? Or would sprawl supporters defeat it? Laura Oppenheimer of *The Oregonian* noted: "The Metro Council rarely deviates from a forceful message sent by its advisory group." But supporters were uncertain. Only time will tell.

ELECTED OFFICIALS MUST LISTEN TO VOTERS

Nothing is more important than understanding how sprawl politics control the housing market. The only way to give consumers more alternatives to sprawl is to stop the influence of the sprawl lobby. Otherwize consumer demand for alternatives to suburban sprawl will not be satisfied. Pity those elected officials who publicly castigate and oppose sprawl. They face brutal attacks by very powerful sprawl interests. Despite taking $1.5 million from developers in his campaign to become governor, New Jersey Governor James E. McGreevey courageously spoke out against sprawl in his 2003 state-of-the state address:

Congestion and sprawl threaten our quality of life. It is time to draw the line and say 'no more' to mindless sprawl.

There is no single greater threat to our way of life in New Jersey than the unrestrained, uncontrolled development that has jeopardized our water supplies, made our schools more crowded, our roads congested, and our open space disappear. Will we take on the special interests, and finally end the cycle of unchecked development that is destroying our quality of life?

Wealthy developers use their deep pockets and expensive legal talent to take towns to court if those towns dare oppose their development efforts. They can effectively bully unwilling taxpayers into submission.

The days of builders saddling taxpayers with the costs of development are over. We will establish impact fees so that developers, instead of local taxpayers, bear the burden for the cost of added roads and new schools. Let me say to those who profit from the strip malls and McMansions — if you reap the benefits, you must also take responsibility for the costs.

No governor has ever been so explicit about the sprawl threat, but what McGreevey said applies to almost every state in the Union. And like in most other states, after McGreevey delivered this address, the sprawl industry struck back.

At New Jersey's 2003 annual builders' convention with over 8,000 attendees, petitions were circulated to express opposition to the governor's anti-sprawl campaign. Attendees cursed the governor as television monitors played an endless loop of the speech in which the governor declared war on runaway development. And the head of the New Jersey Builders Association warned of the impact of the state's growth management efforts: "There will be no place outside the ghettos for middle-income and low-income New Jerseyans." It was a not so subtle scare tactic. Control sprawl and people will have to live in dangerous inner-city ghettos. Suburban sprawl or urban hell is the choice offered by home builders.

Some nine months after the governor's address, *The New York Times* ran a story, "War on Sprawl in New Jersey Hits a Wall." The governor's ambitious proposals were stalled. Why? Home builders used their muscle with the state legislature. A McGreevey official was quoted: "I don't think anyone was under any illusion that the Legislature was not and is not under the thrall of the builders' lobby to a large extent." Legislators stooped to the sprawl industry. In March 2004 *New Jersey Monthly* quoted a senior McGreevey official: "We got killed by the builders. The power of that lobby, the fear they strike into the hearts of legislators of both parties, is enormous." David Pringle, head of the New Jersey Environmental Federation, said the builders, "have no interest in smart growth and comprehensive planning. The building association has very slyly used politicians' dependence on money to tilt the playing field in their favor. You'd have to be a blind idiot to think builder money doesn't control the Legislature." Ironically, but predictably as we'll see later on, the website of the Builders Association contains a toolbox section with the heading, "Building a Smart growth State."

In 2004 the McGreevey administration adopted storm-water regulations to stop development within 300 feet of more than 3,000 miles of protected rivers and streams. More than 200,000 acres could be out of bounds for development. So the New Jersey Builders Association started a legal challenge, calling the governor's anti-sprawl policies "anti-housing."

Sprawl politics in New Jersey suppresses smart growth despite consumers' pain from stubborn sprawl and their desire for HEALTHY PLACES. A 2004 survey found that 64 percent of New Jerseyans believe there's too much commercial and housing development where they live. Annual permits for new homes for 1998 to 2003 were nearly twice that in 1990. Sprawl is the spam of the built environment; it keeps coming, people bitch and moan about it, but nobody seems capable of stopping it. Not even governors.

> SPRAWL: (verb) to grow, develop, or spread irregularly, carelessly, or awkwardly and without apparent design or plan, as in "the city sprawls down the whole coast;" noun, haphazard growth or extension outward, especially that resulting from new housing on the outskirts of a city.

> SMART GROWTH: (noun) sensible growth: economic growth that consciously seeks to avoid wastefulness and damage to the environment and communities.

So what makes up this powerful but ignored sprawl industry? Look for companies that make money directly or indirectly from sprawl development. Most important are land developers, land speculators and builders. Add a large army of architects, real estate agents, investors, planners, traffic engineers, construction companies, engineering firms, land use attorneys, and consultants. Plus powerful trade associations, notably the National Association of Home Builders, the National Association of Realtors, and the National Association of Industrial and Office Properties that also have local and state groups. Then count the automobile and road building industries, their suppliers, plus their trade associations (see Figure 1-1).

On the side of sprawl is much of the retail industry that feed off roads, especially national fast food and big box chains. Do not ignore the pharmaceutical industry that benefits from selling drugs to manage the ill effects of physical inactivity and sprawl stress. Home lawn care businesses also benefit from sprawl. Then there are all the industries making electronic products for making home refuges more comfortable for couch potatoes. And note the new and expanding business of making products for bigger people that sprawl helps create, including plus-size clothing, super-size towels, seat belt extenders, home scales handling up to 1,000 pounds, and devices to help the obese put on their socks and wash their bodies.

Sprawl politics are everywhere. Many governors trying to fight sprawl and support smart growth have been stung and sometimes prevented from even trying to do anything. Some have attempted to avoid opposition by using terms other than smart growth, including quality-growth, balanced growth, sensible-growth, livability, and grow-smart. It does not work. Governors have often taken the safe route of stressing land conservation and brownfields (areas of land reclaimed from pollution) programs. The sprawl industry has little problem with these, because public funds cannot buy enough land to significantly diminish sprawl development in most areas, nor has urban brownfield site redevelopment siphoned off many customers from sprawl.

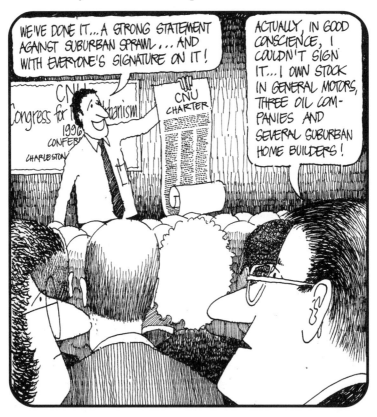

Figure 1-1. Many parts of the American economy prosper from sprawl development.

Stressing urban revitalization is also a safe route. Actions aimed directly at sprawl bring out the sprawl lobby, including: compelling local governments to adopt effective planning, requiring them to have urban growth boundaries, and enabling them to levy impact fees on developers to pay for public infrastructure like roads and sewage and water lines. Limiting new highway construction is also dangerous for politicians.

Consider these cases:

In the fall of 2001 Missouri Governor Bob Holden announced his intention to issue an Executive Order establishing a task force to examine growth issues. But vicious right-wing opposition caused him to back down. A group called the Missouri Eagle Forum utilized traditional conservative scare tactics and put out a lot of nutty rhetoric: "If implemented, Smart growth will necessarily lead to diminished individual freedom. …The end result will be total government control of all Missourians' lives." A group called Restoring America warned "this is a really huge attack on freedom and individual rights." Other opponents said that the task force would control private property rights. The efforts of a number of groups supporting the governor and smart growth were no match for such fear-inducing rhetoric.

Years of studies had identified the need for growth management initiatives in Michigan, but former 12-year governor John Engler did little. In 2002 Jennifer Granholm was elected governor of Michigan and said: "We don't want a state adorned with strip malls and wearing only gray pavement," and, "Agriculture, forestry, mining and tourism are all threatened by urban sprawl." The head of the Michigan Association of Home Builders was moved to counter that if smart growth proposals gain momentum, "Twelve thousand members of MAHB will get very active in the Michigan Legislature." A state senator confessed, "Builders do have a lot of influence. There are so many of them. Everybody in the Legislature has friends in the building industry." Friends armed with hefty campaign contributions.

So Democrat Governor Granholm with the Republican Senate Majority Leader Ken Sikkema formed a 26-member bipartisan "Michigan Leadership Land Use Council," that included ample representation from the sprawl industry. No surprise then that the Council stayed away from recommending explicit actions to curb sprawl, such as impact fees paid by developers for public infrastructure, such as roads and schools. They preferred to focus on revitalizing urban areas to attract people away from sprawl. This common political compromise ignores demand for suburban living and unmanageable costs for urban revitalization. If smart growth is limited to just urban revitalization, it will fail.

In 2003 Frank Cagle wrote a column for *KnoxNews* entitled "Bredesen double-cross promotes urban sprawl." It turns out that Tennessee Governor Phil Bredesen had garnered lots of votes by promising to address suburban sprawl, but then supported construction of a beltway that would open more land for sprawl development. Cagle noted, "It would appear the Knoxville business community's fund-raisers for Bredesen...had more influence than voters. ...Those of you who foam at the mouth about urban sprawl should get ready. You ain't seen nothin' yet. ...The Bredesen administration has evidently decided that the voters...are expendable."

In Hawaii large land developers have always been extremely powerful. No surprise then that former Governor Benjamin Cayetano vetoed a modest smart growth bill in 2001 that many parties, including me, had worked hard to get passed by the legislature. In that governing body, the sprawl lobby was not able to overcome citizen outrage about rampant land development wiping out the natural beauty of the islands and harming tourism. But it won in the end by reaching the governor.

Arizona's then-Governor Jane Dee Hull faced rising discontent with sprawl in 1998 and a strong grassroots smart growth effort, but she caved in to sprawl interests in business and the legislature. Compromise became concession. She backed "growing smarter" legislation crafted by sprawl lobbyists that public interest group Common Cause said was "a new low mark for deceptive ballot measures designed to pull the wool over the eyes of Arizona voters. It is a fraud, and the Governor of Arizona should withdraw her support of it." It passed and she became part of a well financed conservative effort to defeat smart growth. She stacked the Growing Smarter Oversight Council with friends of sprawl. Developers avoided requirements for impact fees and urban growth boundaries.

Normally, the sprawl industry focuses on local governments to maintain its market domination. As Hunter College Professor Tom Angotti said: "Land use controls are poorly coordinated and it is easy for large real estate developers to play local politics and manipulate them. Local real estate developers tend to control local governments and use their influence there to negotiate the terms of engagement with the global and regional investors."

With more attention to smart growth, sprawl politics are getting uglier. In Readington Township, New Jersey, a developer hired private investigators masquerading as a pro-environment husband and wife team seeking to buy a horse farm. The town was trying to preserve farmland after massive sprawl development had already eaten up too much open space. Over a three year period the couple secretly taped numerous conversations with town officials to gain evidence for a lawsuit claiming that the developer was being treated unfairly.

Community based planning and design, presented in Chapter 7, and citizen activism, discussed in Chapter 8, must offset the sprawl industry's hold on government. When elected officials hear that voters want real communities they may listen less to developers and home builders. Public officials must see sprawl as a public health threat and a way to control spending on infrastructure and limit taxes.

CITIZENS MUST OFFSET THE POLITICAL INFLUENCE OF THE SPRAWL INDUSTRY.

"Prosecutors showed that Collier County [Florida] government in the 1990s was basically a developer-run criminal enterprise, with politicians enjoying free golf, envelopes stuffed with cash and even a free wedding reception while rubber-stamping developments and waiving fees."So concluded The Washington Post in 2002. Land development is the engine of economic growth in Florida and developers keep it fueled with money to government officials.

Across the nation in California, according to the *Mercury News* in 2004, sprawl-fighting Ventura County Supervisor Steve Bennett summed up his experience: "The development industry is just too good at buying the votes they need at the local government level. It's too tempting. It's too easy. There's too much money involved. There's too much political pressure involved." Too few elected officials can resist that pressure.

The sprawl industry removes choice from the housing marketplace through a powerful "sprawl lobby." Few people know that the sprawl lobby is one of the most influential in the nation. But experience has revealed the truth to some citizens. Listen to three of them:

In Washington, Alex Steffen wrote, "Fashioning Smart Growth from Mindless Sprawl," in the *Seattle Post-Intelligencer* in 1999: "Sprawl, unlike crime, pays. Powerful interests – big developers, land speculators, construction corporations – get rich off sprawl. The sprawl lobby is strong and ruthless. We need to demand that our leaders find the courage to stare down the sprawl lobby and get to work on a statewide 'Smart growth' initiative."

In Texas, Roger Baker wrote in *Bicycle Austin* in 1999: "It is clear that the City Council is terrified of the sprawl lobby or they would stand up for the interests of Austin in opposing sprawl through publicly funded subsidies for highways conducive to sprawl."

In North Carolina, Dottie Coplon wrote a comment on a 2003 article in *The Charlotte Observer* titled, "Why Sprawl Lobby Has Clout:" "We thought City Council and the county commissioners actually have some say in rezoning. Our naiveté didn't allow us to recognize the source of influence on public officials."

Because of broad public support for smart growth principles and anger about sprawl's impacts the sprawl lobby occasionally visibly supports smart growth through publications and policy statements. This public support is disingenuous. Rather than publicly attack smart growth outright, they redefine it and sprawl to suit their own business purposes. They blur the distinction between sprawl and true HEALTHY PLACES. They subvert true smart growth attributes and messages with lies and distortions. They say most Americans don't want smart growth, but for those who do they claim they provide it. What the sprawl lobby really works at is instilling fear about smart growth, often through their conservative and libertarian surrogates – sprawl shills.

I use the terms "un-place" and "blandburbs" for sprawl developments because place and place-making matter so much. Community is sacred, and calling a sprawl development an un-place or a blandburb reminds us that true community is missing. A collection of homes and roads does not make a community. Land-taking is not the same as place-making. When private space is cherished and public space undervalued there is no real community, it is an un-place. Sprawl un-places are the psychic slums of suburbia, where people seek refuge within their home, where land is not enjoyed but endlessly traversed in cars, and the built environment does not nourish residents and community. Of course, here too, people may unite when terrible circumstances arise, but sprawl does not support that spirit in everyday life.

The conservative Heritage Foundation noted that the National

Association of Home Builders is "laboring to refine the meaning of the term." This is how they do it: "Smart growth is planning for the future." What fatuous rhetoric. All planning is planning for the future, including decades of planning that gave us the sprawl world. Similarly, the Urban Land Institute, an association for developers, defines smart growth as "development that is environmentally sensitive, economically viable, community-oriented, and sustainable." Nice feel-good rhetoric that makes it easy to apply the label of smart growth to projects and places that do not deserve it, which the sprawl industry often does. Compared to the ten smart growth principles given in Chapter 6, such statements say nothing meaningful or substantive about the attributes and goals of smart growth.

Sprawl supporters portray the market as fair by saying "people, not government, not planners, and not builders, choose where they live." This is classic sprawl-speak. Hundreds of years ago when pioneering settlers could go into wilderness areas lacking other people and government, they could live wherever and however they wanted. Americans nowadays can only choose what government allows to be built and what developers and builders provide in the market, except for the very few who buy their land and hire their own architect and builder.

In truth, the sprawl lobby has victimized everyone who has had little opportunity to buy a home in a HEALTHY PLACE. In the spirit of "you have to spend money to make money," big money is spent on campaign contributions and lobbying to protect sprawl. There is outright influence- peddling by the sprawl lobby through payments to office holders for favors, which are not always illegal. Real estate industry personnel hold many appointed and elected positions in government, allowing them to shape project and policy decisions, despite conflicts of interest. Sprawl industry leaders assert that their big spending is needed to protect the American dream, which is actually their dream of more easy money from sprawl development. By becoming a shield for sprawl the phrase "The American Dream" has become the most dangerous and dishonest cliché in history.

In 2001, *The San Francisco Bay Guardian* said the city of San Francisco "needs to turn its planning process completely around and shift away from developer-based planning and toward community-based planning." It noted contributions of $3 million to Mayor Willie Brown's reelection campaign from developers who "called every single shot" in a planning process that "was completely out of control." In 2002, citizens approved a new system to reduce the influence of developers. It was opposed by the mayor and gave the Board of Supervisors the right to reject any appointee of the mayor to the Planning Commission and Board of Appeals.

In 2003 *The Los Angeles Times* detailed the ways that U.S. Senator Harry Reid (Democrat, Nevada) had helped pass legislation that "promised a cavalcade of benefits to real estate developers, corporations and local institutions that were paying hundreds of thousands of dollars in lobbying fees to his sons' and son-in-law's firms." The bill freed about 18,000 acres from federal protection near Las Vegas and North Las Vegas for development and annexation. The consulting firm of the son-in-law was paid $300,000 by the Howard Hughes Corporation securing a provision allowing the company to acquire 998 acres of federal land in the sprawl-mushrooming Las Vegas area. An appraiser working for the company valued the federal land at $24,448 an acre or $24 million before passage of the bill, but after the bill passed nearby federal land sold for six times that amount, or almost $150 million.

Years of local news stories from just about everywhere detailing the political influence of developers have not stopped sprawl. Sprawl politics continue to distort the market. Sprawl projects roll downhill, despite some speed bumps and pot holes. Most project-related land development decisions are at the town, city and county levels of government. Projects are viewed relative to comprehensive plans. Recommendations move from planning departments to some type of commission, whose decisions can be overturned by a city or county council of elected members. As Charles Lee of Florida Audubon correctly observed, "You find few officials willing to do anything rather than slide down the slippery slope. The days of appropriate relations between commissioners, developer lobbyists and staff personnel are gone." Political campaign contributions by the sprawl industry pay off. Spending thousands of dollars in local elections is a small cost compared to the millions of dollars at stake for sprawl projects. As University of California, Davis Professor Robert Johnston and expert on the impact of politics on local land planning said: "The rate of return for developers is amazing. They're masters of this game: They find cheap agricultural land, put paper on it, and then they make campaign contributions to get the zoning they need."

In contrast to sprawl development, HEALTHY PLACES face steep uphill battles on a slippery slope lubricated by the sprawl industry. HEALTHY PLACE developers and smart growth advocates cannot come close to matching the money and influence of the sprawl industry. Smart growth advocates have neither the money nor political power to be coercive. Corny but true, the housing market will only work better when American democracy works better. Citizens as voters and consumers must counterbalance developer dollars.

Sprawl supporters also focus on state government, where many policies and programs have considerable impact on development, often through highway building and school construction spending, for example. With some state governors promoting smart growth, activities to influence state legislators have become more important to the sprawl industry. By keeping the role of the state as small as possible, it is easier to influence decisions of local governments.

Campaign contributions to local politicians by developers have long been a source of concern regarding conflicts of interest and influence peddling. With this influx of legal payola can you trust land development decisions? Is the local market where you live working fairly? Are developers who are trying to build HEALTHY PLACES where you live finding a level playing field? The more you know, the more likely you are to say "no" to these questions.

In 1998 T. Christian Miller wrote the award-winning article, "A Growth Plan Run Amok" in *The Los Angeles Times*. He revealed corrupt planning and land use management by Los Angeles County and said that "the Board of Supervisors and county planners repeatedly manipulated the growth plan to favor developers." In nearly 20 years, 40 percent of subdivisions were allowed to grow bigger than the county plan allowed; 2,200 homes were built on land designated for 1,000. Valleys and hillsides were swamped with sprawl subdivisions. One powerful Supervisor received $225,000 in campaign contributions from developers seeking to exceed growth limits, often within days and weeks of key decisions. County planners repeatedly allowed developers to count the area of nearby public streets as part of their projects so that more homes could be built. Excessive development caused 20 percent of residents to be devastated by natural disasters such as landslides, mudslides, flooding, fires and earthquakes. Disaster relief claims were 2.4 times higher in subdivisions that exceeded the county's plan than in those complying with it. "In the past, the county forgot who the customer was. Our customer isn't the developer. Our customer is posterity," so confessed one Supervisor. Amen.

Here are more illustrations of the magnitude and scope of the sprawl industry's political activities at the local government level, taken mostly from newspaper investigative reports. Until now these "local" stories have not been seen as a national pattern of corruption of government by the sprawl industry. It is important to present a considerable amount of evidence to document this pattern.

In October 2002, Ocean Township, New Jersey Mayor Terry Weldon, also a planning board member, pleaded guilty in federal court to taking $64,000 from three land developers.

In a 2000 article in *The Sacramento Bee*, Sacramento County, California Supervisor Illa Collin said this about land developers "They have the money to give to campaigns, and they also have the ability to shut money off to campaigns. They just have a very powerful influence, and anyone who says they don't isn't really being honest with themselves." Another county supervisor was fined $290,000 by the California Fair Practices Commission for secretly accepting $256,700 from a leading developer. At about the same time the supervisor voted in favor of two of the developer's projects.

In Louisville, Kentucky in 2001 it was revealed that the County Planning Commission Chairman solicited campaign contributions from developers who appeared before the commission. He stopped raising money from developers after the public attention.

The Tampa Tribune reported the long history of Hillsborough County, Florida, commissioners helping developers. In 2000 the county set up six zones where developers escaped impact fees designed to cover new public infrastructure costs, reducing their costs in areas that would have attracted development anyway.

Eugene, Oregon, has a powerful sprawl lobby called "The Gang of 9." An analysis of Lane County campaign contributions from 1998 to 2003 for all local races and ballot measures found that at least 50 percent of the funding came from the sprawl industry, about $500,000. In return, they received a growth-friendly mayor and city council majority, low impact fees, moved hospitals out of Eugene's downtown, and passed a 2001 ballot measure for a new pro-sprawl highway. Pro-sprawlers continue to push for expanding the urban growth boundary despite a 2003 survey of residents that found only 9 percent thought more land was needed for industrial development. Eugene, Oregon, City Councilor Bonny Bettman said in 2003: "The top agenda item for the local and state right wing is expanding the urban growth boundary. There are land speculators out there that will profit obscenely depending on where the UGB is."

For the Detroit, Michigan area, a 2000 study found that developers, builders and others in the real estate industry were the largest special interest source of 1999 campaign money for mayor, city council and other municipal races. The head of a Michigan public interest group said: "The development community in Michigan is receiving billions of dollars in benefits for thousands of dollars of investments."

In the fast-growing City of Novi in the Detroit area, a mall-builder was the largest source of cash for council and mayoral campaigns in 1999. The firm received approvals to build a new mall and an expanded 12 mile road to serve its shoppers.

Fredericksburg, Virginia, is a high growth sprawl area. *The Washington Post* reported in April 2003 that the former city manager and the chief planner had taken jobs with the area's largest sprawl developer that had benefited from many approvals and concessions from the city that the two had provided. The public had already voted out most members of the City Council over the developer's preferential treatment. One citizen said that the moves "raise questions about decisions made during the time those people served in an official capacity."

Berkeley, California, city council members vote on development projects that come to them on appeal and take campaign money from developers. During the 2000 city council campaign a successful candidate took $4,350 from four development companies, all with projects that could come before the council for a vote. Another elected official called this person "the most blindly pro-development in my memory."

In 2003 *The Kentucky Post* revealed an email and phone campaign by home builders in sprawling Boone County aimed at derailing the reappointment of a planning commissioner. They did not like his advocacy for safer roads, more landscaping, and greenspace preservation. The top elected county official said, "Any time a group has that much influence, it really concerns me." He called the loss "a tremendous setback to the county."

In 2002 the Planned Growth Strategy Ordinance was passed in Albuquerque, New Mexico. The mayor loaded the required task force with real estate and development people favoring suburban sprawl and not the mixed-use urban development advocates that had stimulated the ordinance in the first place.

Angry about Polk County, Florida, commissioners not imposing sufficient impact fees to cope with new school needs, school board member Frank O'Reilly complained in 2004 that the commission has been "bought and paid for by the developers."

In Durham, North Carolina, one of the two leading candidates for mayor in 2001 was an executive with the Home Builders Association of Durham and Orange Counties. About 60 percent of his contributions came from real estate interests. He raised $66,500 compared to $42,200 by his rival, who was an advocate of slower, thoughtful growth and development. The slow growth candidate won, but only because of a large last-minute effort by the Democratic Party which helped him win by the tiny margin of 485 votes.

In early 2004 *The Washington Post* reported how the previous pro-development mayor of Frederick, Maryland, had signed an agreement with developers that required them to pay only $3.7 million toward constructing a road necessary for a large office complex that would cost the city $22 million. The mayor did not get the agreement approved by the Board of Aldermen. The new mayor said: "It isn't fair that taxpayers should bear the burden for the road when most of the benefits go to developers."

In early 2003 in Nevada, the *Las Vegas Sun* revealed that the Clark County Commission had, for several years, ignored the county's master plan, which they were legally obligated to support and protect. Four of the seven commissioners gave developers many waivers, allowing them to move rapidly ahead with sprawl projects. Three commissioners supporting sprawl projects were frequent recipients of campaign contributions from developers and their law firms, and the outgoing chair of the commission had taken a job with a group of development companies. The new chair had supported the actions disregarding the master plan. One of the three commissioners fighting the waivers acknowledged: "Far too often nonconforming zone changes are approved and the wishes of the residents are overridden." In fact, 96.5 percent of nonconforming changes sought by developers were approved in 1999 and 2000. In 2004 one of the commissioners said that the county's approach was "what developers want, developers get."

In Hillsborough, New Jersey, the Planning Board approvals for a 3,000-unit housing project were voided and set aside in 2001 by a State Superior Court Judge because they had been tainted by conflicts of interest. The president of one of the developers was also chairman of the local Municipal Utilities Authority, and had loaned $20,000 to the former Planning Board chairman. The judge spoke of influence peddling.

A 1999 *Newsweek* article recounted how Fulton County, Georgia, officials had declared a moratorium on new development in an area where the sewers were overflowing. A day later the moratorium was lifted for hundreds of developers with a land disturbance permit, which prompted resident Julie Haley to comment: "We're in the middle of a moratorium, and there's twice as much building as before."

The mayor of the small town of Erie, Colorado, had fought rapid growth because of spiraling costs of providing municipal services. According to a 2003 story in *The New York Times*, developers financed a recall campaign to remove her and another town official from office. The campaign failed and the mayor said: "Citizens here want to run the town for their own benefit, not developers."

In early 2003 the *Orlando Sentinel* talked about three commissioners of Lake County, Florida, who "never met a subdivision they didn't like. They talk 'smart growth.' ...Then they vote with developers – the same ones that pour thousands into their campaigns." They had voted to build a sewage treatment plant that would allow 10,000 new homes in an area where every elementary school was already overcrowded.

Much attention has been given to smart growth policies advanced by Maryland's then-Governor Parris Glendening. But are they working? The key concept was Priority Funding Areas (PFAs) where growth is desired and state spending for infrastructure is focused. But a 2002 study by the Baltimore Regional Partnership found that in the five-county Baltimore region some 22.7 percent of projected household growth will be outside the PFAs from 2000 to 2020, exceeding the level before PFAs were created. New census data prompted *The Baltimore Sun* in April, 2004 to say: "Despite the Smart growth policies that then-Governor Parris N. Glendening instituted in 1997, people are still moving to communities far from Maryland's cities, to places without the infrastructure to handle the influx." Commenting in *The Washington Times*, Anirban Basu wrote, "It suggests that Smart growth doesn't have as much teeth as we had thought it might; that it has not interrupted this tendency toward sprawl that has been in place now for decades in Maryland." In August 2004, a Washington Post investigation reported: "no significant shifts in Maryland's development patterns since the passage of Glendening's smart growth package." As before 1997, 75 percent of new development in 2001 was still on greenfield sites outside of PFAs. Developer David Flanagan commented: "I think the rate of sprawl is faster today than I've ever seen it."

In 1998 *The Washington Post* ran the story "Builders Giving Big in Campaigns." It documented the influence of the sprawl industry on county officials. Developers were becoming increasingly concerned about smart growth policies and "growing public concerns over the pace of suburban sprawl." In 2002, Maryland sprawl interests were the third highest source of spending by lobbyists. A 2002 memo from Glendening's planners to the incoming new governor said that the smart growth program was not overturning sprawl. Policies that take too long to implement allow sprawl to irreversibly devastate the land and quality of life. In 2004, the head of the Maryland Association of Counties said: "Smart growth is inconsistent with the American dream of a big home on a five-acre lot." Lesson: You can lead a local official to smart growth but you can't make him or her support it. Consider these two Maryland cases:

In 2002, in his last year in office, the Prince George's County Executive, a sprawl shill, tried to sell thousands of acres of public land for waterfront homes, which drew criticism because it ran counter to decades of county and state planning and policies. Before elected office he had been a land development lawyer and partner in an exclusive development where he lives in a 19-room mansion on 24 wooded acres. One of the three candidates for that office ran a television ad asking, "Do you want developers running Prince George's County? Stop the developers. Support Jack Johnson." After winning, in the first 15 months in office, fully a third of Johnson's campaign money came from the sprawl industry, some $200,000. In late 2003 he vetoed a bill to restrict development in areas with congested roads. A Council member suspected Johnson vetoed the bill after the builders association visited him and presumably asked for his veto. The county has been called a "developers' mecca."

The Montgomery County Executive in 2001 vetoed a bill to impose impact fees on developers to pay for traffic relief. The Washington Post reported that at least one-third of his campaign dollars came from developers and related interests, over $100,000, in a non-election year. In 2002 a law passed that would raise only half of the funds needed for traffic relief from that of the previous proposal. Developers escaped impact fees dependent on house size, eliminating any incentive for building smaller homes in compact communities. In early 2003, *The Washington Post* reported on possible violations of campaign limits by developers and their associates in the 2002 election cycle, when they gave $1.3 million to county politicians. In 2003 the County Council gave developers what they lusted for, freedom to build in areas previously out of bounds because of traffic congestion. Despite requiring higher impact fees to defray some new public infrastructure costs, one Council member commented that the action "was a gift for developers and a booby prize for our residents."

Note that in a dozen states legislators can take gifts and trips from business interests without any disclosure required. Even when there are disclosure laws, they are often very lax with no meaningful information required. Consider some other states.

The non-partisan Wisconsin Democracy Campaign, in "Realtors Do More Than Buy and Sell Houses in Wisconsin," revealed that realtors achieve "success through a sophisticated system of campaign contributions and lobbying. They peddle influence and they peddle it well." For statewide candidates from 1993 to 1997, $1.4 million came from real estate interests; they gave the most money to legislative candidates.

The Center for Analysis of Public Issues determined that from 1993 to 1997 developers gave more than $8 million to New Jersey legislative candidates. They were the largest special interest source of money, 50 percent more than lawyers and their firms.

The Progressive Leadership Alliance's analysis of campaign contributions to 1997 Nevada legislature candidates found that the sprawl industry had given over $225,600 and achieved their highest priority. The urban growth boundary bill to limit sprawl development in Las Vegas and surrounding Clark County was defeated in committee. The Southern Nevada Home Builders Association said: "The boundary, if enacted, would be a noose, not a ring." Vegas sprawl is a sure bet and keeps paying off for developers.

The Center for Public Integrity revealed that 25 Florida legislators had outside financial interests in real estate and that campaign contributions to state candidates in 1998 from the real estate sector totaled $2.5 million.

In 2000, at least 36 of 211 New York state lawmakers who routinely voted on real estate and land use matters were real estate executives, brokers or salespersons.

Democracy North Carolina reported that in the 2002 election cycle the North Carolina Realtors PAC and the North Carolina Home Builders Association PAC ranked No. 1 and No. 2, respectively, for contributions to legislative candidates. The total was over $478,000, compared to $310,000 in 2000 and only $100,000 in 1999. The escalating amounts correlate with the creation of a strong smart growth movement in the state.

The sprawl lobby did really well in 2000. Colorado Constitutional Amendment 24 would have reduced the influence of developers on local government officials by allowing voters to evaluate the costs and environmental impacts of growth on their communities before it happened. Voters rejected Amendment 24 by nearly 2-to-1, even though a few months earlier 78 percent of voters favored it. What happened? Sprawl interests spent some $6 million to defeat the measure, compared to about $1 million spent by pro-amendment groups. Development interests falsely painted the measure as anti-growth, saying it "could push our Colorado economy into chaos," and called their group Coloradans for Responsible Reform to confuse itself with the pro-amendment Coloradans for Responsible Growth. Ed Quillan noted in the *Denver Post* that anti-amendment groups did not identify any reforms and used "exaggeration, name-calling and unsupported assertions." Eric Fried wrote the *Coloradoan* about four lies of the pro-sprawl special interests, namely that they wanted reforms and claimed that building would cease, the economy would crash, and affordable housing would no longer be built. The sprawl status quo was saved. But in early 2002 growth remained the top issue in Colorado with 64 percent of voters believing the state legislature was doing too little or almost nothing to address the state's growth issues.

Similarly, Arizona Proposition 202 was initially favored by 70 percent of voters but went down to defeat with 70 percent voting against it. Financing the flip-flop was $4.5 million, with $3.5 million coming from home builders. The initiative required urban growth boundaries which are despised by the pro-sprawl gang. Sleazy, dirty tricks were used to defeat the measure. A web site "www.yeson202.com" presented anti-202 propaganda. To scare people about growth management, a television spot showed a family using a porta-potty near their desert dream house. And $50,000 was used to hire two pro-sprawl academics and darlings of developers – Peter Gordon and Harry W. Richardson of the University of Southern California, authors of the article "Why Sprawl Is Good." Their sham report predicted economic collapse if the proposition passed. Two legit professors spoke out. Demographer Tom Rex of Arizona State University said the work was "based on faulty assumptions, so the results are skewed." Economist William Hildred of Northern Arizona University called the study "bizarre," said it used "arbitrary premises" and that its "results obscure issues and mislead the public." Gordon criss-crossed the state telling audiences that over 1 million jobs would be lost, which was ludicrous and found nowhere in the report.

Hiding from public view is the American Legislative Exchange Council. It purports to be a membership organization for state legislators, but business interests account for 98 percent of its revenues and greatly control what the group does. Right-wing members are not made public. The group has fought land use and planning reforms. It says that "Smart growth policies limit freedom of choice and raise the cost of living at the local level." Not true. It also says that sprawl results from the absence of planning. Also untrue. The group says "Smart growth proponents strive for a fantasy community in which everyone lives within walking distance of their job, school and any other miscellaneous destination." That "fantasy community" must be the HEALTHY PLACES so many Americans want and will remain a fantasy as long as pro-sprawlers have their say.

The sprawl lobby is also active at the federal level, lobbying for road building subsidies and fighting some environmental regulations, such as pro-wetlands and endangered species. The National Association of Home Builders took the lead in 2002 to defeat the Community Character Act. It was falsely painted by Tom DeWeese, president of the American Policy Center, as "a very clever mix of socialism and fascism," though it only offered federal grants as incentives for states and communities to improve their land-use planning. Federal campaign contributions from real estate interests increased from $12.3 million in 1990 to $79.6 million in 2000. In the key "soft money" category, where money goes to political parties and not specific candidates, in 2000, real estate ranked second, behind the financial sector and ahead of third-place lawyers and law firms. The National Association of Home Builders' political action committee was raising $2.8 million for the 2003-2004 election cycle; one of its major issues being smart growth. In Fortune's 2001 ranking of the top 25 most effective lobbying groups in Washington, D.C. the National Association of Realtors was #9 and the National Association of Home Builders was #11, much higher than groups representing the pharmaceutical industry, bankers, teachers, farmers, and governors; both had become more powerful over time. The biggest retail beneficiary of sprawl is Wal-Mart and in 2003 it became the biggest corporate donor to federal parties and candidates, not to mention the largest company on the planet.

CORRUPTION IS A TOOL OF THE SPRAWL INDUSTRY.

Either you feel dizzy and depressed after reading all this proof of the power and influence of the sprawl industry, or you feel good because your beliefs have been verified. Have no doubt; the sprawl industry is willing to do and spend whatever is necessary to maintain the sprawl status quo. Sprawl's political tentacles reach into every part of the nation and every part of government. Business as usual means sprawl as usual. But who really pays for sprawl's grip on society? You do. The untold millions of dollars spent every year by the sprawl lobby to control government are passed on to people living, shopping and working in sprawlspace. Think of it this way. Every one of us pays a "sprawl lobby tax" that costs much more than dollars; it costs our quality of life, physical and mental health, and choice in housing, transportation, and shopping. There are also higher taxes to pay for public infrastructure for expanding sprawl. Does this make any sense?

Yet there is cause for cautious optimism. State and local government officials seem to be getting the message; a 1999 survey of the group found that 78 percent ranked "livable community" concerns as either the most important or a very important issue. The most serious issues included traffic congestion and suburban sprawl. A few elected officials are making strong commitments to fight sprawl and support smart growth.

"Maine's special quality-of-place is in danger. ...Maine's way of life, our countryside and communities, are being changed for the worse by sprawl," so said Maine's Governor John Baldacci in 2003. He made the fiscal case for smart growth by noting that sprawl was causing the state to spend about $50 million annually for new roads, schools, and water lines to service blandburbs while established towns and cities were decaying.

In 2003 Massachusetts Governor Mitt Romney said, "The bottom line is that smart growth is good for Massachusetts. With smarter development, we can build more housing, create a better tax base, nurture active communities, create shorter commutes, and protect precious land resources."

Early on, California Governor Arnold Schwarzenegger also showed support for smart growth, which his predecessor Gray Davis did little to advance. William Johnson, Mayor of Rochester, New York, advised the U.S. Conference of Mayors in 2004 to find ways to stop developers from gobbling up land and said that mayors "now understand the consequences [of sprawl] and they don't have the resources to pay for it." Senator Hillary Rodham Clinton said in 2004: "We should also be looking at sprawl – talking about the way we design our neighborhoods and schools and about our shrinking supply of safe, usable outdoor space – and how that contributes to asthma, stress and obesity."

Will these politicians walk the anti-sprawl talk or take limo rides with sprawl lobbyists? Without stronger citizen support political leaders may succumb to the sprawl lobby, be hamstrung by legislators shilling for sprawl interests, or use do-nothing strategies to avoid taking a stand in the debate, thereby perpetuating sprawl and all its negative aspects.

Sprawl opponents confront "Home Rule" states, where local governments control land use and planning, or "Dillon Rule" states which limit local governments' control of land use and planning. For example, Virginia is a Dillon Rule state and New Jersey is a Home Rule state. In reality, no state keeps all power or devolves all of its authority to localities under the United States Constitution. Smart growth can be advanced or thoroughly thwarted in both types. In Dillon Rule states the sprawl lobby must corrupt state legislators; in Home Rule states it must corrupt local officials. The sprawl lobby is adept at both. Even in Dillon Rule states that try to spur smart growth, flexibility allows localities to pursue sprawl, creating openings for sprawl interests. Similarly, Home Rule state governments can use funding (such as for school and roads) or regulatory permitting decisions to spur smart growth, which sprawl lobbyists try to prevent.

Here is more proof of sprawl-industry power. Fifteen percent of buyers of new homes discover serious defects in construction. And the problem is getting worse as builders speed up house construction from 120 to 200 days a decade ago, to 90 to 120 days today, and use cheaper materials. The respected *Consumer Reports* reported in 2004 that municipal, state and federal governments offered few consumer protections. For example, 40 states do not regulate home-warranty programs; 23 states do not regulate home inspections; 18 states have "right to cure" laws that give builders a chance to fix defects and block suits by homeowners. An insidious problem is the sale of "buy-back" homes that builders buy back from original owners because of serious defects, but do not disclose to the second buyer.

How could the largest expense and investment of Americans be so vulnerable to low quality? *Consumer Reports* explains it: "Builders, developers, and real-estate companies are among the most influential political constituencies, and often heavy campaign contributors." There is also corruption. In 2003 New Jersey's State Commission of Investigation revealed many municipal code officials and inspectors had been illegally taking gifts of meals, liquor, parties and golf outings from builders and developers to look the other way when inspecting their properties. And yet the Federal Trade Commission had not filed suit against any home builder for defective construction in more than a decade!

Billion-dollar Enron-type scandals of corporate corruption rightfully grab the headlines. With the sprawl industry, there are a thousand points of thousand-dollar corruption spread nationwide. For decades, multitudes of companies and politicians have maintained sprawl through local land use decisions and billion-dollar government spending on roads, schools, and other public infrastructure necessary for sprawl land development. Sprawl corruption has made Americans pay higher taxes, suckered them into expensive and risky automobile dependency, and slyly seduced them into an unhealthy sedentary lifestyle with high medical costs. Because there is no single "catastrophe" involving a huge dollar or death figure, there are no headlines about sprawl corruption, but there should be. Untold local sprawl tragedies add up to a national catastrophe.

Tom Garner of Pensacola, Florida, where 80 percent of citizens wanted little or no additional growth, made a strong case in 2004 for voting "for the candidate who has accepted the least amount of pro-growth money." What I call the sprawl lobby, he called the "growth lobby" as others do. But sprawl interests use dirty tricks to prevent citizens knowing before they vote about sprawl lobby contributions, such as providing contributions on Election Day or after a candidate wins election, and funneling the money through a seemingly non-related organization. A Placer County, California, pro-sprawl supervisor candidate won in 2000 with the help of over $80,000 from sprawl interests, nearly 60 percent of his total, but $40,000 arrived in the six months after the election, mostly from sprawl interests. In the Sacramento, California, area the county's deputy sheriff's association gave more than $70,000 to pro-sprawl candidates in 2000, but its revenues from dues was less than $8,000; the rest came from sprawl interests, according to The Sacramento Bee.

CONSERVATIVES AND LIBERTARIANS LIKE AN UNFAIR MARKET.

Sprawl shills say that smart growth is "coercive" and will "force" Americans to live in apartments and "force" them out of their cars, with the inference that people should fear government. Baloney! Smart growth advocates are not trying to do that, nor are they or government agencies capable of doing that. Sprawl has the power, not smart growth.

There is no evidence whatsoever that smart growth is coercive, anti-American, or promoting just city apartment living or that it is trying to require everyone to use public transit. In truth, smart growth means providing more housing and transportation choice. More market choice means a stronger democracy. Conservatives have a hard time seeing the difference between individuals freely and voluntarily reducing their car use and choosing public transit or walking to serve their own interests, versus government actions that compel such choices.

Conservatives like to speak of attacks on the American dream, to anger people that their dream is being threatened. The National Center on Public Policy Research published, "The Campaign Against Urban Sprawl: Declaring War on the American Dream." Never mind that the traditional dream is a well nourished creation of the sprawl industry. Conservatives ignore the many people seeking an American Dream Community.

The support of sprawl is indeed ironic. Conservatives and libertarians profess to believe in the private sector market, but do not support a fair market, a competitive market where many consumers would not choose sprawl. They are not defending suburbia. They are defending sprawl. They wail against government regulation, but not against the zoning ordinances that support sprawl and block smart growth development. They do not complain about government subsidies for road building. They rail against infringing upon property rights, but not against the denial of housing choice to consumers who want to own land in a place that is not part of sprawl. Call it sprawl hypocrisy.

Sure, suburbia has received a bum rap through writings and motion pictures. Attacking suburbia is easy, but it has not curbed sprawl. Suburbia is just geography, not the geography of nowhere but the geography of anywhere. The enemy is not suburbia; sprawl land use and the sprawl culture are. Smart growth will never reach its full potential if it is perceived as the enemy of suburbia. A true HEALTHY PLACE in a suburban area is remarkably better than a typical sprawl subdivision. We must have suburban HEALTHY PLACES because urban revitalization by itself cannot provide enough housing for the expanding population.

Conservatives are dead wrong when they say "anti-sprawl policies are profoundly anti-suburban." They conflate sprawl and suburbia, with the aim of instilling fear that smart growth will ban the suburban option. Here is more combative sprawl-speak: "People are not ready to embrace a vision of 'smart growth' that would deny them the opportunity to enjoy a suburban lifestyle." Smell the sprawl lies. Smart growth does not mean outlawing the "suburban lifestyle." To the contrary, smart growth offers a better quality suburban lifestyle. Sprawl took the "urban" out of suburban and smart growth puts it back in. Many of the HEALTHY PLACES given in later chapters are in suburban locations, because their developers overcame zoning obstacles, and because so many people want to live in suburbia. Smart growth gives consumers a non-sprawl housing option in suburban locations, not just better urban neighborhoods. Discourse about cities versus suburbs should be replaced by talking about blandburbs versus HEALTHY PLACES.

Sprawl developers and builders prefer to stay in the background, out of sight of the public. They let think-tank and academic shills publicly defend the sprawl status quo and attack smart growth. As the conservative Heritage Foundation said, "conservatives and libertarians find it hard to be card-carrying members of the smart growth movement." Gripped by sprawl rapture, conservatives and libertarians defy the gravity of their principles and nurture a government-distorted market. Why are they against giving consumers more choices for housing and transportation? Who are they serving, if not consumers? Card-carrying members of the anti-smart growth cottage industry serve certain business interests, particularly large land owners who want free reign to plunder land and natural resources. These include land developers and corporate road building, logging, mining, petroleum, and drilling interests. Sprawl shills get speaking fees from pro-sprawl groups; their talks aim to defeat local smart growth efforts.

By using sprawl-speak the sprawl industry's rhetoric is intentionally confusing and deceptive. So too are the steady stream of reports and opinion articles from sprawl shills, who increasingly avoid the dirty s-word – sprawl – in favor of generalities. They would rather define the American dream with vagueness to avoid distinguishing sprawl from smart growth. Sprawl shill-meister Randal O'Toole talks about the American dream as "mobility, affordable housing, and a clean environment with accessible open spaces." Who could argue with that? Sprawl supporters increasingly prefer to talk about public policies rather than the dissimilar design attributes of sprawl subdivisions versus smart growth communities. They fear public policies that support smart growth. They talk about freedom of choice while ignoring market distortions that thwart attempts to build HEALTHY PLACES.

Conservative authors have developed a "footnote fetish" to make their documents look researched and professional, as if footnotes prove accuracy. The aforementioned paper illustrates this tactic; the ten page paper is loaded with some 40 footnotes on two pages. Do not be fooled. Nearly 70 percent of those footnotes are the works of other sprawl shills. This reflects the intellectual incest among what one writer dubbed as "the sprawl boys." They share their data and thinking, write for each other's publications, quote each other, and hold positions in each other's organizations. Believing each other's lies and distortions, dogma replaces truth. Like fertilizer, they fling malodorous disinformation and misinformation to cultivate their pro-sprawl party line. They fabricate facts from false assumptions, twisted logic and bad data, and often ascribe to smart growth and its advocates things that are absolutely false, and then criticize their own lies.

Here are some typical malevolent statements repeatedly trumpeted by conservatives and libertarians to instill fear about smart growth:

+ "Smart growth is great if your dream is living in a noisy apartment, taking a crowded train to work, and never seeing a tree."
+ "Smart growth planning means confining family life to dense cities with little privacy."
+ "Smart growth's real goal is to increase congestion, not reduce it."
+ "Smart growth is coercive."
+ "Smart growth 'would force us out of our cars and make us live on

top of one another.'"

At a meeting held by Kentucky's Smart growth Task Force in 2001, pro-sprawl advocates sat in the first row holding small flags of the former Soviet Union. Despite the end of the cold-war, right-wingers portray smart growth as a socialist or communist movement, such as the assertion, "unless you really like the way Moscow looks and works, you should celebrate urban sprawl." Sprawl shill-meister Wendell Cox wrote an article titled "Nickolae Ceaucescu: Father of Smart growth." Ceaucescu was the ruthless communist dictator of Romania. It was published by the Heartland Institute that receives funding from the American Highway Users Alliance, the American Petroleum Institute, the Alliance of Automobile Manufacturers, the Asphalt Institute, Exxon Mobil, General Motors, and many home builders. Cox had the cheek to say that smart growth "would tell people where to live" and that it "would require no less than forced abandonment of much that is currently developed." He is warning suburbanites that if smart growth succeeds they will be forced out of their homes. This ridiculous right-wing rhetoric is an act of desperation, because sprawl has become vulnerable. Sprawl shills would much rather attack smart growth than have to defend sprawl.

Sprawl shills have a "don't fence me in" mentality and proclaim that "the automobile is an instrument of freedom and pleasure." But smart growth offers Americans more opportunities to freely reduce personal car use to get more freedom and pleasure. A pet target of conservatives is public transit, which many Americans want more of. Conservatives circulate data on how little Americans use public transit compared to cars, as if there is something about transit itself that explains its lack of use when the truth is that too few Americans have easy access to public transit because of decades of rampant sprawl development. Talk about faulty logic and incomplete analysis.

Are Americans willing to change? According to a national survey by the National Association of Realtors, transit options for commuting to work would be used if they were convenient, safe and available: 62 percent would use rail or train, 57 percent would use a combination of public bus and rail or train, and 52 percent would use public bus. Conservative propaganda that Americans will never stop driving is just so much hyperbole. By fighting efforts to make transit convenient, safe and available, they hope to make their propaganda self-fulfilling.

Sprawl shills know that improved transit can shift development from outer suburbs to land available within cities and the original, close-in suburbs – "infill development" or the filling in of land in older, urbanized areas. They condemn government spending to build light rail, but conveniently ignore the huge amounts of public funds spent on roads that service their blandburbs. They ignore how infill development can reduce traffic congestion, if transit is provided for higher population density areas. When people live near transit they are 5 to 6 times more likely to use transit to commute to work, according to research. Road lovers also ignore the benefits of transit and focus only on costs, a sure sign of bias. A cost-benefit analysis for a transit line in the Cincinnati area found that the cost of $750 million was offset by $1.5 billion in benefits. The Victoria Transport Policy Institute analyzed rail transit in the U.S. and found that the total national subsidy was offset by more than four times higher economic benefits — $12.5 billion versus over $53 billion. In particular, the 2004 study noted how the rail-bashing work of sprawl shill Randal O'Toole was "flawed and biased," ignored many rail benefits, used outdated and inaccurate information, and misrepresented other information. It comes to this: Sprawl shills' religious conviction is "in roads we trust."

Sprawl shills blame congestion on too little road building. They reject "induced demand," how expanding road capacity leads to more traffic and worse congestion. They are wrong. More road capacity outside cities promotes more dispersed sprawl development requiring more vehicle use.

Conservatives and libertarians ignore incontrovertible data that prove personal car use is reduced by applying smart growth principles to community design, and that just a small reduction in cars on a road can greatly reduce congestion. Conservatives discount mixed-use communities where many routine non-commute trips – constituting 85 percent of trips – can be done by walking or biking. The data for "The Metropolis Plan" released in early 2003 to guide growth in the greater Chicago metropolitan area, showed that when non-vehicle transportation increased from 15.3 to 28.9 percent, from a number of land use and community design actions, the average time lost in congestion delays would drop from 27.2 to 8.7 minutes per person per day. So, close to a doubling of walking, biking and transit use was predicted to cut average congestion delays by two-thirds.

With lower public support for road building, sprawl shills advocate greater use of tolls to reduce traffic congestion. Local governments like toll roads more than raising taxes. And only about one-third of road spending nationally comes from gasoline taxes, something that few Americans appreciate, and politicians resist increasing them. Many Americans will face expensive tolls that vary with the time of day for some lanes – so-called 'congestion pricing.' Freeways and superhighways did not solve traffic congestion. Billions spent on road building did not work. Will tolls reduce congestion? Time will tell. Sprawl shill Randal O'Toole believes, "WE CAN TOLL OUR WAY OUT OF CONGESTION." He also says that "We're not auto-dependent, we're auto-liberated." Remember that the next time you are stuck in traffic. Do you feel liberated? Only this is certain. More tolls will be a financial incentive to reduce personal vehicle use. And with the right alternatives, that is good.

Traffic congestion is likely to stay, no matter what. The best solution to traffic congestion is personal, what you do, not what government does. It is projected that if current sprawl trends continue, national vehicle miles traveled from 2000 to 2025 will increase annually at over twice the rate of population growth. Based on past data, only 13 percent of this mileage growth will be from population growth, with 87 percent resulting from the same people driving more. So during nasty stuck-in-traffic times don't blame immigrants or vacationers for traffic madness. Demand alternatives to sprawl and oppose more road building. Blame sprawl pushers who care more about protecting auto-related business interests, road builders, automakers, and the petroleum industry. There is a better way. Let those Americans who stick to heavy vehicle use deal with traffic congestion and high costs, and let others have an opportunity to slash their automobile addiction. Those who want help with their addiction need something that might be called "Automobile Addicts Anonymous," which could complement the powerful pro-car AAA with 46 million members. Formerly known as the American Automobile Association, it supported 50 years of sprawl for its growth and success.

To attack smart growth for raising home prices and wasting money on public transit, conservatives talk about Portland, Oregon. They think Portland is smart growth paradise. While Portland has been at the forefront of smart growth many other places have used similar policy approaches. Vicious attacks on Portland are based on intentionally wrong and misleading analyses and information. The Congress for the New Urbanism commissioned a distinguished panel of experts to look at the material being widely circulated by some prominent conservatives.

According to the CNU report "Correcting the Record," the leading conservative spokesperson "has used incomplete, incorrect, and deceptive numbers to convince people that cities should be more like Atlanta, and less like Oregon." CNU got it right. Smart growth policies in Portland have helped create a high quality of life and place that many people eagerly seek.

In early 2003 there was a conference held by conservative and libertarian groups in Washington, D.C. entitled "Preserving the American Dream." The air was thick with false information. Conservatives in conversations and speeches consistently talked nonsense about smart growth. Speakers spread fear that smart growth will drive up housing costs, increase traffic congestion, and rob property owners of their rights. The conference should have been called "Fighting Smart growth — How to Limit Housing and Transportation Choices for Americans." Aside from conservative organizations, financial supporters included an association of property owners, a road builders group, a home builders group, a development company, and the leading conservative foundation.

Beware of pro-sprawl op-ed articles in your local newspaper. Articles written by some group or public relations company may be the basis for opinion articles submitted to local newspapers. In October 2003 the Editor of *The Columbus Dispatch* in Ohio described cases of "journalistic fraud." In one, two people from the Buckeye Institute had published an op-ed article prepared by a public relations firm; in another an article from the Reason Public Policy Institute was the basis of a guest article. The contributors were banned from publishing in the newspaper.

Despite sprawl's record, shills like Wendell Cox get attention. He testified before the U.S. Senate Committee on Environment and Public Works in 2002; his testimony was titled "Dangers of Smart Growth Planning" and contained his usual litany of fabrications about smart growth, namely that it is "coercive" and "rations land and development." Cox's politics provide such opportunities. He advised the first presidential campaign of George W. Bush, and Newt Gingrich appointed him to the Amtrak Reform Council which has helped him fight public transit.

Anti-smart growth extremists are more like snake oil salesmen than scholars. Other than outright lies, they are masters of stretching the truth, telling half truths, and using sound bites that promote unwarranted fear and distrust. Their attacks against smart growth aim to thwart consumer choice in the marketplace. Pro-sprawl intellectual litter clutters the path to truth; it is more than repulsive, it is dangerous. The Footnote Fascists with their intellectual incest are deceitful. Forget less government and a free market. Sprawl shills welcome government money for infrastructure and road building, their favored corporate subsidy and handout. They fear more direct citizen control of government land use decisions, now perverted by sprawl developers and their business allies. They want to keep you subservient to sprawl. Take it personally. Remember that the evil done by sprawl shills and developers lives after them, long after them.

Here are conservative and libertarian groups that provide venues for sprawl shills who have a one-sided, extreme positive view of sprawl development and are also anti-smart growth:

+ Allegheny Institute
+ Buckeye Institute
+ Cascade Policy Institute
+ CATO Institute
+ Commonwealth Foundation
+ Foundation for Economic Education
+ Georgia Public Policy Foundation
+ Heartland Institute
+ Heritage Foundation
+ Independence Institute
+ James Madison Institute
+ John Locke Foundation
+ Mackinac Center for Public Policy
+ Maryland Public Policy Institute
+ National Center for Policy Analysis
+ National Center for Public Policy Research
+ Pacific Research Institute
+ Political Economy Research Center
+ Reason Foundation/Reason Public Policy Institute
+ Thoreau Institute

As shills for the sprawl industry and property owners hoping to cash in on sprawl development, their materials having anything to do with sprawl and smart growth should display the following:

CONSUMER WARNING: Believing pro-sprawl propaganda may be

hazardous to your health.

The Dallas-Fort Worth Star-Telegram in 2004 published an article by sprawl shill Pamela Villarreal of the National Center for Policy Analysis. Her extreme pro-sprawl commitment was shown by her attack on smart growth; she warned about falling for "what is really a pipe dream: people living close together in harmony with one another, embracing mass transit and bicycles, and businesses of all sorts locating to a vital and robust urban community." The American Dream Community is not a pipe dream.

A POPULATION OF 400 MILLION REQUIRES CHANGE.

Look out for land-lies. Conservatives' abundant land argument is their most misleading, foolish and dangerous argument, namely that development has hardly consumed any of the nation's land. Sprawl, they argue, can keep sucking up land as if there's no tomorrow. Their intellectual disgrace, however, is defining current land supply as the total land area of the nation minus the fraction already developed. This is misleading and just plain stupid. Do not be fooled when sprawl shills say only a small fraction, about 5 percent, of the entire nation's land has been developed, with the inference that we have sooooooo much land to sprawl in. This is a general statistic for the whole nation. What matters from a market perspective is land where development is technically possible and where people want to live, not a simplistic and misleading statistic. That kind of land is being rapidly consumed. These sprawl shills want you to believe that unchecked development can continue without any government controls.

First, think about deserts, canyons, mountain ranges, steep hillsides, frigid northern plains, wetlands, barren and desolate regions, and flood plains, for example. There are also federal lands, tribal lands, and contaminated lands. Federally owned land is 83 percent of Nevada, 65 percent of Utah, and 63 percent of Idaho, for example, and overall is about 25 percent of all land. Significant land is also preserved as parks, forests, wetlands, scenic vistas, and natural habitats, as it should be. Some historic land is precious because of cemeteries and old buildings. Already, 20 percent of historic civil war battlefields have been lost to development. Considerable land near railroad tracks, power lines, cell phone towers, and underground pipelines is undevelopable.

Other land is agricultural, and most Americans want to keep it that way. A survey of Seattle, Washington and Portland, Maine residents found that 91 percent believed it was important to preserve productive farmland. But one million acres a year are being lost to sprawl development. Do Americans really want to depend even more on imported foods that receive little government testing?

Now, think about 50 million or more people needing housing in the next 20 years, and 100 million or more by 2050. All over the country single acres are already selling for $500,000 to $2 million, because they are in land-scarce areas with strong housing demand. Do conservatives want to deny Americans the right to live in geographic areas they choose? Unbridled land development will do just that, especially for Americans who are not wealthy. In the long run, low density sprawl reduces housing affordability.

In contrast to land where development is impossible or unlikely, consider that some 53 percent of the United States population lives on just 17 percent of the land, excluding Alaska and Hawaii. The most desirable land is in coastal counties. Americans like living near oceans, the Gulf of Mexico, and the Great Lakes, even when natural hazards exist. Coastal areas are suffering major impacts from development. Sprawl by the sea is usually made up of small (very expensive) lots with huge houses.

The 2003 report by the Pew Oceans Commission emphasized the many negative impacts of sprawl on coastal resources and their contributions to our society and economy. If there is any place where smarter development is urgently needed, it is on coastal lands, which contrary to the thinking of conservatives, is limited. Someone who wants to live in a coastal area is not likely to see living in Missouri or South Dakota as equally attractive.

It matters not that towns in rural Kansas are giving away land for new homes as well as other incentives, such as free water and sewer hookups, to lure new residents. The tiny town of Marquette with some 600 residents had 80 lots on former wheat fields to give away, worth about $1,200 each. In the first year only 21 lots were taken by people seeking real community and neighborliness. Not that there's anything wrong with Kansas, but few people want to live in rural Kansas, but if sprawl continues, some people may have to. Even in Canada and Australia, with enormous undeveloped land areas and low population, the anti-sprawl movement is very strong, because of rapid sprawl expansion around cities. In Canada, the Ontario

Provincial Minister of Public Infrastructure said in 2004: "We've got to stop this whole sprawl-type manner of growth and do something that's more effective."

California is the most populated state and the third largest after Alaska and Texas. Right-winger Randal O'Toole looks at the world through sprawl-tinted glasses and spreads the propaganda that California "is hardly running out of land," because only 8.6 percent of all land is developed for urban and rural living. The Association of Environmental Professionals said: "Growth in California has always been outward toward open land. The paradigm is shifting as we realize that we have just about used up all the new developable land out yonder." The 2002 "Invest for California" report said that the high growth counties of Los Angeles, Orange and Santa Clara will lack sufficient land to accommodate projected household growth through just 2010, if current development patterns continue. In high-growth San Diego, 88 percent of the land is developed.

The Los Angeles Times ran a story in 2003 about Orange County reaching its final build-out and quoted a real estate analyst: "We're outta land. We don't have any dirt left." It was noted that the county was known "as fertile ground for developers" and that "the political playing field still favors the developer." In 2004 the paper said "Orange County is running out of land to build on – and the signs are most evident along its most coveted stretch of real estate, the coast [where] nearly every acre of the 42-mile shoreline that isn't formally set aside for open space is developed or about to be developed." In one coastal development the lots alone were going for $2.5 million and more. As activist Mark Massara said, "People are partying while Rome burns."

Reflect on these other examples of voracious land consumption and, in some areas, land scarcity:

With 32 percent of land developed, New Jersey is the most developed state. "Measuring Urban Growth in New Jersey" reported that all remaining available land in the state will be developed in about 40 years, even with preserving one million acres. This could drop to 20 years if sprawl development is mostly 5-acre or larger residential lots, which is currently popular or mandated by local government.

In four key southeastern Michigan counties, only 27 percent of the land was developed in 1965; by 2020 it is predicted that 60 percent will be fully developed, without major population increases.

On Long Island, New York, by 2003 80 percent of Nassau County and 64 percent of Suffolk County were already developed.

In 2000 the *Boston Business Journal* discussed the additional costs of development on contaminated land, like Superfund and brownfield sites. But "with developable land growing ever scarcer…more developers are willing to assume the extra risks, costs, wait and complexity" to use this type of land. The fraction of developed land in Massachusetts increased by 50 percent during the 1980s and 1990s.

In reflecting on the home building boom in 2003 an economist at the National Association of Home Builders said, "The only complaint I heard from builders last year is that they can't get enough land."

It helps to see land development as a classic zero sum game, or a fixed-size "land pie" that gets sliced up. Developers want a bigger slice and what they consume cannot serve other purposes. According to the Michigan Land Resource Project developed land nearly triples from 1980 to 2040 if current trends continue. Developed land increases from 6.4 to 17.7 percent. The additional 4.1 million acres comes from reductions in farmland (17 percent), forestland (8 percent), wetland (10 percent), and open green-space (24 percent). Massachusetts data for 1985 to 1999 showed 40 acres a day developed with 78 percent coming from forests, 17 percent from farms, and 5 percent from open space, according to the Massachusetts Audubon Society. Nearly 60 percent was used for low density, large-lot sprawl.

An exception to the land pie model is infill projects in areas already developed. Millions of acres in cities, on average about 15 percent of city areas, sit vacant or abandoned. In Columbus, Ohio, there are 2,700 vacant buildings. By redeveloping such areas for affordable housing, mixed-use projects and parks, some greenfield development can be eliminated.

Michigan's Public Sector Consultants provided these shocking historic trends in housing-unit density. Before World War II, Michigan cities averaged 5.5 dwellings per acre. The immediate postwar suburbs have 4.7 dwellings per acre, which dropped in the 1960s to 3.8, then in the 1980s to 2.6, and then in suburbs developed in the 1990s, to an average of less than one home per acre. From 5.5 to less than one home per acre in half a century; this is data of the absurd. In some areas of the state one home per ten acres is common, not counting farms. Declining home density explains why the annual number of acres lost to suburban development jumped 67 percent from the five year period of 1987 to 1992 to 1993 to 1997.

Children should learn this in school: Land developed is land lost. A future with little greenspace and farmland is unpopular. A Michigan poll in the summer of 2003 found that 84 percent of adults favored "giving funding priorities to infrastructure in existing communities rather than encouraging new growth in the countryside." And 80 percent agreed "we need more communities in Michigan where people can walk from their homes to their stores and offices." Sprawl really does sow the seeds of its own destruction when it ruins what people value.

Sprawl is spilling over from one state to another. When an area gets saturated with sprawl or actions are taken to limit sprawl, developers jump to adjacent states with cheap rural land and tax advantages for residents, at least in the short term. "Sprawl export" is growing. Importing areas get sprawl housing and big bills for creating new infrastructure and public services, and original residents get higher taxes. Exporting states keep the jobs and workers. Sprawl developers shrewdly market large homes to lure people into commuting long distances. Sprawl is being exported, for example, from the metropolitan Washington, D.C. area into Pennsylvania and the panhandle of West Virginia, from the Minneapolis-St. Paul metro area of Minnesota into rural areas of Wisconsin, and from the Boston metro area into New Hampshire and Rhode Island. People moving from Portland, Oregon into Washington are causing a backlash. As editor Tom Koenninger observed in *The Colombian* in February 2003: "We have over-population problems, a plethora of strip malls and too much urban sprawl already. ...the last thing we need is a bunch of Oregon people who have already fouled their own nest coming north across the Colombia River to foul ours." Get ready for interstate sprawl wars.

Think sprawl perfect storm. Just as population is increasing by large amounts and land wanted for development is dwindling, sprawl developments are getting less and less dense. More land is used for each housing unit, and because subdivisions are more dispersed, more land is used for roads, water lines and other infrastructure. Population growth is unrelenting – one more person every 11 seconds. Every 11 seconds! As the nation approaches a population of 400 million, sprawl's land consumption is unsustainable. By 2050 total national land developed would more than double, if current sprawl patterns of development continue. The sprawl industry's continued political influence will make us feel like the Crowded States of America.

How does low density sprawl create the Crowded States of America? An enormous fraction of open space would be gone in regions where most people live. Nothing but ugly repetitive sprawl subdivisions, strip malls, office parks, big box stores, and roads, in large patches of the nation. Metropolitan areas would increasingly merge into other metropolitan areas, a trend that is occurring daily. People would constantly feel like there were too many people and not enough room. Traveling by car would be even more painful than anything now experienced. Think traffic congestion is bad now? Another 100 million people in traffic will imprison Americans within their cars or their homes, or both. Americans will receive this bleak future unless more people act now. Time-blind Americans today will cause land-poor and time-poor people tomorrow.

This is the choice. Cover land with endless individual private sprawl spaces and ribbons of roads. Or have islands of compact HEALTHY PLACES with distributed public greenspaces between them, including open space, parks, farms, wilderness areas, greenbelts, natural habitats, and forests. If spaciousness is sought solely in large sprawl homes on super-size lots, then there will be no outdoors spaciousness for many more people to enjoy near their homes.

Real estate agents say "they're not making land any more." They are right. Building land from trash in coastal areas has not worked and, with rising ocean levels, never will. In fact, rising sea levels and poor land management cause considerable coastal land to be lost, with much more loss predicted for the future. For example, along the Louisiana gulf coast about one football field size area is being lost every half hour, with thousands of square miles already lost. The Chesapeake Bay is expected to rise 4 to 12 inches by 2030. Buying a home near the shoreline and adjacent to coastal wetlands is shortsighted, and building even more homes in such areas is madness.

Imagine a future where your descendants live in a very sub-urban built environment. Just as in many science fiction books and movies, development could go underground. Land consumption and scarcity has gotten to the point where there is serious thinking about building down rather than up and out. The cost of building large tunnels and caverns can become competitive to costly surface land use. Already, a number of cities have underground retail complexes.

Also think about large holes in the ground, such as old quarries and surface mines. Land scarcity is driving developers to use them, despite engineering challenges. In a few cases HEALTHY PLACES are being built. In Bay Harbor, Michigan, a century-old limestone quarry site with five miles along Lake Michigan is giving way to a 1,200 acre community with 800 houses, a town center with shopping and dining, a marina with yacht club and a golf course. Outside Chicago a former 650 acre stone quarry site is becoming Cantera, a mixed-use community with 330 apartments, 170 townhouses, offices and light industrial plants. So when the sprawl shills tell you that there's plenty of land ask yourself why we're going down into caves and using mines for suitable housing.

Gregg Easterbrook, an influential author and editor, wrote in *Housing Policy Debate* in 1999: "Despite its negative image, sprawl is efficient and reflects consumer preference. In a nation where so much developable land remains, sprawl is hardly the environmental threat it is made out to be." He referred to "the mythology of vanishing land" and said "From a national land-availability standpoint...sprawl is a non-issue." He remains sprawl-blind. In his 2004 *The Progress Paradox* he said this about the upcoming population of 400 million: "If 50 percent more Americans are on the way, that means there must be 50 percent more suburban subdivisions, 50 percent more malls, 50 percent more of everything—unless anyone thinks it is fair to deny to newcomers the physical space and comfort that current Americans enjoy." Think about this.

This linear time-blind thinking with all its "musts" embraces the sprawl-stuff culture. No land problem, no traffic problem, no environmental problem, no social capital problem, no cost of infrastructure problem, no sedentariness problem, so let sprawl beget more sprawl, and according to Easterbrook we'll have a non-renewable source forever despite our rapid consumption of it. It doesn't even pass the laugh test. To not "deny" future residents the same kind of "physical space and comfort" now enjoyed is a recipe for collective self-destruction. What would our world look like today if, in 1960, consumers had started to expect suburban homes on 5-acre lots because homebuyers had the right to get all the land they wanted? Rural Kansas would be getting crowded. What is "fair" to future generations? Saving some land and nature for them is the right thing. Easterbrook is blind to sprawl's negative impacts and the inability of the culture of consumption to truly satisfy human needs. The limitless land-lie must be exposed.

Of all things, death may bring land-truth to sprawl shills. They should not count on getting a burial site where they want one. Despite so much unused land in the nation they may have to be buried in land distant from family and where they have lived. There is a grave shortage of grave sites. About half of the nation's 100,000 cemeteries no longer sell grave space or allow burials. Some only sell plots where the dead are buried on top of each other, two or three coffins deep. Things are getting worse with little land available for cemetery expansion or creation. This is good for the cremation business, but for personal or religious reasons many people reject this option, and they probably will not want grave sites in land-rich places like Oklahoma and North Dakota unless they live there. A new option is a "green burial" that protects land rather than consuming it. Without embalming, people are buried in biodegradable caskets or no casket at all, offering cost savings. In a wooded memorial preserve people can picnic, hike or take nature classes. As one family member who chose a preserve said "It's full of life, not death."

Sprawl's expansion is out of control. Greed drives land gluttony. By developing and consuming excessive amounts of land, the current pursuit of happiness by the few denies the future pursuit of happiness by the many. In that sense, sprawl is unconstitutional.

Someone who remains unconcerned about rapid U.S. land consumption after learning the truth about sprawl is like the person who falls off a 60-story building and upon passing the 20th floor still thinks "everything is okay." This is extreme time-blindness, where the future is blocked out. Very "in the moment," very Zen, but often dangerous. For facing death, present-centeredness works, but we still have time to act and prevent wall-to-wall sprawl. Do not succumb to land-lies from sprawl shills. An even uglier, crammed sprawlspace is rushing at you.

BEWARE FREEDOM TO SPRAWL.

In 2004, Ben Brown wrote in *USA Today* that the "consequence of unlimited individual freedom [is] more sprawl, a pattern of disconnected subdivisions and strip malls that clogs roads and turns unique landscapes into annexes of Anywhere, USA."

Sprawl often hides behind protection of property rights. Sprawl shills cloak their attacks on "un-American" planning in general and smart growth in particular as noble protection of sacred constitutional property rights. They defend the benefits of the few at the expense of the many. They guard land owners' right to take big money from sprawl developers and keep the "self-replicating" machine producing look-alike blandburbs. They whine against illegal "takings" of property by big, bad government. Know this. The sprawl industry is not protecting the rights or choices of the vast majority of Americans.

Winston Churchill wisely said: "Land, which is a necessity of human existence, which is the original source of all wealth, which is strictly limited in extent, which is fixed geographical position – land, I say, differs from all other forms of property in these primary and fundamental conditions." Seeing land ownership too narrowly and selfishly is as treacherous as believing that the air we breathe and the water we drink can be owned and denied to non-owners.

Overemphasizing property rights opposes community and social connectedness. Property rights must do more than serve the owner's need or greed. Landowners have obligations to the community and should cause no harm to others and their legitimate interests. Property rights – like all individual freedoms – are limited to protect the rights of others. There has never, ever been a time in the United States when land owners could do whatever they wanted with their land. A 1999 national survey by the National Association of Home Builders found that only 11 percent said people should be able to use property solely as they see fit. Conservatives should remember land value connects to the quality of the surrounding community, the actions of many other land owners, and the needs and values of the public. Victoria University of Technology Professor Colin Clark correctly observed that the development value of land depends on "its proximity to opportunities for employment, shopping, education, etc. In other words, the seller…is mainly selling the fruits of other people's labor."

Our constitution and courts provide ample protection of private property rights. Greed is another matter. The courts consistently reaffirm that landowners are not guaranteed the maximum economic return on their land. But their reasonable economic interests are protected. Nor are landowners being forced to keep their land pristine or agricultural simply to benefit society as a whole. Various approaches financially compensate landowners for preserving their land.

THE SPRAWL INDUSTRY CAN CO-OPT
CONSERVATION EASEMENTS.

An "only in America" story: North Carolina developers buy 4,400 acres for $10 million, and by placing restrictions on using 3,000 acres through a conservation easement get a federal tax deduction of about $20 million and keep the land. More data of the absurd.

Saving land for environmental purposes through conservation easements is promoted by many environmental organizations. They have become popular among rural landowners who can retain ownership but donate development potential. Financial benefits include a charitable deduction under federal law when the easement is donated to a non-profit entity, typically called a land trust, or sold below its full value. There can also be property tax savings and in some cases a state tax credit. But there are issues. Exactly what will be allowed on donated land and how will restrictions on land use be monitored and enforced forever? Valuations of the economic worth of land are problematic. The Internal Revenue Service and the General Accounting Office found that easements are often over-valued. The land may have little development potential. Or it may be of dubious environmental value. Protected land may not be accessible to the public.

Similar to easements are Purchase or Transfer of Development Rights programs by which land owners sell their development rights. Using public funds for preventing development on certain land can be cheaper than paying for new public infrastructure. In Loudoun County, Virginia, through 2003 $8.9 million was spent to prevent more than 500 future homes on more than 2,500 acres that would have cost the county about $19 million for schools and other infrastructure needs. In some places developers buy the rights so they can build in areas designated for growth.

Know this. For all forms of land conservation, the amount of land is miniscule compared to the land being consumed by the sprawl industry.

Recognizing that easements are donated and development rights are sold voluntarily and for financial benefits, what do conservatives say about them? Henry Lamb of the Environmental Conservation Organization, a conservative group whose name is far greener than its values, said:

> When a person fragments the title to his land with a perpetual conservation easement, or by selling development rights, he is, in effect, robbing future generations of the opportunity to make their own decisions about how to use the land. What right do we have to deny future generations the use of prime real estate? ...Not only are we stealing our children's birthright, we are condemning them to eventually live in a socialist state, where government owns all the sources of production.

There you have it — pure right-wing apocalyptic prose. We get a "socialist state" if we save some land and greenspace for future generations. Contradictorily, the rights of current property owners are disregarded by people who supposedly prize property rights and a free market. What these right wing patriots prize is land development. They have no problem with land owners profiting from selling their mineral rights, exploration rights, grazing rights, water rights and air rights, but not development rights. Something else makes little sense. If conservatives believe that America's endless amount of usable land removes any need to control sprawl, then why are they so negative about landowners donating or selling their development rights? Their attitude should be, "who cares, there's more where that came from." Protecting the sprawl industry is the only logical answer.

Do easements limit sprawl? Sometimes, but sometimes the sprawl industry benefits and sometimes taxpayers subsidize sprawl development through easements. Even without public funds, developers surely pay lower taxes and shift tax burdens to the public. Developer profits increase or sprawl is made even more attractive through increases in lot and home size or reductions in home prices. Developers have recognized that easements providing green infrastructure near sprawl homes allow them to charge higher prices for land and homes. As one developer said, "I call it enlightened self-interest." But many developers and builders see easements as reducing cheap land for sprawl. When the state of Indiana was considering spending public funds to preserve farmland it faced opposition. Builder Mark Wynn's view was that, "All farmers have to do is not sell their farm." To be fair, developers of HEALTHY PLACES and conservation design communities can also create easements and benefit from them.

Legally binding land use restrictions are not always what they seem to be. Developers can get changes. An easement set aside 22 acres of a 70-acre 140-home sprawl subdivision in Ohio. But about five years later a very large house was built on 4.5 acres when a majority of the landowners near the conservation area approved the change. One of the residents observed, "These builders do what they want to. If it's a conservation easement, it shouldn't have been built on."

In December 2003 *The Washington Post* ran a front-page story with the headline "Developers Find Payoff in Preservation." In one case a Pennsylvania developer built a new sprawl subdivision on a historic 450-acre farm. On 100 acres there are 163 home sites surrounding an 18-hole golf course. He created an easement for 131 unusable acres, not contiguous land, but a dozen islands, as well as an easement for the 220 acres of the golf course. The developer described the federal tax benefit he received as "a shocker" and "a bonus." A local township ordinance required that at least 60 percent of the land had to be open space anyway. The township manager said, "He shouldn't have gotten anything."

In the North Carolina case mentioned above, which yielded a $10 million profit while letting the developers own all the land, there are 350 home sites and an 18-hole golf course for which another easement and tax deduction may be obtained. All the land covered by easements provides a green amenity for the residents, allowing the developer to charge more money for lots.

Another twist on the easement benefit for developers occurred in California. The Sierra Club brokered a deal that let a developer overcome opposition to a large sprawl project for 11,000 new homes called River Islands. The developer agreed to provide $8 million to a local land trust to purchase conservation easements, a good deal for a $125 million project.

Here is another approach used to keep land from development that also backfires. Owners of agricultural land in some jurisdictions get taxed only on the basis of current value, not accounting for future development potential. This is supposed to help owners stay on the farm, especially on the fringes of metropolitan areas. However, land developers often buy such agricultural land and are able to qualify for the favored tax treatment, allowing them to hold the land at low cost until using it for sprawl development. They may even create a conservation easement for parts of the land unsuitable for sprawl development. Are such land purchases speculative and risky? Not really. Considering a 50-year sprawl trend they are safe bets.

The tax break scam is widely used in North Carolina where land owners can get tax breaks by growing some limited amount of crops or trees even if they have concrete plans for development and the property is already zoned for typical sprawl development. In Wake County, with only about 250 full-time farmers, there were more than 2,000 landowners getting tax breaks amounting to $7.5 million in a recent year. The legislature made it easy by requiring landowners to make only $1,000 yearly from farming or horticulture and this figure had not been adjusted for inflation in 30 years, nor is there vigorous enforcement.

Often times all you have to do is follow the water. Developers need land with water. No water? Buy annual water rights from farmers to make relatively cheap rural land in water-poor regions useful. Either developers or local governments under the influence of the sprawl lobby do this. Some farmers can make much more money selling water than farm products, and they stay on their land. Of course, this defeats the goal of nearly all states to maintain their agriculture industry. This is happening, for example, in Colorado. One owner of a 300-acre farm sold his water rights for $1.2 million. Three generations of family farming ended, so that the Denver suburb of Aurora could sprawl even more. In California, a shift of water from desert farms will support sprawl in San Diego.

In all three cases of easements, agricultural taxes, and transfer of water rights, the sprawl industry works to get laws they can benefit from.After a 1999 pro-sprawl report from the National Center for Policy Analysis attacked anti-sprawl efforts for limiting the ability of land speculators to develop more sprawl, Larry Bohlen of the Sierra Club observed, "Why have land speculators traditionally been the largest contributors in political campaigns? They must think that they are getting something for their money." In 2000, Keith Schneider, of the Michigan Land Use Institute, wrote that then Governor John Engler, a friend of sprawl, supported an agricultural tax, but "the governor's aides entered into closed-door negotiations…with home builders and realtors." They prevented a significant recapture fee used by California and other states to get part of the windfall when farmland is developed after receiving tax breaks.

It comes to this. The first imperative of sprawl developers and home builders is: GET THE LAND. As one Florida county official said, after developers had bought an enormous amount of agricultural land: "The barbarians are at the gate." The second imperative is: GET GOVERNMENT

TO REMOVE ZONING OBSTACLES, PUT IN INFRASTRUCTURE, AND
ASSURE WATER.

Sprawl developers use super-size homes to lure people from older suburbs and cities to drive longer distances. Gluttonous land consumption
marches on and on, with a little help from its friends, often unseen. A perverse program in upstate New York to save farmland from development
actually motivates land owners in other parts of the country to sell out. As
Marty Broccoli of Oneida County explained: " They're selling farms for
$15,000 to $50,000 an acre to housing and commercial developers, and
we're saying, 'Hey, you can buy a good working farm for $800 to $2,000 an
acre in upstate New York." Take the money and run….to upstate New York.
One such farm family moved from South Dakota and explained that they
selected New York land with a river view because it could be sold someday
for housing development. Imagine one of those giant mazes of dominoes
falling in a chain reaction after just one is knocked down. Landowners are
falling down one after another. Too few landowners and too few consumers resist sprawl.

AN INVISIBLE LAND USE PLANNING INDUSTRY.

The Public Policy Institute of California found in its 2002 survey of
adult residents that an amazing 77 percent believed that local voters – not
government – should make local land use and development decisions at
the ballot box. This is a clear no-confidence vote in developer-influenced
planning boards and commissions. Considering who is making land use
decisions, it is not surprising that citizens are so cynical about local government.

What does the planning system that affects our lives consist of? Though
many local jurisdictions lack any planning apparatus and sprawl has free
reign, here are the key parts in most places:

PLANNING DEPARTMENT: Towns, cities, and counties have professionals to manage the local planning effort. They typically feed information and recommendations to the Planning Commission. Planning
staff provide technical assistance and guidance, and manage regulatory oversight and enforcement.

PLANNING BOARD OR COMMISSION: Following state law, they typically prepare and revise the required comprehensive (or municipal) plan and local land use regulations such as zoning or subdivision codes. They also review development proposals. Most states require that a board of zoning appeals or adjustment be created, which may be the same as the commission, to handle requests for variances. Most formal public participation and lobbying for sprawl take place here.

LOCAL GOVERNING BODY: The city or town council, or board of county commissioners, and/or the top elected official, appoint the members of the board or commission, whose actions must be approved by the governing body, or overturned by it. More political influence of the sprawl industry occurs here.

METROPOLITAN PLANNING ORGANIZATION: These are non-elected regional bodies that focus on transportation planning and, increasingly, integration with broader land use issues.

There is a large and mostly invisible urban and land use planning industry. There are planning departments in universities and local governments, local planning boards and commissions, journals and magazines, and professional associations. Here is the sticky problem. The dominant form and methods of urban and town planning conflict with human needs and the environment. Tens of thousands of highly credentialed professionals have collaborated with government to create a system that pumps out sprawl un-places. New Urbanism pioneer Andres Duany captured the truth: "It is the professionals of recent decades that have ruined our cities and our landscapes."

How did we lose real communities with high social capital from decades of so much professional land-use planning? Somewhere along the sprawl highway land-use planning became separated from community design. For too long planners have focused on plan-making rather than place-making. The planner's mantra should be: THE PLAN IS NOT THE PLACE. Planners are too subservient to the political and government systems that pay them directly or indirectly, and that are under the influence of the sprawl lobby. Planners who care too much about accommodating all and any growth do not preserve and enhance quality of life and quality of place.

The public is blind to the tricks played in creating a comprehensive, master or general plan, the key legal instrument to guide local land development, and associated regulations. Local governments spend big money making plans that no sane person wants to read. The public deserves a reliable vision and plan for how their community should develop. It does not work out that way. Developers want and get flexibility. Loose language is cleverly built into documents to undermine seemingly strict requirements. As Charles Lee of Florida Audubon observed: "The plans and the regulations are written in a way that one can use weasel words that allow you to justify any decisions under them later." Exactly the point. Another trick is to get governing bodies to pass "zoning text amendments" to make a project legal and avoid public scrutiny through rezoning. Despite developers' complaints, strict control of development is often a sham.

Picture a bunch of developers getting together, grumbling and strategizing over drinks. A Colorado court has just found that comprehensive plans could be used as the basis for denying permits for development. What to do? Within minutes the answer is clear. Get the state legislature to pass, and the governor to sign, a law making comprehensive plans advisory only. This was done in 1997. It may have helped that from 1996 to 2002 development interests gave $2.7 million to state elected officials. The top recipient by a huge margin was Governor Bill Owens with $454,000. A 2001 survey of Colorado registered voters on the governor's performance in several main areas revealed the lowest grade for managing growth.

Zoning regulations have been called the DNA of land development; they implement general or comprehensive plans and have promoted sprawl. Back in 1968, William H. Whyte observed in *The Last Landscape* that "zoning has so far been used principally for the protection of property interests. …The administration of zoning has been terrible. …it is an elaborate mechanism for insuring a satisfactory status quo, or a future reasonably similar." Satisfactory to the sprawl industry and its supporters, of course, not the increasing numbers of Americans suffering the effects of sprawl. Planning and zoning efforts have grown bigger but not better.

A 2000 survey of employees in the King County, Washington, Department of Development and Environmental Services, found that nearly two-thirds believed that management viewed its primary customer to be developers that seek permits, not county citizens. In 2003, five county transportation planners filed a whistle-blower complaint about bad data being used to decide whether or not new developments cause unacceptable traffic congestion. An independent study confirmed many of their charges. As in a 1998 decision by a hearing examiner and a 1999 county auditor's report, all the errors favored developers.

According to a 2002 survey of planners and planning commissioners by the *Planning Commissioners Journal*, an amazing 21 percent of planning board members came from the sprawl industry, including homebuilders, building contractors, developers, appraisers, surveyors, architects, landscape architects, and planners. Another 7 percent were attorneys, many of whom likely worked for developers and homebuilders. So, probably at least a quarter of planning board members are likely to favor sprawl development that serves their financial interests.

Additionally, survey respondents commented frequently about the political nature of appointments to boards. When politicians appoint sprawl supporters, such boards do not serve the public. Planning boards and commissions should be fair, objective, and unbiased decision makers and advisors to elected officials. But that probably is more the exception than the rule.

Interestingly, medical professionals constitute only one percent of planning board members. We need more health professionals and public health officials directly involved with planning and zoning. The situation is equally bad in planning departments. A 2003 survey of 10,000 government planners by the American Planning Association found that only 8 percent said they had collaborated with the public health office in their jurisdiction. One exception is the Tri-County Health Department for Adams, Arapahoe and Douglas counties in Colorado; it worked to get active living objectives considered in building and zoning decisions.

Governors have done no better when they have formed various kinds of task forces, commissions and cabinet groups on growth management. State health departments have not been at the table. This was the case, for example, with Michigan's Land Use Leadership Council and Florida's Growth Management Study Commission.

The sprawl industry lambastes government for impeding their efforts. Yet sprawl is ubiquitous. The sprawl industry is not the underdog fighting a hostile government; it feeds the fox guarding the sprawl hen house. Sprawl shills say consumers cause sprawl, which only is logical if Americans have had something other than sprawl to choose, but they rarely have had competitive options because the sprawl industry has effectively blocked them. The "we just give them what they want" defense is garbage – sprawl shills want to shift responsibility and blame to consumers.

There is some way out of this. We must shift power from the sprawl industry and the politicians it controls, to citizens. Distrust in government caused Florida Hometown Democracy in 2003, to launch a petition drive for a constitutional amendment that would give local voters control over land-use changes through referenda, instead of local and state politicians. Lesley Blackner, one of the group's founders, made the case thusly: "We have government by the developer and for the developer. Too many of Florida's elected officials only define the 'public interest' as keeping the development industry happy." The group may win, despite opposition from the already panicked Florida Home Builders Association, local politicians, and Governor Jeb Bush, who said the initiative is "a great name but a bad idea." Strange that an elected member of the state government would suggest that decisions based on citizen choice would be "a bad idea." Most Floridians are unhappy with gluttonous land consumption. A 1999 state survey found that only 8 percent thought the state was very effective in managing growth, 57 percent thought suburban quality of life had declined, and over 75 percent wanted more public involvement in planning and development decisions. Now, these Floridians must act.

Substantial developer money was spent to defeat Colorado's Amendment 24 because it transferred to citizens the traditional land-use and planning powers of local government. The National Association of Realtors said: "Transfer of decision-making process from trained planning staffs and elected representative government to citizen vote is likely to create uncertainty in the market and unpredictability and delay in the land use and development process." Meaning: citizens cannot be controlled as easily as government bureaucrats and elected officials. It was recommended that the "building community, including REALTORS should not be visible in the campaign" against smart growth. Interestingly, the U.S. Supreme Court sanctioned referenda on land-use in a case where a developer sued the city of Eastlake, Ohio, because of an ordinance requiring approval by 55 percent of voters for changes to its comprehensive plan.

More recently, Peter Q. Davis, a local California politician, supported the 2004 Rural Lands ballot initiative that would limit sprawl on nearly 700,000 acres in San Diego County and give citizens the right to vote on development. He said, "This initiative is necessary because the political establishment has made a mess of the planning process." A similar initiative failed in 1998 when, like the second effort, developers, builders and realtors plowed money into defeating it. In 2003 and 2004 much of the money was "laundered" through the local Farm Bureau, in favor of farmers getting rich by selling out to sprawl developers. Some $450,000 was spent on television ads; the initiative was defeated on March 2, 2004. An initiative leader said, "We think the opposition, with its big developer money, ran a very deceptive campaign and it confused the voters." Indeed, the opposition said that the initiative promoted sprawl. Sprawl kills truth.

A 2004 poll by Peter D. Hart found that 46 percent of people do not believe they have any say about what government does, compared to 32 percent 50 years earlier, which explains why 65 percent favor greater use of referenda and ballot measures. S. Mattox from Florida observed: "Why do we, as citizens, bother to vote for our so-called representatives if all they do is the bidding of the lobbyists? We, the citizens, are no more represented than the people in some Third World country." After a "greedy few land speculators and developers" lobbied the Volusia, Florida County Council to back-off urban growth boundaries, some citizens started a campaign in 2004 for a ballot measure to amend the county charter. In 2004 Sycamore, Illinois residents voted more than two to one in favor of a referendum to stop new subdivisions, but it was only advisory. Joyce Smith said: "Now we will see how the city council and government act and if they start listening to the people." Sprawl lobbying aims to protect the sprawl industry from people when government should be protecting people from the sprawl industry.

Long ago President Teddy Roosevelt said: "I believe in the Initiative and Referendum, which should be used not to destroy representative government, but to correct it whenever it becomes misrepresentative." Misrepresentation happens when elected officials are nothing more than shortsighted shills for sprawl. Our nation began with a revolt against taxation without representation, now we suffer from taxation with misrepresentation....to pay for sprawl. But sprawl shill C.C. Kraemer sees referenda that cut the power of the sprawl lobby as "the rule of the mob, not the rule of law." That's right-wing belief in democracy.

VOTES MUST BEAT MONEY.

Know this. In the political arena, the underdogs are citizens fighting sprawl projects and the sprawl lobby. However, voters do not necessarily prevail even when they win. For example, in early 2003, a judge in Douglas County, Nevada tossed out the growth limit that voters had passed the previous November, which cut in half the rate of new house construction. A local developer and home builder was happy about the decision, he had been chairman of the county's planning commission that enacted the sprawl-friendly master plan that the judge ruled should prevail. A leader of a citizens group indicated their intent to appeal the verdict to the state Supreme Court.

On the good news side, the Pennsylvania Supreme Court upheld the right of multi-jurisdictional planning and zoning to prevent development in one part of a total area while steering it to areas already developed. Toll Bros., a major developer and homebuilder, and eight owners of 312 acres of farmland seeking a financial windfall from selling land for development had sued local government. After seven years they finally failed with the argument that the agricultural land was in the path of growth and should not be off-limits to development.

Professional planners now speak of "planning rage" among citizens, which surfaces in public meetings with local officials. People fighting the system get flushed with anger, then get in their vehicles and confront traffic congestion. As discussed in Chapter 7, conventional public participation events held by government are next to useless. Planning rage is an expression of people suffering from "sprawl rage." There is some way out of this. Smart growth advocates are winning elections.

In April 2003, three smart growth advocates were voted into office in Lawrence, Kansas – yes sprawl is alive and well in urban Kansas. Along with the mayor, four of the five city commissioners became a smart growth supermajority that sent chills through the "growth machine" of builders, real estate agents and developers.

In Loudoun County, Virginia, a high growth area near Washington, D.C., anti-sprawl candidates won eight of the nine county supervisor positions in 1999. They enacted policies for a more enlightened style of growth, including open space preservation and HEALTHY PLACES. But attempts to get new powers to better manage growth from the state legislature, prompted the Home Builders Association of Virginia to threaten, "You would be giving local governments a weapon of mass destruction on

＋　　＋　　　　　　　　　　　　　　　　　　　　　　＋　　＋

the economy of the commonwealth." What ridiculous rhetoric to call smart growth a weapon of mass destruction. As the Loudoun Board chairman said: "Evidently, they are concerned more about the rights of developers than the rights of the taxpayers."

Pro-sprawl groups planned to reverse things in the 2003 election, mounted more than 200 lawsuits to gut the smart growth reforms, and gave $460,000 to supervisor candidates, seven times what they gave in 1999. The pro-sprawl candidates often confused voters by seeming to embrace growth controls while more than 50 percent of their campaign funds came from development interests. It paid off. They became the six to three pro-development majority. At their first public meeting in January 2004 they rewarded their sprawl backers by extending water and sewer services to a wide area, committing to a major new highway, opposing state legislation allowing local governments to levy impact fees, and stopping funding of a land preservation program. Hold-over pro-smart growth supervisor Scott K. York said this about the new pro-sprawl majority: "So far, they've shown nothing in terms of managing growth, other than managing to let developers off the hook and to leave taxpayers saddled with millions to make up." In five years 20 new schools must be constructed to handle the sprawling developments careening across the countryside. York described their policy as "Leave No Developer Behind."*The Washington Post* editorialized: "With a build-away majority now in command on the Loudoun County Board of Supervisors, developers are having a field day. ...Growth can't be stopped, but reckless ruination can and should be."

Sprawl interests are the leading business source of money to Virginia politicians and keep the state under constant sprawl siege, despite strong citizen support for smart growth. A survey of Virginia voters in early 2003 found that 77 percent supported the adoption of smart growth legislation by legislature; 82 percent supported the legislature empowering local communities to adopt impact fees; 75 percent rejected the notion that building new roads would solve traffic congestion and agreed that road building results in more sprawl and congestion; and 56 percent rejected the property rights argument that zoning and land use policies hurt land owners and the development industry. In 1999 27 bills to help localities control growth were introduced in the General Assembly; after they all failed, Stafford County Supervisor David Beiler noted: "The developer lobby got everything it wanted, the local governments got nothing they wanted to control growth." He attributed this to the $2 million developers put into that year's elections.

Face sprawl politics. For more housing choice and a chance to live in a HEALTHY PLACE, fight the political influence bought by the sprawl industry. Vote for ballot initiatives and candidates supporting smart growth, community based planning and design, and public transit. Remember that government spending on new roads is essential for sprawl expansion, so pay attention to road spending. Learn whether candidates take money from land developers, home builders, real estate interests, and road building companies, or their trade associations.

Sometimes votes beat money. In November 2003, despite big spending by developers and home builders, Ann Arbor, Michigan, voters approved a ballot initiative by a 2-to-1 margin to tax themselves to preserve land outside the city to stop sprawl. Pro-sprawl groups had committed $400,000 for their campaign and used a popular sleazy tactic, groups with deceptive names to mislead voters with misinformation, a typical dirty trick of the sprawl lobby. Two of these were the Washtenaw Smart growth Initiative and Washtenaw Citizens for Responsible Growth.

Be an informed and conscientious voter to get more opportunities to live in a quality neighborhood and community. Or, do it for your children or grandchildren, who may not enjoy living in the Crowded States of America, where they see the natural world on their plasma screens, because the real thing has been gobbled up by gluttonous land development.

THE RIGHT SOLUTIONS WERE GIVEN IN 1981.

Most anti-sprawl Truth and Wisdom were revealed long ago in a forgotten 1981 report. Even the title was noteworthy: "The Affordable Community: Growth, Change, and Choice in the '80s." It was produced by the Council on Development Choices for the '80s that had a distinguished, diverse group of 35 members, including some notables, such as Bill Clinton, then-Governor of Arkansas, several other governors, and a number of mayors, architects, and developers. What I call HEALTHY PLACES, the report called "urban villages," a few of which existed in 1980. Here are samplings of Truth revealed years before the Congress for the New Urbanism was formed in 1993 and "smart growth" was coined in the late 1990s.

On mixed-use development: "Instead of separating houses from everything else, the Council urges localities to create a mix of land uses in their neighborhoods and communities. ...Residential developments that mix attached housing, detached houses, and apartment buildings can be marketed profitably. ...New reasons for mixing uses – to save energy, to save money, to make communities more convenient – explain why mixed use developments are spreading now and should become prominent in the '80s."

On compact land development: "The more dwellings per acre in a residential area, the more effectively land costs can be kept in bounds. The more spread out a development pattern is, the greater the costs of personal transportation and public services and facilities. ...Compact housing does not mean crowding or discomfort; well-designed, it offers privacy, ample room, open spaces and amenities. ...The Council believes that the market would support much greater amounts of affordable, compact housing than is now being produced."

On transportation: "Americans will never willingly give up their cars, nor should they. But...they may well want to drive less, and they should have that choice. People seem to want more transportation choices... More homebuyers are seeking housing located near to their workplace."

On affordable housing: "[Housing] must suit a greater variety of needs and preferences, and it must be located reasonably close to where jobs are."

On urban villages: "An urban village may be thought of as a form of development or redevelopment that combines the other Council recommendations – compactness, infill and revitalization, transportation options, mixed use, and affordable housing. ...Urban villages can be planned and developed in central cities, suburbs, small towns, or rural counties. Their development helps to achieve the goals of a balanced mix of housing and jobs and economic and efficient delivery of public services and facilities."

Urban villages did not displace sprawl development (called "haphazard," "ad hoc," "scattered," and "wasteful development" in the report.) Americans did not get the greater choices the report repeatedly emphasized. State and local governments did not heed the message about ways to reduce infrastructure spending. The profitable business opportunity was not acted upon by the nation's development and home building industry. Affordable housing became more of a problem.

Listen to the Council's three co-chairs from that 1981 report: "[Americans] need to be made aware of new forces in the marketplace and the choices that could and should be theirs." "Could and should," not "will." Few jurisdictions changed zoning laws to help industry pursue the recommended forms of development. But, logically, there was no inherent reason why local governments should not have been persuaded, as the Council was – one third of which were local government officials – of the many benefits of mixed-use urban villages. The fact is that sprawl domination remained because the sprawl industry blocked change.

A more widely read report was released in 1994 by the Bank of America and others. "Beyond Sprawl" forcibly made the case against continuation of the sprawl pattern of development in California. The need to move beyond sprawl "has never been more critical or urgent. ...we must move beyond sprawl in the few remaining years of the 20th century. ...We cannot afford another generation of sprawl. [The state] is increasingly characterized by a limited supply of developable land. ...A do-nothing approach, in effect, constitutes a policy decision in favor of the "Beyond Sprawl" status quo. ...We must act now." But the urgent call for curbing sprawl was not heeded in California, or anywhere else. Only the power and influence of the sprawl industry can explain the inaction by government and the private sector. We must learn from history.

For too long the sprawl lobby has escaped scrutiny. One exception was a political analysis by Merrill Goozner, then with the *Chicago Tribune*, published in Salon.com in July 1999. A member of the Council behind the 1981 report had become President Bill Clinton and had a "livability" initiative that Al Gore focused on. Here is Goozner's incisive observation:

Unfortunately, the Clinton administration's anti-sprawl program....doesn't pose a serious challenge to the sprawl lobby. ...Like most of the [state] smart growth initiatives around the country, the Clinton plan is doomed to fail because it doesn't reckon with the powerful development interests that have a stake in sprawl – most notably the home builders and road construction lobbies, which dominate every state capital and are already mobilizing to oppose smart growth plans.

Smart growth advocates salivated over a major anti-sprawl element in Al Gore's campaign. But the opposition became active. Right-wing sprawl shills portrayed livability as anti-American Dream. The Heritage Foundation released "The President's New Sprawl Initiative: A Program in Search of a Problem." Gregg Easterbrook, Michael Kelley and other writers asserted that the livability agenda protected the values and privileges of more wealthy Americans while denying suburban housing for lower income people. Smart growth was falsely smeared as undermining upward mobility. Gore backed down— beneath the surface something else was going on.

In July 2000 the *Associated Press* and others ran stories on sizable contributions to the Gore campaign from employees of a development company just days after it had received favorable support from the Clinton White House for a contentious shopping mall project in New Jersey. *The American Prospect* ran a major story on the New Jersey victory for the developer and the "eyebrow-raising coincidence." Another story talked about Gore's promotion of "sleazy real estate deals that would move industrial jobs away from urban Miami onto farmland between two National Parks." Even the most liberal politicians can get corrupted by sprawl money.

Ron Gurwitt wrote about Gore's support of smart growth in Salon.com in January 1999: "It all sounds good, until you begin to think about who might be arrayed on the other side. There are, for instance, state highway departments, which…are unremitting asphalt lovers. There's the construction lobby. There are engineers, financiers, developers and land-use lawyers. There are state legislators who count all those people among their closest friends and contributors." Enough said. Livability lost and the sprawl lobby won, again. We do not need more reports. We need effective action that recognizes the power and influence of the sprawl industry.

THE SPRAWL INDUSTRY PROTECTS THE STATUS QUO.

The sprawl lobby may be stronger than ever. When President George W. Bush spoke in April 2004 at a large fundraiser in Coral Gables, Florida, the first person he thanked was "long-time friend" Armando Codina, the developer who hired brother Jeb in 1981, made him rich, and took him back after he was Florida's Secretary of Commerce and after he lost the governor's race in 1994. The second person thanked was Al Hoffman, another developer. Codina and Hoffman had been Florida electors in the

Electoral College that made George W. Bush President.

Governor Jeb Bush has not used the state's legal framework to limit the ravenous sprawl consuming Florida. As The Washington Post observed in 2002, Florida's governors' "growth management efforts have failed for decades, and Jeb Bush's administration has been especially close to real estate interests." A former attorney for the state, Ross Burnaman, summed it up: "Jeb and his lieutenants are by and large selling the state out."

And Al Hoffman is buying land and politicians, making him the most influential Florida developer. He has headed an exclusive council of CEOs advising the governor, been the finance chair for the Republican National Committee, and been a prodigious fund raiser for the Bush brothers. In November 2003 Hoffman hosted a reception for President Bush at his sprawling Fort Myers mansion; some 700 guests provided $2.5 million. As a "Ranger" for President Bush's re-election campaign he has bundled at least $200,000 in contributions; he made Super Ranger status by also raising $300,000 for the Republican Party. Amazingly, in early 2004, out of 165 such Rangers at least 40 percent were connected to the sprawl industry! In May 2004 Hoffman put Jeb Bush's former chief of staff on his company's board of directors, where she would earn $40,000 or more yearly.

"You can't stop it. There's no power on earth that can stop it," so boasted Hoffman about land development. Presumably in his mind that includes voters and government officials. In October 2003 Governor Bush and his Cabinet approved a project for a marina that could handle 100-foot yachts and a 15-story condo with 48 units selling from about $4 million to almost $9 million. Jim Baltzelle, editor of the *St. Augustine Record,* who attended the meeting, reported "Bush did not mention during the Cabinet meeting that his campaign finance chairman was the developer on the line. Neither did anyone else." In late 2003 Hoffman got Governor Bush to create the new state Office of Destination Florida; state funds are used to attract even more senior citizens to retire in Florida, providing even more business for developers like Hoffman.

Hoffman was behind a scheme to transport water from the northern panhandle to southern Florida. But after that failed he switched to fighting a state rule that would allocate water first to the Everglades cleanup and possibly limit development in his neck of the woods. When Congress approved the $8.4 billion Everglades restoration it required that the environment would have first rights to the new water captured in reservoirs and well fields, and in January 2002 President Bush and Governor Bush promised as much. Time will tell whether Hoffman and his cronies unravel that promise.

Carl Hiaasen has been writing about Florida sprawl for many years. In a 1985 *Miami Herald* column he said: "This year the Legislature passed a 'growth management' law, supposedly to impose order on the state's tumultuous development. Frankly, the notion of 'orderly growth' is about as tangible as the tooth fairy. Growth that is orderly would break a century-old tradition of lust, greed and wantonness." In 2004 Hiaasen said: "Selling out to wealthy developers is a grand tradition in Florida politics. Those who are paving and malling the state throw more money at candidates than do any other groups." Others have echoed these sentiments.

+ A *Daytona Beach News-Journal* editorial in 2002 got it right: "If 'growth management' was an oxymoron in Florida prior to 1985, it has since been exposed as a bald-faced lie. This state doesn't manage growth; it plays it, staking finite resources on a Ponzi scheme's final payoff." The editorial noted that research had shown that Florida's unique and fragile natural resources could only sustain a population of 6 to 7 million, but that local and state government had already approved developments to handle 100 million.

+ St. Petersburg Times writer Bill Maxwell opined in 2003: "The Sunshine State, one of the nation's great treasures, is fast becoming the Asphalt State. What we are doing to our paradise is criminal and, well, stupid."

+ Joe Newman of the *Orlando Sentinel* reported in 2003, "When it comes down to it, no matter how much lip service state and local planners offer against sprawl, they rarely do anything to stop it."

Newspaper truth has not dented Florida developer power. Long ago developers and their political allies pushed Florida off the 60th floor of sprawl-central. Florida keeps tumbling toward social, fiscal and environmental disaster in bright sunshine for all but the time-blind to see. Laws are passed as window dressing and the sprawl blitzkrieg continues. Perhaps the grassroots Florida Hometown Democracy initiative will wake up Floridians before the sprawl hits the fan, before most Floridians are surrounded by sprawl instead of natural beauty, and fighting brutal traffic to get everywhere. Meanwhile, sprawl developers will be enjoying their waterfront McMansions and yachts in the state they developed to death.

And when Jeb Bush leaves the governor's mansion is there any doubt that he will join his bulldozer buddies and profit from development?

Pro-sprawl gang member C. Kenneth Orski proclaimed: "In the end, the verbal skirmishes fought over 'smart growth' are of little practical consequence, for the 'smart growth' movement has no power to reshape America's urban landscape in any significant way. The 'smart growth' movement is likely to go down in history as yet another planning ideology that has foundered for lack of a realistic understanding of demographics, market forces and consumer preferences." He's counting his sprawl subdivisions before they hatch. Also in 2003, sprawl shill Chris Fiscelli said: "In the end, the smart growth flame will likely burn out... Then we'll think back and remember this smart growth vision was just another bad dream."

Sprawl is the bad dream. If smart growth is losing, why keep fighting it so viciously? Because smart growth will succeed if Americans have more choice. Sprawl dominance needs more than willing consumers; it requires the market distortions obtained by the sprawl lobby and its shills to deprive consumers of choice.

Listen to economist Thomas Sowell, an intellectual idol of conservatives: "Urban sprawl is today's contrived crisis." Contrived? Is all that traffic congestion people are suffering through imaginary? Are all those hillsides in Colorado and California covered with sprawl subdivisions a mirage? He also said: "This is a culture war – and the only thing worse than being in a war is being in a war and not knowing it, while the other side is carrying out a Jihad." He said this in 1999 when the smart growth movement was not nearly as strong as today. He was right about the culture war, but wrong about the "other side."

I say this to smart growth advocates and all Americans: Wake up and smell the bulldozers! Learn from history. Do not fall into the trap of believing that sprawl developers will come around and respond to demand for HEALTHY PLACES. Do not think that environmental groups or regulations are blocking HEALTHY PLACES. Do not ignore the corruption of government by the sprawl industry. Do not be duped by superficial support from business groups. Do not pin too much hope on what some elected officials may do. Focus on the mass housing market and satisfying consumer demand for HEALTHY PLACES. Engage the enemy. Do not hesitate to blame the sprawl industry, sprawl shills, and corrupt politicians. Heed the wise words of history professor Laura McCall: "Cooperation works for the status quo, the vested interests, the big money, the established, the well-positioned, and the spin doctors in government and the media. …What works is not compromise, but finding ways to insure that the status quo eventually understands – that they 'get it.'"

The sprawl industry sees current attacks as replays of a long string of battles it has won. Sprawl stakes are high. Unless smart growth advocates and health professionals take this long term war more seriously it will be lost, like the wars against drugs, poverty and polluters. Smart growth advocates must stress the politics of sprawl and the personal benefits of choosing an alternative, rather than sprawl's environmental and social equity impacts. We need a more pragmatic market approach.

Our nation had clear warnings decades ago from prescient thinkers like Lewis Mumford, William H. Whyte, and John Keats. The right solutions were revealed in the 1981 and 1994 reports discussed above. Yet we remain stuck in sprawl. How do we finally get unstuck? First, we need to shed light on the sprawl battle and the forces aligned against a fairer housing market with more choice for consumers. Second, we need to inform citizen-consumers about why they should choose HEALTHY PLACES and demand more of them.

Satisfying pent-up consumer demand requires unleashing citizen power. We need consumer muscle in the housing market and citizen power in the political arena. The housing market and our political system have failed consumers, because the sprawl industry has used politics to distort the market. Americans must help themselves secure more housing and transportation choices. You must take sprawl personally. To paraphrase Edmund Burke: "The only thing necessary for the triumph of sprawl is for good people to do nothing." Resistance is not futile. But it is difficult and requires courage.

Tom McCall was courageous. The acclaimed governor of Oregon inspired a state law in 1973 to control sprawl through urban growth boundaries. He is the true father of smart growth in America. He said sprawl put "cancerous cells of unmentionable ugliness into our rural landscape" and was "a shameless threat…to the whole quality of our life." He wisely recognized that land "is our most valuable finite natural resource." Despite its anti-sprawl tradition, in 2000, 54 percent of Oregon voters were persuaded to pass a constitutional amendment that would have busted that tradition if the state's Supreme Court had not tossed it out. Property-rights activists continue to push their agenda to reimburse land owners if regulations reduce property value, even though it could bankrupt the state. Current Governor Ted Kulongoski has been tagged "Kulonsprawlski" for wanting to expand urban growth boundaries; the *Eugene Weekly* wryly observed "The sprawl prospect has local land speculators drooling."

Too many good people have done nothing. Sitting in suburban traffic congestion on the weekend and thinking "I wish someone would do something about this" is not enough. As novelist and ecologist Edward Abbey said, "Sentiment without action is the ruin of the soul." Civic inaction and physical inactivity go hand in hand in blandland. A war rages in the United States, the people against the tyranny of relentless, runaway suburban sprawl. America's silent majority does more than live in sprawl, it lets the sprawl juggernaut keep dividing and isolating us.

Time to choose a side.

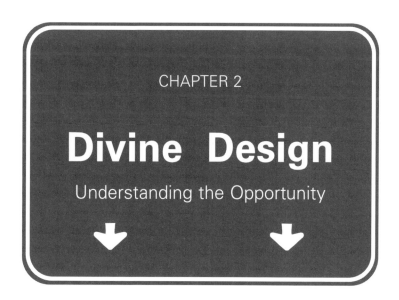

CHAPTER 2

Divine Design

Understanding the Opportunity

Sprawl is unhealthy at any price.

Helter-skelter suburban sprawl clutters the American landscape. But more and more Americans realize the terrible price being paid for the sprawl lifestyle. The real issue is community design. Sprawl is bad design; bad for people and bad for the environment. Smart growth is all about better community design.

Listen to a mother in an outlying suburb of Kansas City as she reflected on her need to drive to do just about everything, including grocery shopping, taking her kids to a park, dining out, renting a video, and going to the post office. She observed "I used to live in an urban area in Independence, and I walked all the time, and I didn't have this extra 10 pounds. My son, after we moved out here, he put on 50 pounds." She made the right connection. Living in automobile-dependent sprawl is unhealthy.

"Life is too short to spend it commuting or cutting grass." So said a man who moved from Virginia sprawl, with a two hour commute, to a new high density infill project near Washington, D.C. that required an eight-minute drive. He made the right connection. Time is too valuable to spend so much of it in vehicles.

In the sprawl capitol of Atlanta an insightful resident observed: "There is no question that sprawl is wrong and we are wrong by purchasing houses that contribute to it. The market only brings us what we will buy. If we refused to buy into this stressful lifestyle, something would have to change. But for every person…who would gladly give up the burbs to live in a smart growth community, there are 20 other people who would choose the status quo because of complacency or ignorance or both."

She grasped the nature of the housing market. Do not expect people to choose something other than sprawl if they do not see a real alternative to it. Do not blame people for choosing sprawl. Do not condemn suburbia just because sprawl has taken it over. With sufficient information about the negative impacts of sprawl, consumer complacency can be conquered. Consumer power can transform the housing market. The same consumer power that has sustained sprawl can embrace and advance HEALTHY PLACES. As architect Karen Harris said, "You don't have to go along with the consortium of homebuilders and realtors who keep building the same thing because people keep buying it."

So here is the good news. You do not have to spend so much time inside your home and car. There is, indeed, a healthy alternative to unhealthy sprawl. HEALTHY PLACES are designed for people to live together in a community with real neighbors and an inviting public realm. It is not some theoretical concept. Nor is it new. This type of community was invented long ago. It was the *normal* way human beings lived together in this country. It was what we had before sprawl and its mirror image – urban decay, because sprawl thrived by sucking the lifeblood from cities.

Decades of promoting exercise and fitness by health, wellness and exercise professionals and organizations have failed, as evidenced by rising levels of sedentariness, obesity, overweight, and many related diseases. Seventy percent of Americans do not get enough regular physical activity for good health. Medical and public health professionals talk about various kinds of interventions, but the one intervention they have ignored is the personal decision to choose a community that supports everyday, active living. The right built environment can help a person accumulate at least 30 minutes of moderate-intensity physical activity on most days of the week.

You should live in a place that is *intentionally designed* to provide a higher quality of life. To get a higher quality of life you must seek a higher quality of place. People are not just what they eat but also where they live. Place really matters, not so much house as community. You cannot maximize your health and quality of life if you live in a poorly designed built environment. Living in suburban sprawl may seem infinitely better than living in an urban slum, but you can do better. That is not the right comparison, nor the choice facing consumers, as you'll appreciate once you learn about true alternatives to sprawl.

A true sprawl alternative is a community that improves physical, mental, social, and economic health. It is a HEALTHY PLACE. This term encompasses many other expressions that you may have read about or seen used in advertisements for housing. These include: New Urbanism, Traditional Neighborhood Development, compact development, livable communities, healthy communities, new towns, transit-friendly development, smart urbanism, sustainable communities, garden villages, master-planned communities, urban villages, close-knit communities, transit villages, and neo-traditional design. While projects described by such terms may offer benefits over sprawl development, they may not be fully consistent with HEALTHY PLACES and smart growth. With the exception of smart growth, none of the many terms has reached widespread understanding or acceptance in the public and private sectors. The Centers for Disease Control and Prevention (CDC) has used the term HEALTHY PLACES for communities designed for active living. Chapter 6 provides a simple checklist so that all this semantic confusion does not stand in the way of finding a true alternative to sprawl.

To save greenspace we should put as much development as possible in areas already developed. Hence, the hierarchy of preferred locations for HEALTHY PLACES is: (1) rebuilt or new neighborhoods in cities, (2) improvements in older suburbs, and (3) new communities on greenfield sites. The term "infill" is used for the first two categories. Regardless of location all HEALTHY PLACES must share basic smart growth features.

A mounting problem is intentionally misleading terms being used by the sprawl industry. Sprawl-speak perverts language to mislead consumers and keep the market safe for sprawl. In sprawl-speak strip malls are often called "town squares," major six-lane suburban roads without trees are called "parkways," and cookie-cutter suburban subdivisions are called "villages" and "towns." "Community," "neighborhood," "historic" and other catchy words are often used in advertisements to appeal to consumer desires for something other than typical suburban subdivisions. There are no legal requirements for "Oak Hills Village" to contain any oaks or hills, or "Green River Forest" to contain a river or woods. What consumers usually get is an automobile-dependent place that does not have good geographic genes.

The sprawl culture has perniciously "dumbed down" and "defined down" the meaning of community and neighborhood. The terms have been trivialized and turned into clichés, perfect for sprawl-speak. This has protected sprawl by undermining the search for true community and neighborhood.

Here is a basic truth. Living in sprawl where people are physically separated from other people, and from their jobs and virtually all other destinations and needs, is fundamentally unhealthy. Like swimming upstream, people can try many different strategies to be healthier, but find themselves still stuck with an emptiness that may defy complete understanding. Sprawl limits even the best of intentions to be healthy. *Sprawl exhaustion results not from healthy physical activity, but from the stress of sprawl living*. Physicians can advise their patients to get more regular physical activity, but be totally unaware that the habitat where the person lives does not support physical activity, and in fact may actively work against it. Schools may encourage kids walking to school, but not understand that street designs do not provide safe routes, and if they do know this, they must get some other government agency to make street and sidewalk improvements, not easily done.

Most people find that sprawl life is not exactly what they hoped it would be. Increasingly, people ponder their quality of life. Often, while suffering in traffic congestion, not just during commutes to or from work, but in the evenings and on weekends. Is life getting better or worse? Is it what I had hoped for? The conclusion for many: "Despite my success, prosperity and possessions, something is missing."Already, for millions of Americans, the sprawl has hit the fan.

Disillusioned and stressed-out, Americans try religion, plastic surgery, the Internet, more stuff, new jobs and mates, and drugs – legal and illegal. But what is right there in their physical surroundings is usually not seen as the culprit or the solution. Few people look down their street and connect what they see in the bricks and mortar world to their quality of life.

Take a moment and look down *your* street. A lot of what you see or do not see may explain much about your quality of life and your health.

Hardly anyone has learned about the impact of community design – or what professionals call the "built environment" – on the quality of their lives. School curricula do not include this subject. In a highly mobile society, people do periodically reflect on the special attributes of a general location, particularly its climate, access to whatever amenities they value – like theaters and beaches – and of course, employment opportunities. Closeness to family, cost of living, and quality of schools are also among the many factors captured in the calculus of relocation.

There are two levels of the geographical and geo-social landscape. There is the regional or metropolitan level, and the smaller scale community and neighborhood. Research has found that people put more weight on the community than their specific residence. When faced with the dilemma of a less desirable house in a more desirable community, or a more desirable house in a less desirable community, which do you choose? People overwhelmingly choose the better community. According to Fannie Mae Corporation (the nation's largest source of home mortgage financing), Americans prefer a good community over a good house by a margin of three to one. But what is a better community? We need to raise expectations about community if more consumers are to get truly better communities.

Focusing on your immediate neighborhood is difficult. Over time, more and more routine needs are met within the larger regional or metropolitan area. These include jobs, visiting family and friends, medical services, shopping, parks, and even schools. As involuntary members of the automobile-dependent culture, typical Americans meet these needs by driving, repeatedly. The more dependent you are on far flung destinations, the less vital is your local neighborhood and community. As your sprawl universe constantly expands, so does your driving. Like some new law of physics, sprawl fills space until all land is developed (see Figure 2-1). Development consumes land, replacing natural environment with built environment, on, above, and below the land surface. Each of us is a land consumer, but not necessarily a gluttonous one. Sprawl may be highly organized in the form of a large subdivision that one land developer creates, or disorganized in the form of large numbers of individually purchased lots and homes in an area. The former is more visually pungent because of its well defined pattern, but the latter is still sprawl. High land consumption is a critically important characteristic of sprawl with serious consequences.

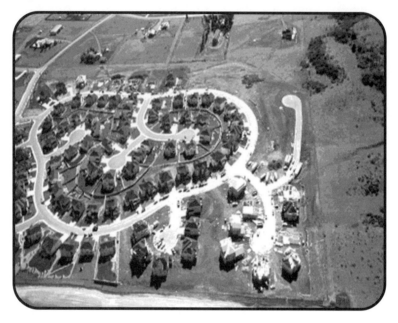

Figure 2-1. Suburban sprawl development consuming farmland.

WE MUST DECREASE LAND CONSUMPTION PER NEW RESIDENCE.

Just as too many Americans are eating too much food and becoming increasingly obese, and consuming enormous amounts of energy to fuel their automobile habit, they are also consuming more and more land. Some land consumption is driven by population growth – more than 25 million people per decade! Talking about population growth, or worse yet controlling it, is not politically correct, even though the rate in the United States is the highest of all the industrialized nations. Every *year* another Chicago-size jump in population hits the country. But that is not the whole story. *Annual increases in land development and automobile use are typically three or more times greater than population growth.*

There are times when you need statistics to tell the story.

Brace yourself.

Between 1982 and 1997 urbanized land in the U.S. shot up by an amazing 47 percent – another 25 million acres – while population grew by only 17 percent. In Northeast states, where the population rose only 7 percent, developed land jumped 39 percent. The most responsible region was the West, with a population increase of 32 percent and a 49 percent increase in developed land.

Something besides population growth is going on. The amount of land used per person has been increasing with sprawl development. Average home size has increased over 100 percent since 1950. According to the 2000 census, between 1970 and 2000, the average size of all new homes increased by about 50 percent. But from 1970 until today the average size of just single family houses has increased about 70 percent. Bigger homes mean bigger lots. Lot sizes outside metropolitan areas are almost twice those within the metro areas. Average lot size has increased over time to almost 2 acres, mainly because of "large-lot sprawl." Nationally, the Department of Agriculture found that lots of 10 or more acres in largely rural areas have accounted for an amazing 55 percent of the growth in housing since 1994. This is data of the absurd and powerful evidence of land use inflation, or land gluttony that drives more car use.

As house size has increased, household occupants have decreased. Household size has dropped from 3.7 people in 1950 to 2.6 today, creating need for up to 30 percent more housing. Just from 1970, household size has shrunk about 25 percent, with single-person households skyrocketing. Before sprawl, in 1940, less than 8 percent of Americans lived alone. With the current much larger population, nearly 26 percent live alone. Fewer persons living in homes generate more business for the sprawl industry.

As household size shrunk, the average number of cars per household increased from 1.2 in 1969 to 1.9 in 2001, according to the Federal Highway Administration. Paralleling the explosion of developed land, from 1960 to 1997, when the U.S. population increased 49 percent, the number of vehicles increased a whopping 181 percent. Census 2000 data revealed that 34.2 percent of Americans live in households with one car, 38.4 percent with two cars, and 17.1 percent with three or more cars, leaving just 10.3 percent with no car. More cars mean larger garages and more parking spaces requiring more land. In 1985, only 55 percent of all new single-family homes had space for two or more cars, which increased to 75 percent in 1998 and is still rising. For the first time in history the number of vehicles has exceeded the number of licensed drivers, according to an August 2003 announcement by the Department of Transportation.

Many older urban areas experience no population growth, but land gluttony still occurs and is the most obscene type of sprawl. Consider the Pittsburgh, Pennsylvania metropolitan area; it lost 1 percent of its population between 1982 and 2000, but its urbanized land area increased by 49 percent. In the same period, Buffalo, New York, gained 3 percent in population, but developed land jumped 53 percent. What's happening? People are moving from central cities and old suburbs to new sprawl subdivisions in once rural areas. Each new sprawl residence uses more land. So understand this: population growth is not the entire problem. Sprawl's rising rate of land consumption for new housing is just as important.

In a smart society with rising population, land consumption per new residence would not be increasing sharply. This is not unjust; it is necessary. In fact, this has been accomplished, at least in a few places. In Santa Clara County, California, between 1984 and 2000, the population increased 22 percent, but urbanized land area increased only 7 percent. Meaning that newly added population consumed less land than earlier residents had. Average residential density in 2002 was 5.3 homes per acre, compared to 11.4 units per acre for the newest residential development, the fifth straight year in a row when new development was denser than the area as a whole. Land scarcity and high land costs drove higher density, without which housing costs would have been higher. Similarly, in Colorado Springs between 1980 and 2000, when population increased by 68 percent, developed land area increased by only 32 percent, which helped reduce per capita city spending by 7 percent. Everyone in these areas benefited.

Perhaps things would be different if the government officials making land use decisions had learned in school that quality of life depends on sensible land use. Watching what is going on around them, listening to their complaining constituents, and honoring their commitment to serve the public interest are not working for most "public servants." Likely because they are serving a more financially rewarding master, the sprawl industry. Our elected officials should recognize that though a pretty flowering plant in the wrong place is a weed and an exotic animal in the wrong place is a threat, there is no right place for sprawl, not if you believe in true community.

PEOPLE DESIRE TRUE COMMUNITY.

The noted author and conservationist Wendell Berry captured the sense of community: "Essential wisdom accumulates in the community much as fertility builds in the soil." Residents committed to place-making nurture and grow a community. Sprawl is more like dry sand in which nothing grows, certainly not neighborliness.

A yearning for neighborhoods with less dependence on cars is bubbling up in the hearts and minds of millions of Americans, as it should. After a half-century of a soul-less sprawl society, there is clear evidence that the start of the 21st century is at the edge of housing history. But moving from sprawl to HEALTHY PLACES is more than some technical shift in housing and planning – it is a *cultural* paradigm shift. Professionals, politicians and bureaucrats will not make it happen. Consumers must make different choices when the market gives them real choices, and demand more choice when the market fails them. But the catch-22 is that 50 years of dominant sprawl culture blocks most consumers from making anti-sprawl decisions.

Most Americans no longer value or remember smaller scale neighborhoods and communities where people live well without a car. These are only seen in movies set in past times, like *It's A Wonderful Life* set in the pre-World War II small American town of Bedford Falls, or in old television shows like *Leave It to Beaver*. This smaller, more intimate scale of living prevailed here historically, until the end of World War II, and still does globally. By embracing sprawl and cars, American culture has greatly destroyed the soothing social fabric of real neighborhoods and communities. Pre-sprawl American society was more united, healthier and safer. Now we have too little social cohesiveness. Sprawl-disconnectedness has dehumanized society. Americans now have more possessions and information, but fewer human relationships and connections that really matter. *The sprawl culture supports consumption and telecommunication, not community and face-to-face conversation.* Think of the sprawl built environment in terms of Marshall McLuhan's memorable "the medium is the message." Sprawl is the message, a very disturbing message.

Sprawl has also given automobiles the power to dehumanize; they provide transportation but devour the time needed for active living, families, friends, community neighborliness and civic engagement. Minutes per mile may be just as significant as miles per hour, as in "it took me 30 minutes to move one mile on the beltway tonight!" Civic, public spaces that once were designed to facilitate contacts among people and neighborly relationships have been replaced by isolation dressed as privacy and the myth that constant car travel is something people enjoy, or worse yet, that it is inevitable. You have a right to choose a different lifestyle. You have a right to more options for housing and transportation. You have a right to get your time back. Too many people are time-poor, despite owning so much stuff. Time-poverty erodes quality of life.

There is hope. Within most people, like an ancient animal instinct, lies the desire for true community. It is an amorphous desire to be and *feel* positively connected to both the built and natural elements of a place and the other people who share the place. You can be more than an occupant. You can feel attachment to a place because you have special feelings for it, pleasant memories of it, or positively interact with it and its other residents. To desire community is to want to be with others who share *common* interests, values, and responsibilities. There is desire for a collective identity, not just a personal one. Sprawl residents may have personal wealth, but in a real community there is also common wealth. [Four states are legally commonwealths, meaning that citizens are united for the common good.] When people share commitment to a place they are active residents, rather than passive ones. A genuine community and its residents shape one another and benefit from each other. Consumers who want a true community value:

+ A place that residents take *pride* in.
+ A place where some neighbors are part of an extended family.
+ A place where people recognize a shared future and work on supporting a shared vision of that future.
+ A place with strong social networks, where people vote, volunteer, host block parties, join neighborhood watch, and organize open-air markets, and community festivals and gardens, for example.
+ A place where the "home" is seen as much more than the individual house or apartment, because it includes public spaces in the neighborhood and community.

The latent need for community is actualized during crises and emergencies when Americans rise up to join together and support each other to protect the community and, if necessary, repair and rebuild it. A historic example of this, on a national scale, is what occurred in response to the terrorist attack on September 11, 2001. That spirit of solidarity and mutual concern is the *everyday* goal of real neighborhoods and HEALTHY PLACES. Real neighborhoods support that special sense of community without requiring a common threat, enemy, or catastrophe to ignite it. A real community is greater than the sum of its parts, because of positive people-place and people-people connections.

Sprawl un-places are broken intentionally by their design. Around them should be posted "Out of Order" signs, warning people that they do not function as real communities. Except for individual houses and dead shopping centers, entire blandburbs cannot be easily fixed-up, renovated and turned into HEALTHY PLACES. Putting in sidewalks, for example, is not enough. Like chemically contaminated industrial complexes, sprawl un-places are here to stay, unless major site demolition and cleanup scrape the land clean. This has happened in a few locations, not because sprawl was rejected or unsuccessful, but because the sites had become terribly contaminated from actual nearby toxic waste sites.

Too few Americans have focused on the physical surroundings outside their homes: the streets – often without sidewalks, the buildings, the limited number of places adults and children can easily and safely reach by walking or cycling, the absence of convenient parks and trails, the absence of vibrant street life, and the coldness of streets where people are feared rather than welcomed as neighbors. People focus on their homes and what is indoors. All too often they have given up on the surrounding built environment because they live in an un-place. Un-places beat down people.

In the past few years the energetic smart growth movement has steered public attention to the negative aspects of the sprawl culture. It has done a poorer job of defining an easily understood and practical solution for consumers. When smart growth advocates talk, what they say is often vague and general, or just loose fragments of fixes aimed more at government officials than individuals. Something is needed that makes sense to millions of consumers trying to maximize their personal benefits through their own action.

Luckily, some land developers with courage and persistence have prevailed. There are suburban and urban HEALTHY PLACES – true communities – that people are living in across America. That animal instinct we have for community may quietly tell us to find what we once had. But exactly where are these HEALTHY PLACES and how can they be correctly identified?

An instinctual desire for community is not enough. Consumers of housing must also understand the impact of the built environment on their lives to become motivated to seek and demand HEALTHY PLACES. Everything you do and feel is affected by living in a place that is unhealthy by design. No matter how big and expensive your house is or how big the lot is, your wellbeing is greatly affected by the design of the built environment surrounding you. Un-places are like having bad geographic genes that program you for poor health. There's just so much you can do. You can try to take responsibility and improve your life, but an unhealthy place constrains you. Suffering the consequences of a sedentary life may not be your fault. Living in a sprawl un-place, trying to be physically active outside work is like exercising on an asphalt trampoline. You cannot overcome sprawl. But you can escape it.

The built environment does not happen by accident, although it seems that way at times. Un-places are purposefully created. Governments have shirked their responsibility to provide a healthy built environment that supports active living. As former Surgeon General David Satcher said: "When there are no safe, accessible places for children to play or adults to walk, jog or ride a bike, that is a community responsibility."

PUBLIC SPACES MAKE HEALTHY PLACES.

Edward Abbey captured the essence of sprawl: "Growth for the sake of growth is the ideology of the cancer cell." Uncontrolled development is like uncontrolled cell growth. Like some land-eating cancer, sprawlspace expands by consuming open land and sucking time and health from people spending more and more time in cars. Think of HEALTHY PLACES as a cancer treatment. In fact, regular physical activity supported by HEALTHY PLACES can help prevent some cancers, as presented in Chapter 4.

So exactly what are HEALTHY PLACES? They have vibrant neighborhoods of housing, parks, and schools within walking distance of shops, civic services, jobs, and transit—in short, a modern version of the traditional American town or old city neighborhood of times past. Creating the look of an old fashioned small town, however, is not the same as creating the experience of it. The point of great community design is to create a set of conditions that diverse people positively respond to. The result is a new social atmosphere in the space outside homes.

With extensive variety and opportunities of mixed land use, HEALTHY PLACES offer reduced land consumption on a per capita or per dwelling basis, ample greenspace, and building designs that reflect the local culture and harmonize with the natural environment. HEALTHY PLACES are also designed to improve public health, preserve open space, and enhance environmental quality. They can be created in cities, old suburbs, and on new greenfield sites, which are sites without any prior development. HEALTHY PLACES can be small neighborhood projects or much larger new communities with several neighborhoods. They are at a human, not automobile, scale. They are walkable, friendlier places.

On the other hand, sprawl differs fundamentally because it is single land use development. Individual parcels of land are used for a single purpose, such as homes, stores and restaurants, or office buildings, or schools, or civic buildings. All conceived, developed, and designed *separately* and separated physically for people using them. From its onset, sprawl development does not have the glue of community planning and design in the public interest and for public convenience. The collection of pieces is not guided by the central goal of building community.

Sprawl results from misguided, piecemeal, or ignored professional and official land use planning. Sprawl presumes that getting anywhere will be in a vehicle, not by walking or public transit. Sprawl regurgitates at the edges or fringes of metropolitan areas and spreads outwards. Older developed areas suffer and can become as blighted as central cities. Sprawl feeds off lower cost land in rural areas.

Aside from dispersed land use, the emphasis on *private* spaces in sprawl un-places contrasts with valuable *public* spaces in HEALTHY PLACES. Sprawl residents inherit the tradeoff between private and public spaces made by others. Inattention to public spaces in blandburbs breeds social isolation and reduces neighborliness; people fear public spaces because they fear strangers. This fear dooms real community. There is little desire to go outdoors to be with neighbors. The final destination of alienation is sprawl.

Anti-social sprawl residents "cocoon" themselves. They insulate and isolate themselves from the outside world inside their residential refuge. Or, as Lewis Mumford said in *The City in History*, 1961, blandburbs allow residents "to withdraw like a monk and live like a prince" inside "an asylum for the preservation of illusion" from which "escape is impossible." Decades later, withdrawal and illusion remain, but escape is possible. Some cities, or at least parts of them, are better. Suburbs are getting HEALTHY PLACES. Just as people once escaped cities because of low quality of life, people are increasingly fleeing from sprawl un-places. Too much of a good thing is wonderful, according to Mae West. But sprawl is a bad thing and we have too much of it.

Most un-place residents see no alternative and just focus on improving their quality of life by embellishing their private space. Wearing headphones outdoors is just one omnipresent sign of this habitual search for disconnection from unappealing surroundings. A more extreme choice is living in gated "communities" built within walls and fences and often guarded at the entrance. They are becoming more popular. It is estimated that some 7 million American households are in over 20,000 gated places representing "fortress America."

Gated un-places are like sprawl on steroids. They no longer are just for the wealthy. Their popularity punctuates the dominance of the sprawl culture. Anyone with an up-and-leave mentality can secede from society and the public realm. Gated places take sprawl to another sick level of alienation. Similar homes mean residents come from a narrow economic class. Racial bias can be promoted by location and design. Concern about security is generally far greater than interest in community life and neighborliness. People on the outside of the walls and tracts are feared. Space outside is someone else's problem. These gated, walled-in and bunkered places exemplify exclusion and civic disengagement. They are the antithesis of HEALTHY PLACES. Their homeowners associations can be more tyrannical than any government; rising association fees are like rising taxes. Association rules are like strict government regulations; noncompliance and unpaid fines and fees often lead to foreclosure. There are few highly participatory processes involving extensive communication among most residents. Boards of directors rule.

The point is that all sorts of public spaces are essential for nourishing social interactions among residents and others in the neighborhood. They are not for decoration; they must be routinely used by residents. The public realm of public spaces is crucial for creating experiences and memories that are place-centered and cherished. Public spaces make or break HEALTHY PLACES.

PHYSICAL SEPARATION BREEDS SOCIAL DISCONNECTION.

Sprawl separation is moving indoors. Indoor isolation is the newest trend in design of home interiors. More rooms so "any family member can go to get away from the rest of us," said Carl Ledbetter who built a 3,600-square-foot house with an "escape room" and special rooms for studying, sewing, and each child. Walling off people inside homes is "good for the dysfunctional family," according to a National Association of Home Builders official. A major home builder said: "We call this the ultimate home for families who don't want anything to do with one another." Couples want separate offices, separate Internet rooms, separate bathrooms. Family members no longer want to watch television together. *Privacy is the ultimate pathology in the sprawl culture.* Cocoons are becoming honeycombs. Indoor space can become as alienating and fragmented as sprawlspace. What does this say about personal relationships and family life?

The movement of people from cities to sprawlspace, from public space to private space, and from cocoons to separate rooms reflects what the philosopher George Santayana said, namely that Americans don't solve problems as much as they just leave them behind. Especially people-related problems. Engagement with technology and consumption replaces engagement with people and society. No surprise that Americans would rather shop than vote. Paradise is not around the corner or down the street or over there in a new suburb. Sprawl paradise is being alone with plentiful comfort food in your own room in front of a giant plasma screen in a big house on a big lot with a Hummer and two SUVs in the garage. Sprawl is not just a suburban locale or a pattern of land use; it is a state of mind, a world view, a set of behaviors, and desire for mucho possessions. The sum of all sprawl is the sprawl culture.

Despite ubiquitous communication technologies, most people are more disconnected than ever before in sprawlspace. People can be plugged in and hooked up almost every minute of the day. Yet even as they communicate more and more, they are disconnected at a deeper human level from other people, from nature, their government, and the places where they live. Nothing is more absurd than people walking outdoors while talking into a cell phone. The worst case is when people do this in beautiful settings, not listening to the birds or the silence, or truly appreciating the surrounding natural beauty. This is technological alienation. When the sounds of birds are masked by the cellular refrain of "can you hear me now?" something is very wrong. Personal technologies that invade public spaces make them less inviting and pleasant for others. It is technology pollution. The disrespect for public spaces that sprawl has spawned is shown by widespread street and park littering.

Living so long without authentic community and without positive social and emotional connections to neighbors makes it difficult for many people to see HEALTHY PLACES as uniquely beneficial. Sprawl has inbred a familiar and accepted social isolation that will be difficult to overcome. Walking to and from local stores and talking with neighbors or family members may no longer be prized by people who have only experienced the sprawl-automobile culture. Sprawl makes loners.

Sprawl is both the cause and symptom of disconnection. It is disconnection by design. Just as sprawl spreads over the land, sprawl spreads disconnection among the people living on it. One thing is certain. Physical separation inevitably breeds social disconnection. Sprawl shill Peter Gordon believes: "Our demands for community are met in many ways. We can use the automobile, or we can even use the Internet." Not so. You clearly should not have to drive to get community.

And the Internet, with its chat rooms, listservs, forums, and email, is not an effective substitute for direct human interaction. Only true victims of the sprawl culture think it is. A cyberspace "community" moves information around, but emails are not the same as conversations with neighbors. A cyberspace relationship is a simulated relationship, more an electrical connection than an emotional one. You get no "messages" from a person's eyes, facial expressions, body language, odor, physiology, or clothes. You get no trust, commitment and loyalty. Cyber relationships are one-dimensional and illusory. You may pretend to be someone else, just as those you communicate with may do. Cyberspace lacks completeness just like sprawlspace. Virtual reality is simulated reality. Cyberspace is a logical extension of sprawlspace, another step away from dealing directly with people, nothing like a place-centered community. Electronic isolation exacerbates physical isolation.

Developments are being wired to provide Intranets for residents as if virtual communities can replace neighborliness. Writing in *The Washington Post* in 2004, city dweller Bernard Ries lamented the loss of old fashioned neighborhoods: "I've scarcely gotten to know my neighbors. I've missed that old sense of communal comfort." Though he praised his community listserv, he confessed that "an e-mail list is no substitute for gossiping on the front porch with folks you really know." An Internet or Intranet "virtual front porch" is settling for less.

So this is progress in our sprawl culture, from couch potatoes to cyber potatoes. The exploding Internet and email world has morphed into cybersprawl; surfing the Internet is like wasting time driving around blandland. The challenge is not letting the Internet become an electronic escape from direct interaction with other people. Use it for getting information. Do not let it be sedentary-enhancing technology.

As Robert Putnam so well articulated in *Bowling Alone*, the sprawl culture has reduced *social capital*. The book created an "idea virus" as the concept of social capital quickly moved from academic circles to widespread conventional wisdom. In contrast to physical capital which refers to physical objects, financial capital which refers to economic resources, and human capital which refers to the assets of individuals, social capital results from valuable connections among people that comprise loose or formal social networks. Interactions among people help them build communities and a sense of belonging, commit themselves to each other, and knit the social fabric. Social capital builds trust and positive working relationships among people. It also has been shown to correlate with improved health. Social capital improves with face-to-face encounters, which the built environment either facilitates or blocks. Social capital may increase as a result of crises, but not necessarily persist without a built environment designed to support it.

HEALTHY PLACES are the means to regain a more communal society and improve social capital in a permanent and sustained way. They are high-trust places. Without real neighborhoods, metropolitan and suburban areas designed for cars rather than people are destined for social isolation. In sprawl un-places people lack a habit of togetherness, and criminals, terrorists, and children who become computer hackers and killers live invisibly, unknown and unseen by neighbors. The combination of physical separation among houses, lack of public spaces, and increasing dependence on cars inevitably undermine social capital. Putnam found that each additional 10 minutes of commuting time cuts all forms of civic engagement, such as attending public meetings and volunteering, by 10 percent.

Sprawl is more than buildings. Half a century of sprawlspace development has shaped our thinking, actions and tastes. Culture is a way of life; it is accepted behaviors, beliefs, values, and attitudes. American culture is dominated by the sprawl culture, which affects everyone, wherever you live. You can choose to ignore sprawl, but it will not ignore you. Sprawl's ideas and behaviors are passed from parents to children. Sprawl is a shared system of knowledge, symbols and preferences. The car and fast-food cultures are byproducts of the sprawl culture. Once strong, place-specific rural, urban, and pedestrian cultures have been smothered by the generic sprawl culture, which is not a New York state of mind, not a Mayberry state of mind, just a bland suburban state of mind. Bland places make bland people. Bland people make a bland culture. We have capitulated to blandburbs in blandburbia. An exception is Tom Miller, the pro-smart growth Mayor of Franklin, Tennessee, who heard residents express their fear that new development would make their historic city bland; he observed that "generic suburbia" is "bland at best and alienating at worst." Bland *is* bad.

In 1985, Kenneth T. Jackson noted in *Crabgrass Frontier* that suburban sprawl "is perhaps more representative of [United States] culture than big cars, tall buildings, or professional football." Fifteen years later the voice of the contemporary and youthful hip-hop world was heard. According to William Upski Wimsatt's *Bomb the Suburbs*, 1999: "The suburbs is more than just an unfortunate geographical location, it is an unfortunate state-of-mind. It's the American state-of-mind, founded on fear, conformity, shallowness of character, and dullness of imagination."

Those who "think outside the box" reject the sprawl culture. They shop outside the box of chain and big box stores, view the world outside the box of computers and television sets, live outside the box of monotonous sprawl subdivisions, and use travel modes outside the box of motor vehicles. For individualism the trick is not getting squashed by organizational orderliness and commercial conformity, hallmarks of the sprawl culture. Just as blandburbia is based on design and architectural mediocrity, the sprawl culture is a meritocracy based on mediocrity. Thankfully, developers who think outside the box build HEALTHY PLACES for consumers who also think outside the box and get rewarded, because people don't make sprawl better, sprawl makes people worse. HEALTHY PLACES make people better.

"Americans will be able to drive at 100 miles per hour on 14-lane super highways and cross the country in one day!" This big car-lie was given at the General Motors 1939 World's Fair exhibit.

There is no mystery in the real America why the biggest quality-of-life complaint is traffic congestion. Most Americans spend one-third of their car time in traffic congestion. As sprawlspace expands more time is required to drive within it. Freeways, beltways and Interstates centrifuge sprawl development outward. Road networks are like the blood circulatory system of society, making nearly all activities possible, if you can bear the pain. Traffic congestion is like artery-clogging cholesterol. Personal mobility should not equate to motor vehicles. But in sprawlspace there are few options beside cars. The light at the end of the sprawl tunnel is from more cars making life more miserable. Mary Jane Baker in Tulsa, Oklahoma expressed her frustration: "Distances that would normally take only a few minutes to drive are jammed with whizzing SUVs and hurried angry drivers. Just the process of going out to dinner is so exhausting that most people I know stay home, or within a few blocks distance of their homes."

By definition, sprawl means relentless dispersion and spreading out of people and destinations. People are compelled to drive more and more, so that even if there were no more people there would be more driving and traffic congestion. People are spending more time *inefficiently and painfully* getting from one place to the next to the next to the next.... And each year gets worse for places already suffering with traffic congestion, with more roads crammed and more hours of gridlock. And each year more places and people start feeling the pain of congestion on their roads. As congestion has worsened, the potential for enjoying the solitude of driving to think about things or listen to music has shrunk. Forget the television commercials showing drivers in a blissful state. Driving is hard, stressful work. And we pay a lot to do it. Nationally, the cost of traffic congestion in wasted time and fuel increased by over $60 billion from 1982 to 2001, according to the Texas Transportation Institute.

This is an immutable sprawl truth: New road capacity both follows sprawl development *and* causes more of it through induced demand. New roads on the fringes of metropolitan areas spur sprawl development. It may seem illogical and destroy your hope, but according to considerable evidence, road building is *not* a solution to congestion. In the short term traffic speeds up and travel times decrease. This draws more motorists, promotes more sprawlspace development, and soon congestion reappears. The worst situation is building new or wider roads in rural areas in anticipation of future traffic. What a gift to sprawl developers. Also, massive amounts of money are made by building roads, meaning there are pressures from businesses and industry associations, not just drivers exasperated with congestion. But the truth is spreading. Expensive new roads quickly reach capacity within months and not the years or decades predicted by traffic engineers. Build roads and cars come. It is an American tradition. What a deal; suffer in two lanes of congested traffic, or suffer through construction and get four lanes of congested traffic.

Street wisdom is that "adding lanes to solve traffic congestion is like loosening your belt to solve obesity." Traffic engineers relish adding car lanes. They are said "to have asphalt in their veins, and asphalt in their brains." Listen to Sam Schwartz, former Traffic Commissioner of New York City: "Traffic engineers have failed. If you compare the accomplishments of our profession over the last 50 years to the medical profession, our performance is equivalent to millions of people still dying of polio, influenza and other minor bacterial diseases that have been cured." Surgeons bury their mistakes; traffic engineers bury drivers in congestion and pedestrians in accidents.

The linkage between land development and traffic deserves the highest attention by the public. Sprawl development is the prime cause of most traffic congestion around, into and out of central cities. Congestion is also a fact of life on roads connecting suburbs.

Research has found that habitual traffic congestion and long commutes also correlate with many physical health impacts, including hypertension, back problems, cardiovascular problems, gastric disorders, hemorrhoids, higher rates of colds and flu, visual impairment and stroke.

The growth of spread-out sprawl development in the past fifty years has produced a mutually reinforcing dependency between cars and ever larger geographical areas, each feeding on the other: more sprawl, more roads, more cars, more sprawl. Who made this deal with the Detroit devil? Who benefits? *Do you?* Better to seek an alternative to constantly darting about within the expanding sprawl universe.

An exasperated suburban resident summed up her sprawl lifestyle: "driving is my life." Like so many others, after getting home from work she is "home for four minutes and then it's off in the car." And in the expanding sprawl universe each trip is getting longer and taking more time on roads that are congested all the time. Rush hours have turned into rush days. Automobile addiction is now so ingrained in American society that it will be difficult to cure. Automobile addicts behave like vehicular sheep taking any road, especially those to sprawl un-places. But sensible car use without automobile addiction is possible.

Physical inactivity is a bad habit that is tough to break. People are not to blame. Routine physical activity has been designed out of daily life by an army of professionals who created the sprawl-dominated built environment. People may not welcome physical activity, because they are not accustomed to it or not physically able to handle it because of longstanding sedentariness. Given a community where one can easily walk to a local grocery store or supermarket, some people will still unthinkingly use their car. Walking home with a bag of groceries or a shopping cart, the way people do in cities, may be seen as a sign of a lower economic status, as if one cannot afford a vehicle.

The major victims of automobile addiction are the elderly when they lose their ability to drive, or at least to drive safely. Stranded in suburbia without mobility defines an aging nightmare – loss of independence – that 77 million aging baby-boomers can contemplate. A community that supports "aging in place" supplies mobility without cars, design for active living, homes appropriate for different stages of life, and opportunities for older residents to contribute to the social and civic life of the community. *In the right place, aging in place is aging with grace.*

In sprawlspace, people may spend money on belonging to some type of spa or physical fitness club, or they may make some commitment to a civic organization. But all too often, after spending so much time commuting by car to work and then having to drive to do just about everything else, they have no time or energy left over to exercise or participate. If you do not routinely experience this, you are unusual. Nearly everyone is spending more time in cars, but only about 15 percent, on average, of trips in vehicles is for commuting.

Big everyday uses for cars include shopping (19 percent), other family and personal business (23 percent), visits with friends or relatives (8 percent), other social and recreation destinations (18 percent) and trips to school or church (10 percent). Millions of Americans do not commute at all, including increasing numbers of retirees, the unemployed, people who work at home, and non-working spouses handling household duties. But they too are on the road incessantly. Also contributing to road clogging throughout the day are all those service workers driving from one work site to the next, plus all those buses, taxis and shuttles, delivery vans and trucks. Road capacity is reduced because of never-ending road repair and maintenance activities, which are mounting because of increasing traffic.

Instead of focusing on the prime causes of losing so much time, companies offer you more high-tech gizmos to make more use of the time spent driving. Who really thinks that ubiquitous use of cell phones, pagers, navigation systems and Internet gadgets really improve the quality of vehicle time? It is a con game. Expect cars to have tiny refrigerators, microwaves, and coffee makers. Automotive futurist Wes Brown opined "Because our lives are so stressful and so busy, we're looking for our cars to be a sanctuary." Cars as safe havens? Wrong. Dead wrong. Cars are not good refuges, they are sources of stress.

American society must choose: seek true community and crack the sprawl culture, or keep sprawl's dehumanizing *automobile apartheid*. It is apartheid because anyone who wants mobility through walking, bicycling or public transportation suffers *discrimination* by a built environment designed for automobiles. First class people are inside cars. Second class people use foot-power or public transit. As sociology professor Stephen Klineberg said about Houston: "No one walks here. This is a car city – it was built by, for and on behalf of the automobile." No better example of the bias for motor vehicles is the short times allotted for pedestrians to cross streets. Even a youthful fast walker can watch the "Don't Walk" light start blinking soon after leaving the sidewalk. New York City's Department of Transportation deactivated 77 percent of the pedestrian walk push buttons at intersections and left the signs telling pedestrians to use them. It was 25 years before it was revealed in 2004 that they had become mechanical placebos. *For 25 years* cars whizzed by hapless pedestrians waiting for a useless walk button to stop traffic. Cars came first.

The automobile no longer connects people. Nor, for the most part, do automobiles routinely connect people to spectacular places. Cars rarely provide pleasure. The car has become the instrument of isolation. The taker of time. The personal polluter. Neighborhood stores have been replaced by malls accessible only by cars. Driveways have replaced sidewalks. Highways have replaced and fragmented greenspaces. Emails and

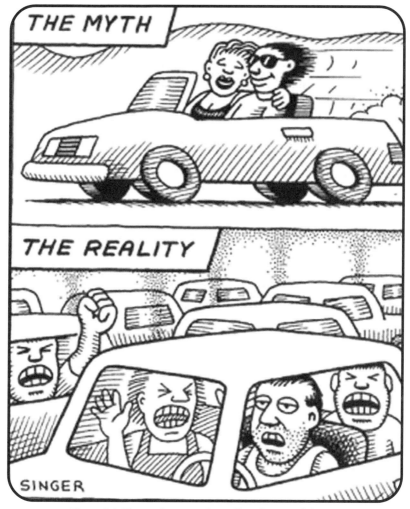

Figure 2-2. The myth versus the reality of automobile use.

cell phones have replaced face-to-face conversation in streets and other public places. Neighborhoods that compel automobile use reduce social ties among neighbors. Close friends who are also neighbors are nearly extinct. Alienation by automobiles produces sprawl rage that breeds road rage and contagious, aggressive driving.

Everyone values personal freedom. But the great sprawl paradox is this: *That big house on a large lot in blandburbia, long touted as the American dream, reduces personal freedom.* As people have more cars, drive more miles to do just about everything, and spend more time stuck in traffic congestion, even on weekends – *especially* on weekends, they lose freedom, because they lose precious irreplaceable time, personal energy, and money. Reacting to the pain of the expanding sprawl universe, people luxuriate with more consumer goods in their private cocoon space.

Personal freedom and independence should mean more than the ability to go where and when one wants. Americans should also have the freedom to travel *how* they want. Right-wing conservatives should value that freedom for Americans. When cars are the only option and people are car slaves, freedom is diminished. When cars dominate lives and harm people they are no longer liberating technology. They are just the opposite (see Figure 2-2). An advertisement for an apartment building near a transit station declared "Own your own life!" Would *you* like to replace some trips in cars with walking or public transit that is convenient, pleasant and safe?

Neighborhoods *designed* to fulfill a wide range of human needs on a human – not automobile – scale are the cure for automobile addiction. If HEALTHY PLACES succeed in a big way it will be a cultural change of historic proportions. Freed from their cars, living in a healthy place, people will be able to slow down to enjoy experience over things, people over technology, smelling flowers rather than auto exhaust fumes. Imagine not spending so much time in *your* car. If you think you are living the life of your dreams, then did you plan to spend so much of it in your car? Over the past 20 years, the time motorists spend *idling* in traffic – getting nowhere – has nearly quadrupled. *Never have so many people spent so much time driving to so many places that they should have been able to walk to.*

While the interest in HEALTHY PLACES is substantial, not all Americans seek them or even know about them yet. Most people, including those who like living in suburban sprawl un-places, have no solid information on HEALTHY PLACES or direct experience with them. To say that they have "chosen" sprawl is incorrect. They have not had an alternative to sprawl with its imposed addiction to cars.

Sprawl developers and residents often justify their locations by comparing them to low quality city situations with terrible schools and high crime rates, as if that's the only alternative or the right comparison. From this perspective, escape to sprawl makes sense. The more valid comparison, however, would be to a suburban HEALTHY PLACE with good schools, in the same region or metropolitan area. Where there are HEALTHY PLACES and people have a true choice, HEALTHY PLACES attract many home-seekers for good reasons.

Imagine having a first-rate home in a place where you walk or bike on safe, well lit and shaded streets, or on a path through a greenway, to your workplace in 30 minutes or less.

Picture yourself walking in 5 or 10 minutes to the local park where you can play with your kids or exercise on the system of local trails running through the entire community.

See yourself walking in 15 minutes to a local restaurant, grocery store, public library, book store, or physician's office in the town center.

Envision your kids safely walking with their neighborhood friends to school.

See yourself walking to the community center building to participate in meetings of local civic groups, or to attend pot-luck dinners and parties with the neighbors, and then feeling fine about safely walking home at night, probably with neighbors.

Visualize living near public transit and not needing a car for commuting and most shopping.

The ugly fact is that most Americans pay dearly for their life-long automobile addiction. They cannot imagine what life would be like without the constant use of cars for nearly all transportation needs. Since they have few real alternatives to cars, it is wrong to say that they "choose" their automobile dependence, or really prefer it. It is more a matter of imposed addiction than free choice. Thinking of the addiction as a "love affair with cars" is misguided, unless you recognize that there is no reason to stay trapped in a bad and unhealthy relationship. It is fascinating that 20 percent of Americans believe that cars reduce the quality of life, compared to 56 percent in France without a car culture, according to a 2003 survey by Market Opinion Research International.

An excellent analysis of the interstate highway system by Justin Fox of *Fortune* magazine in 2004 got things right: "The Interstate system … speeded the trend toward suburbanization at the expense of both city and country. …the auto enthusiasts of the first half of the 20th century had promised something that the Interstate Age was unable to deliver, freedom of movement. … Most of us aren't in love with the car, we're stuck in a long and passionless marriage from which there appears to be no possibility of release." Amen.

Actually, you can escape, if you figure out how costly automobile addiction is, in terms of time, health and money. A family that chooses living in a HEALTHY PLACE can reduce their number of cars as well as their total driving. Just like cigarette smoking, more people will realize that auto-dependent sprawl living is an unhealthy habit. Walk away from it, and keep walking.

CAR CONVENIENCE IS A JOKE.

"A civilization which allows itself to be intoxicated by the madness of mere size, by speed, by quantity, is destined to end in a new type of crass and violent barbarism." Guglielmo Ferrero got it right way back in 1913 in "The Riddle of America" in *The Atlantic Monthly*: Is it far-fetched to consider our super-size, automobile-dependent sprawl culture as crass and violent barbarism? I think not, if you consider the high rates of road deaths, crime, imprisonment, and compulsive consumption in the United States.

If HEALTHY PLACES, smart growth and New Urbanism succeed, quality will triumph over quantity. To fully appreciate the importance of HEALTHY PLACES, it helps to recognize that American society has generally valued quantity and cheapness of goods more than quality and great design. In housing, sprawl is the triumph of quantity over quality, and so too is the sprawl culture. High quality design means a creative blend of functionality, esthetics, materials, cost and, increasingly, environmental consciousness – so called "green" design. The design factor often explains the success of imported goods despite higher prices, but not for American housing and other development, where a low cost, commodity approach produces cookie-cutter sameness of homes, strip malls, and office parks in suburbia nationwide. The sameness and cheapness of the built environment explains why so many of us see a boring, ugly uniformity of virtually all built-up areas in the United States.

Contrast sprawl with older places that have survived with uniqueness and appeal because they retain original historic character, charm, and built environment. New places – with *names* to remind us of old, historic places – seem plopped down from the same sprawl factory. Smart growth critics often claim that it is *merely* a nostalgic attempt to regain the past. But regaining walkable neighborhoods and real communities is being pragmatic. A limited number of people can find homes in older historic places. Most others need new HEALTHY PLACES.

Some argue that the tradeoff of high quality community design for mass production of housing has given Americans lower cost housing and so-called "convenience." But even if sprawl helped give consumers lower home prices, this has come at significant hidden costs for people and government. Car convenience is a joke. Sprawl wastes more and more time. People often say that they move to outlying sprawl locations to get more time with their family, only to get just the opposite because of more time inside their cars. Sure, you can walk a few steps to your garage and car, but then there is the trip, road congestion, and parking. With cars you have access convenience but not usage convenience.

Automobile-dependent destinations do not offer true convenience. Think of all the times you had to get into a car to get to a visible nearby place that was impossible to safely walk to, because of highways or huge parking lots being in the way. HEALTHY PLACES help regain true convenience, because destinations are within local neighborhoods and communities, and many within walking distance of homes and each other. Long car rides are reduced, as compared to suburban sprawl locations.

Moreover, the constant movement within expanding metropolitan sprawl space means very high automobile ownership and operating costs. For most Americans transportation costs are second only to housing, and some 98 percent of transportation spending is on automobiles. Most American families spend more on driving than on health care, education or food. People living in outer suburbs can spend twice as much on automobiles than people living in close-in areas and in urban cores where public transit is available. Automobile expenses are especially burdensome for lower income singles and families, not just for low paid service workers, but also younger teachers, police officers and military personnel, for example. An important economic incentive for living in HEALTHY PLACES is substantially lower car costs.

Sprawl taxes you physically, mentally, and financially.

THE PATH TO GOOD HEALTH DOES NOT LEAD TO SPRAWL.

Sprawl steals your time, health and money. With sprawl and traffic congestion from sea to shining sea, the United States has become "the land of the tired and the home of the sedentary."

Just how unhealthy is the American culture of sprawl and its automobile addiction? Research has revealed that poor physical fitness is a better predictor of *death* than a host of other documented risk factors that the public is more familiar with, including smoking, hypertension and heart disease. Community design really is a matter of life and death, because it determines your capacity to be physically active. Sprawl spawns sloth. And after some 50 years of sprawl sloth, the health care profession now has a new name for the sprawl plague: "Sedentary Death Syndrome." But in unhealthy un-places there are two stages before that: Suburban Blandness Syndrome and Sprawl Stress Syndrome, as discussed in Chapter 4.

Physical inactivity and its related illnesses killed some 365,000 people in 2000, up from 300,000 in 1990, and will soon overtake the 435,000 deaths from tobacco-related conditions. In fact, the CDC projects the death rate jumping to 500,000 by 2005, up another 100,000 deaths in just five years — more data of the absurd. Preventable deaths from the sprawl sedentary lifestyle are five times greater than deaths from microbial agents, like bacteria and viruses, more than three times greater than deaths from alcohol, and two time deaths from firearms, illicit use of drugs, sexually transmitted diseases, and motor vehicle accidents. A sedentary lifestyle is about as lethal as smoking a pack of cigarettes a day. A CDC official remarked that many death certificates that give the cause of death as lung disease, diabetes, heart attack or trauma from car accidents should really say "suburban sprawl." Are you among the 70 percent of sedentary adults? If so, welcome to the world of Sedentary Death Syndrome.

Think for yourself. Consider living in a HEALTHY PLACE for greater physical activity and more free time for family, social and civic activities, for a healthier and higher quality of life. It is not all that risky, as Chapters 4 and 5 will document. Research studies have found that people walk more in neighborhoods with design features making them walkable, versus places without those features. In Austin, Texas, there were over five times as many walking trips in walkable neighborhoods, in the San Francisco Bay area six times, and in Portland, Oregon, four times as many as in pedestrian unfriendly places. Such results show that people do take advantage of community designs that promote walking. Other research found that active people have about half the health care costs of sedentary people.

The sprawl culture will lose its grip on people when they see the sprawl industry as similar to the tobacco industry. However, just as cigarettes and unhealthy foods have not been outlawed, neither will sprawl. Choice is the answer. More choice will follow increased and expressed consumer demand. Until then, with little choice, sprawl will prevail.

The producers of sprawl want you to feel good about their product. But starting with childhood, ubiquitous advertising and more subtle forms of marketing shape habitual behavior patterns – like cigarette smoking – and determine consumer preferences – like driving a car rather than walking. Sadly, hardly anything that is purchased, including your housing, promotes a healthy, active living lifestyle. Walking is the simplest daily form of physical activity offering remarkable health benefits. Why do 70 percent of adults not get enough regular physical activity to maintain good health? Why are over 60 percent overweight or obese? Think sprawl.

The biggest dollar expenditure for most people is housing. Most housing is in suburban sprawlspace, which means about 60 percent of Americans live the sprawl lifestyle. This means living in a built environment that does not support or encourage walking and other forms of regular physical activity. So, about 70 percent of people are physically inactive and about 60 percent of people live in sprawlspace. Yes, the two are connected.

The sedentary-sprawl-consumer lifestyle is lethal for those practicing it, whether you are liberal or conservative, rich or poor, male or female, Democrat or Republican, white or a person of color. Sedentariness is an equal opportunity killer. Living in sprawl is not the only cause of the Sedentary Death Syndrome, but it surely is of paramount importance for most people. Affording expensive health care is not as good as preventing health problems.

Heed the wisdom of Dr. JoAnn E. Manson, chief of preventive medicine at Brigham and Women's Hospital in Boston: "Despite all the technological advances in modern medicine, regular physical activity is as close as we've come to a magic bullet for good health. It's more difficult than popping a pill, but it's worth it." Imagine that – a magic bullet for good health actually exists! But in the consumer society people focus on medicines and other products to get good health. Popping pills rather than active living is what the sprawl culture promotes.

Obviously it is not a question of giving up consumption, but of achieving a healthy balance. The design of the built environment we live in will either help us to achieve that balance or keep it out of reach. Most Americans are sedentary, overweight and living in sprawl un-places. It is worth repeating that their imbalanced lifestyle connects to those 365,000 preventable deaths a year. You do not have to be one of them.

You can, of course, choose to contribute to the nearly $40 *billion* being spent annually on diet and weight reduction products, everything from low-fat and sugar-free foods, to prescription and over the counter pills, to exercise programs and equipment. And you can buy one or more of the 50 *million* diet books sold annually. Joining your fellow Americans on the highway of spending does not lead to health. Better to take the foot path to prevention by finding a HEALTHY PLACE that supports active living. If you have children, their health is at stake, determined by what kind of place you put them in and habituate them to. Oddly, parents worry about how music, Internet sites, and clothes may adversely affect their children, but ignore the short and long term impacts of the built environment on them, or blindly think that a suburban sprawl subdivision is the best they can give their children. It is not.

People need a magic place to get the magic bullet for good health. The magic place is a HEALTHY PLACE. To find such a place you need to connect the dots. Academic researchers want more data. Scientists never have enough data. But there is more than enough information on two central relationships to know what best serves individuals and American society:

1. Regular physical activity promotes health.
2. Superior community design promotes physical activity.

Put the two together and you have HEALTHY PLACES for healthy people. The desire for more data must not stand in the way of shifting from sprawl to HEALTHY PLACES. Common sense and the weight of the available evidence must trump research interests. Get the data, but do not think that there is any downside to immediately recognizing the many negative impacts of blandburbs and culture on people. There is a solution to sprawl. We know how to build HEALTHY PLACES - *now*. Do not let the sprawl industry and its supporters suggest that more data are needed before consumers should reject sprawl and seek an alternative to it. As you will see, there is clear and compelling evidence that sprawl kills. Americans need to demand better community design because they have the right to better health.

WALKING CAN CUT VEHICLE USE.

"Walking keeps us active, trim, fit and medication-free." That's the view of Carroll and Dorrie Pensinger of Waynesboro, Pennsylvania, age 76, who walk everyday for an hour after breakfast, according to a testimonial published in *The Washington Post*. They recounted how a young mother had once stopped them, asking for help getting her young children off to school while she was hospitalized and recuperating from surgery. But they were strangers, so they asked her why she trusted them. Just because she had repeatedly seen them walking by her house, was the answer. She got the needed help. Walking was more than the means to good health, it produced neighborliness.

Walkable communities are very important because, even now without well-designed pedestrian friendly places, walking is the primary way that Americans get exercise, 43.2 percent, versus 10.6 percent for jogging or running, 6.3 percent for aerobics or aerobic dancing, and 5.6 percent for swimming. However, in the past 20 years, when sprawl has run rampant, the number of trips people take by walking has decreased by more than 42 percent. Walking to school has also decreased by a similar amount.

Regular physical activity is the goal of active living. "Exercise" is the wrong way to think about active living. Few people in our sprawl culture have enough free time to exercise almost every day, nor even the mood or energy to do so. *The central idea of active living is to find many different ways of integrating physical activity into daily routines so that physical activity is ordinary behavior and not something special to do.* It would be great if all physical activity was pleasurable, but it is enough if it is just taken for granted as normal behavior. It helps to think of three kinds of physical activity, the three "f's" of fun, fitness and functional.

Fun activities have often been considered "recreational." Any kind of sports activity, for example, may be done primarily for enjoyment. Such activities generally require training, cost, and a significant commitment of time. But there are also less intense activities, such as a nature walk or hike, skating, a brisk walk on a beach or through your community, an energetic walk with a dog, intense gardening, and playing with the kids. And then there is dancing, any kind of dancing is great physical activity.

Fitness activities have a long history. You go out of your way to do them. Pushing people to exercise has not been especially successful, however. For so many people it means tedious, boring, and repetitive activity. People may use various types of exercise equipment, often in special places like gyms and fitness or health clubs that they must drive to, and also in homes. But many homes have largely unused exercise equipment, and many people do not use their membership in clubs. Costs may be an impediment for some people True, there are disciplined runners and bikers who have fitness and wellness goals, but such activities pose issues for many people, such as the need for training and limits imposed by age and health conditions.

Functional activities mean that traditional means of transportation to move your body and electronic communication to move your thoughts are replaced by physical activity, whenever and wherever it is feasible. It also includes doing things without the aid of some type of machine or motor, like opening a can by hand with a simple old-fashioned device rather than with an electric can opener. The big example is replacing vehicle use for getting to stores, jobs, or schools with walking or biking. This requires relatively convenient places to get to and safe and attractive routes to get to them. When you replace vehicle use by walking or biking you are benefiting from "therapeutic transportation." Using motor vehicles is unhealthy transportation. Functional activities also include using stairs instead of elevators and escalators, or when there is no choice except an escalator to climb the moving steps.

At a shopping center, walking increased from 4.8 percent to 7.2 percent when signs were put up near stairs adjacent to escalators to inform people about weight control benefits. At the Centers for Disease Control and

Prevention they discovered that playing music in stairwells upped stair use. But in most buildings stairwells are closed for security reasons or are dark, narrow, dreary, claustrophobic, and unpleasant, instead of open, wide and located more conveniently than elevators. In a new 18-story office building in San Francisco where form follows fitness the main elevators only stop on every third floor, compelling people to walk. In the workplace a different kind of functional activity is walking to someone rather than using email or phone communication. Substituting action for convenience technologies is beneficial, such as walking to a bank instead of using an ATM. Getting up repeatedly during television commercials to have a quick chat with family members or tidy things up a bit around the house is another good habit, as long as snacking is avoided.

These three categories, of course, are not necessarily mutually exclusive, so that you can do something that serves two or three of them; this increases the odds that it will be done regularly.

History shouts one ugly fact. *Despite their many advocates, traditional fun and fitness activities have not been effective for most Americans to avoid the harmful health impacts of a sedentary lifestyle.* Every U.S. president since Eisenhower has had some kind of fitness council. Various statistics show increases in the purchase of sports and exercise equipment. But the larger truth is that there have been greater increases in products that promote sedentary behavior. The problem with "leisure time" activities is that they are usually reserved for special times, places or occasions; often they require other people. Large chunks of time are typically needed, and these can be difficult to get, especially for people spending a lot of time in vehicles who suffer from sprawl stress. You may know intellectually that you should be active, but not have the positive attitude, mood, energy or time for fun or fitness activities. You may be moving through the three stages of unhealthy sprawl life: Suburban Blandness Syndrome, Sprawl Stress Syndrome and Sedentary Death Syndrome, which are discussed in Chapter 4.

Consider exercising with equipment in the home versus using community green infrastructure. Is there any doubt about which is the winner? The developer of the NorthWest Crossing mixed-use community in Bend, Oregon, used a television commercial which showed a mass of indoor exercise equipment offered for free in a yard sale because residents opted instead to use the many trails in the community. A radio commercial had two men meeting on the street; one asked the other several questions about why the other looked so good. The response: "Because I live in NorthWest Crossing and I get out more." The commercials spurred brisk sales.

The advantage of non-leisure time functional activities is that they do not ordinarily require special or large chunks of time, although admittedly they can require more time than the technology or product they replace. For the vast majority of children and adults functional walking integrated into normal daily activities is the easiest way to get routine and effective physical activity, even when it occurs in short spurts. It is likely that the increase in sedentary behavior has resulted more from decreased non-leisure time physical activity than anything else.

This is the key question: How can community design facilitate these three types of activities? Many fun and fitness activities can be supported by diverse greenspaces. When parks, trails, and sports fields are close to homes and workplaces, it is easier for individuals to do whatever activity they enjoy. Substituting vehicle use with walking or biking requires mixed land-use offering relatively close destinations and great street design for convenient, safe and attractive routes. Such places are walkable and pedestrian friendly.

The columnist Ellen Goodman suggested putting warning labels on cars "This Vehicle Will Make You Fat." In sprawlspace walking is inversely related to vehicle use. The more people drive, the less they walk. The more cars in a household, the less walking by its occupants. However, the higher the residential density, the more people walk. And the more people use public transit instead of vehicles, the more they walk. Transit usually means that users walk at both ends of a trip, and often for shopping if there are shops near their points of use. In large cities many people do not have cars, but rely on public transit and walking for all sorts of mobility needs. In New York City, about half of households do not have cars, and in some other cities the fraction is about 25 percent, as in Cleveland. Nationally, it has been found that a 10 percent increase in population density produces a 5 percent increase in transit use, and doubling density can decrease vehicle use by 20 percent. People who live in single family homes walk less than those living in apartment buildings. Development near transit stations usually includes significant multi-unit buildings.

Higher density development around transit stations really does promote walking. The rail line through Northern Virginia suburbs outside Washington, D.C. runs through older inner-suburbs where there has been intentional transit-oriented development and then, further out, through typical low density sprawl areas. In the sprawl areas only 15 percent of users get to the stations on foot, compared to 73 percent in the higher density areas.

A 2002 national survey conducted for the Surface Transportation Policy Project, like many other local and national surveys, showed the strong public support for walkable communities. Consider the following results and think about how you would have voted:

+ 56 percent see their walking as relaxing
+ 48 percent as fun
+ 77 percent would like to walk more for fun
+ 65 percent of Americans see their walking as good exercise
+ 80 percent would like to walk more for exercise
+ 55 percent of people would like to walk more rather than drive more throughout the day
+ 63 percent would like to walk more to stores and other places to run errands
+ 38 percent would like to walk to work

The chief reasons why Americans do not walk more are:

+ Poor community design, including places being too far and too inconvenient to get to, 61 percent
+ Traffic and lack of places to walk, 30 percent
+ Not enough sidewalks or crosswalks, 26 percent
+ Personal circumstances, including not enough time to walk, 57 percent
+ Laziness, 33 percent
+ Physical limitations, 20 percent
+ Dislike for walking, only 17 percent

The poor community design factors describe sprawl un-places, the lack of time correlates with the large amounts of time spent in cars because of sprawl living, and the other factors may result from the effects of sprawl stress. Do any of these factors explain your behavior?

In choosing a community to live in, 79 percent of Americans think it is important to have sidewalks and places to take walks, 56 percent want to be within walking distance to stores and restaurants, 50 percent want to be within walking distance to schools, and 48 percent want to be able to walk to public transportation. As to designing communities so that more stores, schools and other places are within walking distance of homes, 47 percent prefer this *even if it means building homes closer together, which means compact design and higher residential densities.*

To walk the talk you need a sidewalk. Yet so many places lack them. In high growth Charlotte, North Carolina, there are 2,800 miles of streets, but less than half have sidewalks on one or both sides. No wonder that Charlotte has fewer people walking to work than any other metropolitan area of more than one million people. When sidewalks went out of fashion in suburbia a significant misstep was taken, making the built-environment unhealthy. Sidewalks are more than inert concrete. Sidewalks help keep you healthy, if you have them and use them. A resident of a sprawl un-place in the metropolitan Atlanta area said he would like to walk more with his wife and 5-year old son, but he feels unsafe walking along country roads near his subdivision. "I guess we feel a little cheated with no sidewalks," he said.

A place with walkable streets and places to walk to, including a light rail station, is Orenco Station, in Portland, Oregon. The design works. For example, 70 percent of residents spend money in local businesses at least once a week, with many shopping locally on an almost daily basis. This is why: 85 percent said that it was the close proximity of neighborhood businesses and amenities that reduced their need to drive elsewhere for shopping and entertainment. And 18.2 percent of adult commuters walk to the light rail station, an impressive figure, because light rail stations are not near many work locations.

Walking can be so much more than physical activity. Walkers enjoy relaxing experience, visual pleasure, creative thinking, mental rejuvenation, spiritual centering, philosophizing about life, and sometimes being emotionally close to a walking companion. Walking connects you to nature and public space, experiencing and interacting with it. This is why the quality of the public realm is so important. But ear phones, Walkman music players and cell phones, block full sensory connection with the public realm. These products help you stay in private space. You get exercise but not the total experience. Muscles move but the mind stays disengaged with your immediate surroundings, like sleep walking. In quality walking environments, the surroundings – not just the walking – benefit you, if you have a quality walking infrastructure, a network of scenic trails, footpaths and sidewalks.

Listen to Lynn Rabenstein, a resident of Skagit County, Washington, who fit walking into her life to achieve active living: "Walking is a chance to be outside. It's also an opportunity to walk and talk with my husband or a friend. It's become a part of what I do, 45 minutes a day, six days a week, and I have lots more energy now. It's not just for me physically, it's also good for me mentally and spiritually." Beth Walch, a resident of Baxter Village, a HEALTHY PLACE in South Carolina, said: "I can go for a walk and get home three hours later." Why? Because she stops often to chat with neighbors.

Formal exercise indoors does not provide the full range of rewards that walking does. Consider the home treadmill and stationary bicycle, now designed to re-create actual outdoor settings, as if a hill on a motorized device is the same as a real hill that you see and feel under an open sky. Such products fit the sprawl culture perfectly. They allow people to get some physical exercise if they are actually used without, however, compromising a sedentary lifestyle. They safeguard private space and personal isolation. But muscle use alone does not account for the quality of physical activity. Use of such exercise equipment when combined with listening to music or watching television does not offer the many benefits of walking, jogging, running, skating, or biking outdoors. The *experience* is not the same. It is like comparing instant coffee to Starbucks coffee – a very different experience. When the experience is better you will repeat the activity.

Indoor exercise products reflect the suburbanization of the mind; so many people find using them boring because they are. Walking outside is not boring. Directly relating to the outside world is not dull. Even walking repeatedly on the same route outdoors is, amazingly, not boring, as I and other regular walkers know. The path may be the same but the interactions with the outside world constantly change. You do not need technology to make time pass quickly. Walkers feel reenergized not solely because of the muscular activity, but because of the stress-relieving mental activity, often a kind of moving meditation. A roaming, inquiring mind in a body moving under its own muscle power is superior to a bored mind in a vehicle.

Sadly, walking has become a counter-culture activity, counter to the sprawl culture, counter to automobile addiction, and counter to consumption. Dedicated walkers are more a part of an active living subculture than the mainstream sedentary sprawl culture. As Rebecca Solnit said in her excellent *Wanderlust – A History of Walking*: "Walking still covers the ground between cars and buildings and the short distances within the latter, but walking as a cultural activity, as a pleasure, as travel, as a way of getting around, is fading, and with it goes an ancient and profound relationship between body, world, and imagination."

Likewise, an adult bicyclist who reduced car use proclaimed: "When I ride my bicycle, the wind sweeps past me, awakening my body to the fact that I am moving someplace within this world. I am part of my world and community, not removed from it."

It comes to this. More walking and better health equate to less car use. Healthy independence as one grows old results from living in a community where walking can substitute for a lot of car use. Many people want more opportunities for physical activity, particularly walking, that explains the strong actual and latent consumer demand for HEALTHY PLACES. Unimaginative and unhealthy un-places with their constant vehicle use do not support rewarding relationships with neighbors and nature. To get them, reject blandland.

Ideal is a nation of unrecovering walkaholics. They would walk to meetings of Walkaholics Unanomymous where they would brag about walking long distances in extreme conditions, successful battles with cars, and exceptional interactions with other walkers. As part of their 10,000-step program they would recruit friends and relatives who needed support for shaking their workaholic, automobile, junk food and sedentary addictions.

DEVELOPERS MUST RESPECT THE NATURAL ENVIRONMENT.

HEALTHY PLACES are good for people and our natural environment. Very unlike blandburbs that diminish people and degrade the natural world, despite their "green" names. The built-environment should not abuse the natural environment. Buildings don't kill nature, developers do.

If you care about the natural environment, as nearly everyone professes they do, then understand this: Sprawl contributes to loss of wildlife habitat and biological species, loss of forests, loss of farmland, loss of scenic landscapes, increased global warming, increased energy use and air pollution, soil erosion, depleted aquifers, and contamination of water supplies. Sprawl developers all too often exhibit callous disregard for the natural environment.

Consider that the Atlanta region loses an average of 50 acres of trees every day to development. After the state passed a law allowing timber companies to avoid local regulations and permits, sprawl developers clear-cut large tracts of suburban forested land. They claimed they were just harvesting forest products. Why? To avoid requirements to protect trees, to avoid getting a permit for tree removal, and to avoid meeting replanting standards. After the land was deforested and leveled the companies once again became developers so they could build sprawl housing easier and at lower cost without trees getting in the way. They got away with it! Gwinnett County developer Wayne Mason saw his world and liked it: "They ran the environment people out of here a long time ago. You've got no trees. You've got no streams. You've got no mountains. It's a developer's paradise." Sprawl truth hurts. Buildings don't kill forests, sprawl developers do.

Think of science fiction visualizations of future societies, like the 1982 movie *Blade Runner* with its dark, dreary, polluted, built environment devoid of natural environmental features, and you get the correct feel of where unconstrained sprawl development and land consumption are taking us. So too with the future in William Gibson's 1984 classic *Neuromancer*, where much of the action is set in "The Sprawl," a giant unplace. In both cases the natural world has been consumed by unconstrained un-place development, technology flourishes, and people escape the alien and inhuman "real world." Sameness trumps sensibility. Technology serves as an analgesic.

Here and now, sprawling development is not just paving over the natural environment, it is leaving in its path people unmoving in un-places. People do little more than get in and out of their cars and guzzle sedentary-enhancing technologies. When all current un-places link up we reach The Sprawl, which Gibson said in 1989 is "not really about an imagined future. It's a way of trying to come to terms with the awe and terror inspired in me by the world in which we live." Feel the sprawl terror.

MILLIONS OF AMERICANS ARE *FORCED* TO LIVE IN SPRAWL.

We are what we build. We build blandburbs, and we have become awfully bland. Winston Churchill said: "We shape our buildings, and afterward they shape us." Sounds profound and is profound. Except that nearly all of us did not shape our built environment. *Developers, planners, architects, builders, and government officials did the shaping of our sprawl built environment and we are the victims, as surely as we are its consumers.*

I present abundant evidence that in selecting sprawl, consumers are unwittingly voting for a set of unhealthy impacts on their lives. Whether their perceived and real benefits compensate for these impacts depends on how much they know enough about them. Unquestionably, consumers should have a non-sprawl choice. *Condemning sprawl, however, should never be interpreted as condemning people who choose sprawl.* Blame the villains not the victims.

Here is a most remarkable and important fact. According to considerable data, right now at least one-third of home-seekers – millions of people – want the HEALTHY PLACES option, at least intellectually. They want housing that is just one part of a smaller scale, multi-functional community. They want a place that is designed to raise quality of lives, not to satisfy business interests, like fast food places feeding frenzied people in cars fast-forwarding to their next stop. Millions of Americans have suffered sprawl and its many assaults on quality of life so much that they want something else, and the number keeps growing, as it should.

If they attempt to turn theory into action, disappointment awaits most of these people. Should they actually seek a HEALTHY PLACE they are likely to find more of the same old sprawl, often masquerading as something different. The amazing fact is that – although about one-third of people seeking homes want HEALTHY PLACES – *substantially less than one percent* of available homes fit the HEALTHY PLACES model. This is a huge demand-supply gap. In fact, one analysis found that for every 500 new sprawl homes there is just one new home in a HEALTHY PLACE. Millions of Americans cannot find the housing and community product they really prefer in the geographic area they favor. The odds against finding a HEALTHY PLACE are about 500 to 1. You deserve better. The sprawl industry should not control housing type and supply. Sprawl stalks home seekers.

That one-third consumer demand figure comes from data gathered before most people have seen for themselves actual HEALTHY PLACES or known people who live in them. And also before information about the health benefits of living in such places has been widely disseminated. Market demand will surely increase over the next few years, probably to at least 50 percent of home seekers. Latent demand must be transformed into irate demand to make the housing market work. Detailed information on demand for HEALTHY PLACES is given in Chapter 8.

It seems inconceivable and anti-American that so much market demand can be unsatisfied by housing supply. But that is exactly the situation. Millions of Americans want the features of HEALTHY PLACES but are *forced* to live in sprawl, chained to their cars, because they have no other option for housing. Hidden forces cause this. Historical actions by government over the last fifty years have made sprawl the favored, and even subsidized, type of development. Sprawl politics have created and maintained these government policies. As discussed in Chapter 1, the sprawl lobby is your enemy.

There is hope. As explained later, the situation can be changed and consumers given more choices by a fair marketplace where sprawl is not outlawed but made to compete with HEALTHY PLACES on a level playing field. Luckily, no corrupt system is perfect. Consumers in many areas can find a HEALTHY PLACE, if they know what to look for. Know it. Want it. Find it. This is how HEALTHY PLACES will conquer sprawl, and how consumers will get a chance for the magic bullet for good health.

I present a new market-based approach to the sprawl-smart growth debate. It respects consumers who satisfy the totality of their self-interests when they make housing decisions. Previously, people have been urged to support smart growth because it is "the right thing to do," "good for the environment," "good for society," "sustainable growth," or "the way to save cities." Housing is too important to leave to philosophy. The quality of information determines whether someone's decision delivers the benefits they want. With better information different housing decisions will be made. Markets fail when consumers have inadequate information. Consumers do not have sufficient information about the many costs of sprawl living, particularly harmful health impacts, nor about true alternatives to sprawl.

You vote with your dollars, and so far sprawl has won because it has been the only choice on the housing ballot for most Americans. Government in combination with the sprawl industry has rigged the election by keeping out HEALTHY PLACES. In a fair market, large numbers of consumers will displace much *new* sprawl construction, because

HEALTHY PLACES are a better designed product offering greater benefits. In the end, consumers have the necessary power.

When people choose a HEALTHY PLACE, it is as if home and lot sizes are multiplied by a quality of life factor. And it makes sense. People may pay what *seems more* for homes in HEALTHY PLACES because of smaller house and lot compared to what they could get for the same money in a blandburb with cookie-cutter homes. Yet they believe their investment is worth it. Why is the HEALTHY PLACE home worth a seemingly premium price?

At this stage of the game an excess of demand over supply for HEALTHY PLACES is not the major explanation for higher prices. Nor are the higher costs for providing public realm amenities in HEALTHY PLACES the real explanation. Follow this argument. Conventional home builders and realtors use a simplistic financial approach. Home value is defined on the basis of dollars per square foot of inside space. The presumption is that within a certain category of housing, consumers focus on the house itself and will pay more for larger homes, particularly if it seems that the cost per square foot is comparatively low. Besides the home itself, some core location amenities, like the quality of schools, are basically pass-fail considerations. For sprawl housing, consumers focus on the private space they are buying, namely the size of the lot and house, and builders can offer reduced cost because developers have bought cheaper land. For homes in HEALTHY PLACES, consumers use a different economic equation, even if only intuitively.

The ordinary one-dimensional price-private space equation fails to recognize the value of unique *community* features *outside* private homes and lots. Many consumers are willing to pay for a well designed public realm that defines neighborhood and community, including nearby greenspaces, streets designed to promote neighborliness, shopping and school within walking distance, and all the other quality features of HEALTHY PLACES. What is outside homes – called "outdoor rooms" – can be seen as far more valuable than private lawns and yards. When people live near local public greenspace they think of it as their backyard or front-yard. Consumers can also see financial benefits of reduced automobile use and improved personal and family health. In blandland people just buy private homes and not a uniquely valuable public realm. In HEALTHY PLACES the entire neighborhood is your home, not abstractly, but in terms of everyday living.

This much is clear. Many consumers are way ahead of mainstream developers, home builders and realtors. The housing market is bizarre. The law of supply and demand has been retracted. To a disturbing degree *housing supply shapes demand more than consumer demand determines supply*. The annual creation of new housing is so small relative to existing housing stock, in the 1 to 2 percent range, that past home preferences generally constrain the design of new homes. In other words, the people who picked sprawl in the past are constraining the choice for current consumers. Any survey of homeowners will automatically be hugely biased in favor of sprawl. Most people do not know about an alternative to sprawl. How can you say you want something else when you do not know what that something is? Playing it safe, and ignoring the bias in its usual marketing data, the housing industry is very slow in responding to a significant shift in consumer demand. No larger shift can be imagined than from blandburbs to HEALTHY PLACES.

The market challenge facing developers of HEALTHY PLACES is that many consumers must *see* the added community value with their own eyes. Time and time again developers of HEALTHY PLACES discover that sales of homes increase sharply once there has been enough construction of homes and development of public spaces to let consumers see the real live old-fashioned community. Sure, people screaming for something other than sprawl do purchase homes in HEALTHY PLACES before construction, because written descriptions and sketches constituting "plans" are enough for them. But large numbers of people want to see the "real thing." This is a good idea. *Just as the map is not the territory, the plan is not the place.*

Walking down a narrower, tree-lined street with a porchscape rather than a garagescape and reaching a park and town center within a few minutes can convince consumers that a higher quality of life awaits them. They are buying a healthier lifestyle, not just shelter. They are buying community, not just a house. They are buying streets for people, not just cars. When people lose the streets, they lose true community. What turns consumers around? They need to see and feel the irrelevance of higher residential density when design of homes and public spaces is excellent. They need to experience the net advantage of trading some lot and home size for first rate community public spaces that they will actually use and enjoy. They need to sit on a bench in the town plaza or village green. They need to stroll on the sidewalks and greenways that they could regularly walk for pleasure, or exercise, or getting to a community meeting or local shopping.

It pays to remember what some savvy real estate professionals say: "houses don't gain value, land does." And land in a great community has and gains the most value. Rather than getting "more house for the money" in a sprawl subdivision, consumers of HEALTHY PLACES get more quality of life. At Orenco Station, outside Portland, Oregon, 80 percent of surveyed residents agreed that their lot sizes are smaller but more expensive than those in surrounding sprawl suburbs, actually 30 percent more expensive. But of these, over 93 percent would still recommend that their friends or family purchase units in Orenco, despite its high residential density, up to 25 units per acre in some areas. Of nearly 200 people, only one felt that lack of privacy was a problem. In explaining why they were willing to pay more money for a smaller home, after design of individual homes – their private space, the reasons cited related to community design – their shared public space.

The "seeing is believing" constraint may create an initial slower rate of financial return for developers of HEALTHY PLACES. Sprawl has been called "ugly development with early payback." With HEALTHY PLACES, once people can see the total picture there is fast sales and price escalation. In some areas, like Florida, North Carolina, and the Dallas, Washington, D.C., and Denver metropolitan areas, the number of HEALTHY PLACES is large enough for realty to define reality. Excellent design wins when it is seen and felt viscerally.

Pam Sessions and her husband are developing a mixed-use project called Vickery in the Atlanta area, where only a few HEALTHY PLACES have been built, but where "huge demand" for it exists, according to Tom Bell, chairman of a growth strategies task force of the Metro Atlanta Chamber of Commerce. Sessions confessed that she is moving into the project and going from 20 acres to a quarter-acre lot in the hope that others will like the idea of trading a large lot for the opportunity to walk to the market or work. As to future success, she noted: "When you have a good model to demonstrate, it takes a lot of fear of the unknown away."

THE AMERICAN DREAM MUST BE REDEFINED.

Fewer people are California dreamin'. University of Southern California

Professor Kevin Starr framed California's future as "the cutting edge of the American dream – a utopia" or "the paradigm of the dream lost – a nightmare dystopia."

In 2002 Smart Growth America analyzed 83 metropolitan areas and found that the "Inland Empire," of sprawl-rich Riverside and San Bernardino counties east of Los Angeles and north of San Diego, was the most sprawling and least livable area in the nation. Since the 1970s, land developers and home builders have run amok, controlling local politics with their campaign contributions. The result is some of the worst commutes for residents, running anywhere from 100 to 200 miles roundtrip and 2 to 4 hours daily. Two-thirds of the population live over 10 miles from a central business district resulting in considerable non-commute driving. A 2002 survey found nearly 40 percent of commuters eager to take a job within 15 minutes of home even if it meant a 15 percent pay cut. The current population of 3.5 million is expected to increase by 5 million by 2025. Open land is projected to run out by 2040. Children in areas with high diesel truck traffic were found to have 5 percent less lung capacity than kids in less polluted areas. Is this what Californians were dreaming of?

Historians say that geography is destiny. Real estate people preach location, location, location. For neighborhoods and communities, the more important truth is that *design is destiny*. Healthy communities require good geographic genes, and they come from good design.

This much is clear. Lacking a real sense of community, and time and opportunities for regular physical activity, sprawl kills a lot more than people. Sprawl kills greenspace, beautiful landscapes and scenic vistas. Sprawl kills many species that live on open land. As it continues to suck in large numbers of people with no real housing alternative, sprawl kills some old walkable neighborhoods in older cities and suburbs, especially in low population growth areas. Rural towns historically have been compact development surrounded by open space dotted by relatively few homes. Now many towns are surrounded, actually under siege, by sprawl. Sprawl kills the rural "live in the country" lifestyle. First, people consume sprawl; in the end sprawl consumes people and what they once valued – free time, real neighbors, and nearby greenspace.

Sprawl has been a silent serial killer. It is an unseen stalker, invisible because it is ubiquitous. Suburbanites manage not to let their hearts believe what their eyes see. Sprawl does not stand out. It is the norm. It is just there, everywhere, like air. Unquestioned, it seems functional and inevitable. How could Americans be against sprawl? Sprawl *is* America. It is where most people live, work and play. It is equated with progress and economic growth. It is unassailable – except for one thing. With the sprawl lobby's money and sprawl shills' lies, sprawl kills.

Imagine this. Some newly discovered virus has just been determined to cause widespread heart disease, colon cancer, diabetes, obesity, and other health effects among a huge cross-section of Americans, both children and adults. With scientists estimating 365,000 deaths in the United States yearly from this plague, is there any doubt but that this situation would spur a mighty national effort to find a remedy. All citizens would demand action.

This scenario is not some fantasy. It is here now. It is the sprawl lifestyle killing Americans.

Our nation has fought costly and widespread battles against asbestos, lead, radon, and now mold in our homes. Yet sprawl is not that tangible, not something to be cleaned up, but just as lethal and much more sinister. Sprawl is all too visible, but its design needs unmasking.

How could the style of our built surroundings be a silent killer? Something toxic is not entering our bodies. Some radiation is not destroying our cells. Yet the way our communities have been designed is harming us. Why? Sprawl creates a host of unhealthy behaviors. Physical inactivity is a major behavior pattern. Using cars to get everywhere is a major behavior pattern. Spending time inside homes but not outside in public spaces is a behavior pattern. These "normal" behaviors define contemporary American sprawl culture.

Do some people escape the sprawl-induced behavior patterns? Of course. Can strong-willed people resist the many negative influences of sprawl? Of course. They can control their lifestyle, where they live and how they behave. But all the evidence is that many millions of people are victims of sprawl, not knowing how their lives are adversely affected. They – and very likely you – were born into sprawl. Without options and information on true differently designed places, where else to live but in sprawl un-places? Into the vacuum of awareness about sprawl's harmful effects information must flow.

Information drives preventive health care. Consumer power requires good information. You need information about community design and its linkages to good health. It is not enough to retreat inside your home or periodically go to more satisfying vacation places. It is not enough to focus on food and diet. You deserve a magic bullet for good health, as well as a host of other benefits of a HEALTHY PLACE.

Usually presented as a large single family house on a large lot in suburbia, the Bland American Dream is a product of a half-century of sprawl culture. The American dream must be redefined. It should be about the dream *community*, more about *place* than house. An American Dream Community where home size and privacy are replaced by neighborliness and active living. The American Dream Community is designed to be:

+ Family-friendly
+ Activity-friendly
+ Pedestrian-friendly
+ Neighbor-friendly
+ Kid-friendly
+ Elder-friendly
+ Environmentally-friendly,
+ Small business-friendly, and
+ Transit-friendly

Seeking a HEALTHY PLACE can be blocked by the belief of many people that they are already healthy. But good health is not an end-point or a stable condition. It too easily vanishes. By making physical activity a regular part of daily life you reset your life so that you are becoming healthier day by day. *If you take every opportunity, no matter how small, to be physically active because of your spontaneous, automatic behavior, then you have truly achieved active living.* This will help increase your "health span," a new concept from the medical world which means the number of years you feel healthy and are free from serious disease. This contrasts with growing old chronologically with the help of modern, expensive medical interventions, but having a low quality of life because of illness, disease, and physical limitations.

Active living equates to sustainable good health. By design, HEALTHY PLACES maximize the opportunities for active living. It is that simple. It is still your responsibility to make your behavior unhesitatingly responsive to those opportunities. An active living maxim might be "Use your muscles instead of money to buy technology and services." Make climbing stairs a treat.

In the polar opposite sprawl world there are few opportunities for using muscles. Unhealthy un-places are not designed for physical activity. *With a sedentary lifestyle the automatic behavior is to take advantage of every opportunity, service, product and technology that eliminates or reduces physical activity, no matter how small.* Odds are you relate to this tendency. Think elevators, escalators, remote controls, self-propelled lawn mowers and lawn services, drive-through stores and banking, moving walkways, golf carts, leaf-blowers, someone to bring groceries to your car, home delivery of groceries and meals, free trams in downtown centers, emails to coworkers, and Internet shopping.

Habitual sedentary behavior is embedded in our sprawl culture and advanced by a constant flow of innovative products and services. If you want to be a successful inventor, just think of a way to help people avoid using their muscles. Why in the world did someone invent "breath strips" that dissolve in the mouth – to avoid the effort of sucking on breath mints? And what exactly was the pressing need to have so many doors open automatically when you approach them? Did it take too much effort to open doors by hand?

The sprawl booby prize for achieving success and prosperity is a sedentary lifestyle. You choose: The bland American Dream where you consume more and more to be less and less physically active or the American Dream Community where regular activity makes you healthier. For better health take these two steps. Start noticing in your everyday activities all the big and little ways you avoid physical activity. Take control and switch responses, stop taking the "easy way" and, instead, use your muscles the way your body was designed to function. Do not be time blind, see the consequences of sedentariness. Walk to – and in – a better future.

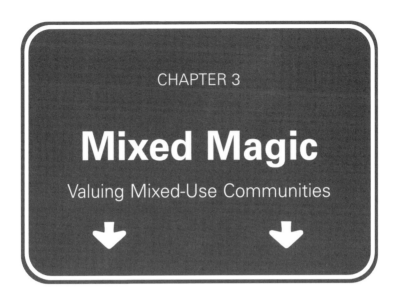

CHAPTER 3

Mixed Magic

Valuing Mixed-Use Communities

Sprawl splinters.

People are hurt by too much physical separation among parts of the built environment.

"We're trying to offer proximity to the water, parks, shopping, entertainment and nightlife. If you buy a condo in our downtown, you can walk to four restaurants, two dry cleaners, the supermarket, video store, two workout centers and a church. That proximity is a compelling reason to live in a more urban context." So said Matt Sloan, master developer of the new community of Daniel Island in South Carolina.

Nature knows. Whether it is trees in a forest, animals in the wilderness, insects in a field, or fish and other living things in the ocean, healthy ecosystems have mixtures of species. Healthy systems have myriad interactions among the components sharing space. Preserving biodiversity is critically important for the natural environment. For the built environment, we must bring the many separated pieces of our daily lives back together to get diversity at the community level.

The cities that people have always favored worldwide to visit or live in have mixtures of housing types and styles, commercial buildings, civic structures, and public spaces. These walkable community systems promote routine interactions among people using their constituent parts.

Single, dispersed uses of land across significant areas where many people live, work and play runs counter to nature and human history. Sprawl is truly unnatural. Dividing up basic human activities so that each is located in dispersed and separate places is fundamentally inefficient and unhealthy. Such separation makes people-people and people-place interactions automobile dependent, painful, and increasingly expensive.

A HEALTHY PLACE has a dynamic, interactive mixture of its built and natural components. Basic live, work and play land uses are within walkable distances or shorter car rides, or are accessible through public transit. We know how to do this. True mixed-use places are *complete, whole and connected* neighborhoods or communities. They bring a feeling of fulfillment and satisfaction to residents that supports better physical and mental health.

Conversely, blandburbs lack completeness, wholeness and connectedness. Something important is missing at any location in sprawlspace; completeness and wholeness are only available at larger geographical levels through extensive vehicle use. Living without completeness, wholeness, and connectedness affects the physical and emotional lives of people in complex, subtle and unhealthy ways. Sprawl is a divide and conquer game with land developers as the players and consumers the objects on the land-board. We the people have been divided and conquered. Our land and natural environment have been subdivided and subjugated. Our social fabric has been shredded by physical separateness.

HEALTHY PLACE developer Bill Bishop believes that "society is more durable, more adaptive and more creative the more diverse it is." Diversity can include many elements within a neighborhood or community:

+ Mixtures of housing types and styles within a common, coherent visual theme.
+ Varied types and designs of commercial and civic buildings.
+ Wide arrays of trees, shrubs, flowers, grasses and other components of a functional and aesthetically pleasing *green infrastructure*.

+ Different types of public spaces, such as plazas and court yards in town centers, picnic tables and benches in parks, walkways, green-ways and trails, waterways and pedestrian bridges, recreational and sports areas, and open air places for social activities.

+ Different transportation options, with parity given to walking, cycling, public transit, and cars.

None of this diversity should get in the way of a coherent look and feel for a place. Effective social fabric and capital require a *visually* elegant and physically connected system which enhances peoples' wellbeing. Pretty much everyone knows from experience that successful places have a special and distinctive local character. Achieving this requires much more than technical land use planning or zoning, and much more than conventional architecture and construction. Creating local character is more an art than science; it may be connected to the special historic, aesthetic, cultural, geographic or ecological features of a place. A unifying *visual* theme prevents the unease that people feel with jumbled architectural styles and building materials, and suppresses eye-grabbing commercial signs and storefronts.

Places are like people. They either have terrific winning personalities or are bland and boring. Think "place personality." Santa Fe, New Mexico, San Francisco, California, New Orleans, Louisiana, and Charleston, South Carolina, offer unique personalities. You enjoy looking down streets while walking. Public space is seductive and interesting. History is celebrated, physical beauty runs deep, and a strong community spirit makes residents feel proud and visitors feel welcomed. There is uniqueness within physical diversity. Great place personality signifies enduring "magic." With it, people want to preserve the place for future generations. Pleasing local character also has real economic value; it attracts workers and business.

In contrast, blandburbs lack distinctive personalities. They are bland to look at and boring to be in. Worse yet, they are ugly, irritating and stressful. Quality architecture and design should be interesting and energize people. Sprawl space has commercial value, but little public value. Why visit such sameness? Why live in it? Would you want to preserve bland-burbs for future generations? If not, then why keep building them?

Where there is place personality people walk and talk. In blandburbs people ride and hide. HEALTHY PLACES have terrific place personality and though they share critical features, they are each distinctive, one-of-a-kind places.

DIVERSITY PROMOTES WIDER CHOICES.

National and state level data usually reveal close elections. But research by the *Austin American-Statesman* showed in April 2004 that American communities had become more lopsidedly Democrat or Republican than at any time since World War II. In 1976 27 percent of Americans lived in landslide counties where at least 60 percent of the vote was for one party; this jumped to 45 percent in 2000. Plus, 40 years of social science research have proved that when like-minded people cluster they become more extreme in their thinking. If blandburb neighbors talk at all to each other, they are unlikely to hear and discuss different views of the world. They have segregated themselves by economic class and political orientation. As a generalization, Republicans and conservatives are more attracted to sprawl's social isolation, private space, low diversity, and focus on consumption; Democrats, liberals and independents are more likely to select urbanized, socially diverse, mixed-use places, with a focus on people rather than things.

These kinds of social and human diversity enhance HEALTHY PLACES:

+ Ages of people, from children to the elderly.
+ Education and economic status, from service workers, professionals, homemakers to retirees.
+ Race, ethnicity and religious beliefs.
+ Cultural and recreational interests.
+ Family status, from young singles to married couples and empty nesters.
+ Political orientation: liberal, conservative, independent, libertarian, progressive, and green.

The extent of social and human diversity desired reflects the "inclusive versus exclusive" preference of people. No community will have the full range of all these aspects of social and human diversity, but HEALTHY PLACES do much better than blandburbs. Diversity is promoted, though not prescribed, through mixed land uses, housing for different income levels, and attractive public spaces that promote social interaction. The community of Russett in Maryland, over ten years old, with some 10,000 residents among 15 neighborhoods, was praised by one of its residents: "Russett is like a mini-United Nations. It has one of the most diverse populations I have ever seen." Indeed, there are Asian, Latino, Indian, Caucasian and African-Americans living beside each other in a variety of housing types, including apartments, condominiums, town houses and single-family houses.

An exclusion mindset shows up in subtle ways. People may oppose putting in sidewalks in older neighborhoods, saying "I don't want people walking in front of my house." They mean strangers. They do not value a close-knit community where there are social interactions among residents in public spaces. The problem is that other residents *are* strangers. Another attitude is "the best neighbors are the ones you never hear from."

Inclusive social and human diversity promotes diverse shopping, restaurants, entertainment venues, and public spaces. People with different backgrounds and tastes can conveniently access places and services they desire. Work on the New Economy has found that young professionals in knowledge-based sectors – part of the "creative class" – place considerable importance on living in places with significant human and social diversity, which contributes to vibrant "street life." Similarly, aging baby boomers and empty nesters are likely to favor high diversity environments. They want wider choices and richer opportunities within a mixed-use community, making diversity a valued community amenity. Sprawl is just the opposite. Sprawl is not just dumb, it is dull. Sprawl makes you seek interesting venues by traveling somewhere, usually by car. *In blandburbs, there's always a dull moment.*

More and more people want to live where they can walk out the front door and into "the action," as long as they feel safe and comfortable. Vibrant street life and diverse activities in the public realm can be found in town centers in newly built greenfield HEALTHY PLACES, and in commercial streets of revitalized neighborhoods in cities and older suburbs. Street life includes the ritual of people-watching, popping into stores, and eating in outdoor patios; it is a social promenade or "passeggiata," as it's called in Italy. The evening stroll remains a part of daily life in many parts of the world, especially places that Americans like to visit. On the other hand, taking a stroll in the blandburbs without a dog may make neighbors suspicious.

Streets in suburbs and cities are getting as ugly as strip mall infested roads. Street life requires good-looking streets. But our crass commercial culture is dumping "visual street spam" on us. Public space is used for commercial purposes, not for promoting people interactions. Stuff put on streets cannot be deleted. You are forced to look at it. Sidewalks are cluttered with self-serve boxes for newspapers and countless other materials, such as real estate brochures. Lines of boxes, often in disrepair, are sources of street litter. Once, original paintings on sides of buildings celebrated the history or culture of a place and were a treat for the eyes. Now walls sell products with huge billboards and faux paintings that are roll-down ads. Kiosks are popping up with still more advertisements. Buses have obscenely large advertisements covering their sides, as do bus stop shelters. People on sidewalks handing out flyers or product samples impede pedestrians. Large ad flags and banners flap from street lights and buildings. Unsightly ads are stapled to utility poles and glued to sidewalks. Local governments sell our souls for paltry amounts of money that ruin streetscapes, even around park areas and plazas. Schlock commercialization is killing street life. This does not happen in true HEALTHY PLACES.

Another aspect of diversity is keeping a place elder-friendly. The number of Americans 65 years or older is expected to climb from 31.8 million in 1991 to over 66 million in 2030. One third of today's Americans over 65 have no leisure-time physical activity, which is very unhealthy. From 1991 to 1998, obesity among seniors age 60 to 69 increased 45 percent. They are victims of their built environment. The dislocation of the elderly from their homes is a major consequence of automobile-dependent sprawl patterns of development. Mixed-use HEALTHY PLACES offer "active communities" for Americans living into their 70s, 80s and 90s — tens of millions of people with the potential for decades of active living. Having amenities, without needing cars, is key to "aging in place" or "active aging," rather than moving to retirement homes or assisted living and nursing facilities.

A study found that older adults want accessible sidewalks, stores and services to walk or bike to, benches to rest on, safe and wide walking and bike paths, trees for shade, and neighbors who can help if needed. Aging baby boomers are redefining what being "old" means and are willing and able to find better places to live. Many "empty nesters" don't need and don't want to remain in large isolated suburban homes. Neighbors to talk to, civic activities to participate in, and interesting places to walk to, are more desirable than looking out of picture windows across large lawns at

silent suburban streets. Given the opportunity, many boomers will move
to HEALTHY PLACES. When baby boomers escape suburban sprawl they
increase the supply of homes for young families with children. Vacating
old sprawl means building less new sprawl.

Southern Village in Chapel Hill, North Carolina, was designed for
neighborliness and active living. It has attracted many retirees. Of the
4,000 residents in 1,500 homes, about 50 percent are over 50 years old and
15 percent are over 65. Diverse housing includes apartments, condos,
townhouses, and detached houses over a price range from just over
$100,000 to $1 million. Features include 13 parks connected by a paved
trail and a commercial center with a movie theater, a co-op grocery, a fitness club, a day spa, a pizzeria, and a church. A 63-year old resident boasted "I never feel my age there." Free buses take residents to University of
North Carolina – Chapel Hill campus facilities. Baby boomers need more
communities like this one.

And demand for them will keep increasing as baby boomers recognize
that sprawl living and sedentariness is unhealthy.

HIGHER DENSITY HOUSING CAN BE ATTRACTIVE.

Boston and Paris are about the same size, considering the city proper,
not the larger metropolitan area. But Paris has four times as many people
living in the same area, about 40 square miles. No matter how you view the
French people and government, it is absolutely clear that Paris is an
incredible livable place with the utmost of personality. There are real
neighborhoods. It is one of the most walkable places on the planet. City
residents everywhere have easy access to a public transit system that goes
everywhere, to marvelous local shopping and restaurants and to remarkable public spaces. Paris has a mixed-use layout of buildings, people living over commercial space, and good urban green infrastructure. The
public realm is as valuable to residents as their private home space.

Smart growth is often attacked because it implies higher population
and residential density. True, authentic HEALTHY PLACES inevitably
equate to higher densities of people living on a piece of land, as compared
to suburban sprawl development, which is characteristically a low density form of living. Yet there is no logical basis for believing that high quality of life depends on *low density* land use. Low density sprawl does not

offer quality social conditions, nor does it guarantee a higher quality of life. Many residents in the sprawling metro Atlanta region feel that their quality of life is in trouble, and another 2.3 million residents are expected by 2025, a 66 percent increase. Yet Atlanta is a very low density area with 3.5 million people living on 1.3 million acres, the lowest density among the top 15 U.S. metro areas. On nearly the same amount of land, 1.2 million acres, 11.8 million people live in the metro Los Angeles area, a 270 percent higher population density.

Higher density has a stigma because of experiences with low quality city living. As James S. Russell observed: "Suburbanites have resisted higher density, multi-family housing, and mixed incomes and mixed uses, because these are emblems of the chaotic and disordered city." However, higher density by itself is not a *cause* of urban social ills or urban flight. Urban decay reduced quality of life because government failed to serve and protect its citizens. Schools decayed. Crime mounted. Slums and empty buildings made streets ugly and threatening.

Nor should higher density be equated with *crowding*. Technically, crowding refers to high levels of residents within homes, not the density of the dwellings themselves. Crowding usually results from poverty or a lack of affordable housing for lower income people; it is found in both rural and urban areas where, for example, several immigrant families live together in order to afford housing. Crowding may also apply to high numbers of people in public places that have not been designed to accommodate them. Nevertheless, people will often use the term to describe the closeness of buildings and higher density housing.

Timing is everything. HEALTHY PLACES are just an old community design whose time has come again. Yet sprawl shills have made density an issue. What do *you* picture for higher density housing? One possibility is block-after-block of high-rise, side-by-side apartment buildings, without any greenspace, often associated with Manhattan and some other megacities. It may be very expensive city housing or low-income, subsidized "projects," many of which have been demolished in recent years because of their hopeless conditions. Another possible mental image is cookie-cutter multi-family buildings like bland garden apartments and cheap townhomes crowded together alongside highways. None of these images holds for HEALTHY PLACES.

To break the negative association between high density and low quality, people must learn that good design can assure higher density residential housing without ugly or unpleasant conditions. More people need to see HEALTHY PLACES, at least through pictures (see Figure 3-1) and computer simulations. Privacy can be protected. Feelings of overcrowding can be prevented. Public spaces that people seek in vacation spots can be provided near homes.

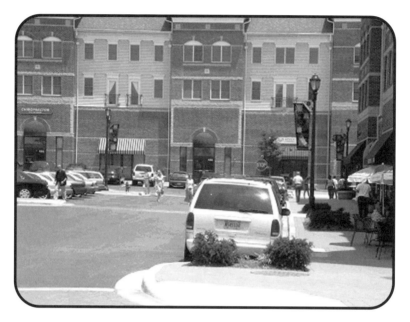

Figure 3-1. Higher density found highly attractive by people
in new town center with homes above stores.

Density numbers help to understand compact, clustered housing and smart growth development. The usual measure is the number of dwelling units per acre, excluding the acreage associated with open greenspaces and other non-residential, public areas. One acre is about the size of a football field, 43,560 square feet. New single family housing sprawl developments often have one or two homes per acre. Older suburbs may have 4 to 8 homes per acre. Levittown, Long Island, often considered the birthplace of sprawl has a density of about 4 units per acre. Rural areas have much lower densities, such as one home on 10 to 50 acres.

Generally, HEALTHY PLACES have densities above 8 units per acre and often run into the 10 to 30 units per acre range because of multifamily dwellings, which does not mean big apartment buildings, however. A mixture of modest multifamily units, such as duplexes and quadplexes, with single family, detached houses can easily produce densities in the 10 to 30 units per acre range. In general, higher densities can be achieved with townhomes, condos, lofts or apartments over stores, and accessory units such as granny flats and in-law units that can be used by a family member or rented out. Large lawns are traded for community greenspaces, like parks and trails, and for more public spaces. Densities will vary within the community, with higher densities around town centers and commercial streets and lower densities on outer streets.

Though it is convenient to use a density measure of homes per acre, such numbers do little to communicate the look and feel of a place. Density numbers by themselves reveal nothing about the quality of the design of the community and buildings. Talk about density of housing provokes emotions. Compactness may be better concept than density. It has been said that density is an emotion masquerading as a statistic. This much is clear. The better the design, the more attractive is higher density to nearly everyone.

To get a better feel for densities, consider these places:

South Beach in Miami, Florida, is a highly successful revitalized and compact older urban area. People love to visit and live in South Beach. It has an average density of about 30 to 35 units per acre, in mostly low-rise, multi-unit buildings of 2 to 4 stories.

Home prices are high in Cambridge, Massachusetts, an older inner ring suburb of Boston. The average density is 13 units per acre in with very few single family units; individual neighborhoods range from 2 to 25 units per acre.

The residential areas in the French Quarter of New Orleans, Louisiana, have a density of about 39 units per acre.

The booming and revitalized urban area of Hoboken, New Jersey, has an average density of about 14 units per acre because of multi-family units.

In New York City, with close to 3 million residences, single and two family residences are the largest use of land at 30 percent and have an average density of about 17 units per residential acre, while multi-family and mixed residential and commercial buildings use 13 percent of land and have an average density of about 100 units per acre. But residential neighborhoods with large apartment buildings can have densities of hundreds of units per acre. This is the case for the Upper East Side of Manhattan, one of the densest urban areas in the nation and one of the most expensive.

The highly praised development of Sailhouse in Orange County, California, has 37 triplex units and 52 small-lot detached homes, with a density of about 12 homes per acre. Dan Nahabedian, working for a homebuilder there, noted "The price of land has forced us into more denser solutions and, of course, what we give up is yard space. We try to give people indoor-outdoor living in various ways. …we're trying to say that the community is your yard."

An even denser California project is Playa Vista in Los Angeles, planned for 13,000 residents with 24 units per acre, and more public space than private. Some other impressive features: 90 percent of parking is underground; neighborhood parks are within a short walk of homes that have wireless Internet access beamed into them.

This is the lesson. *Design determines the acceptability of higher density. Design on any level – community, neighborhood and street – trumps density.* Design is so critical because the numerical figure of density and how residents actually perceive or experience it are two very different things. Consider two proposed projects both meeting a zoning or plan requirement of 25 dwelling units or less to the acre. One with minimal landscaping and little outdoor greenspace may be perceived as being at a much higher density than the better design with multi-unit buildings that look like single family houses and windows facing ample greenspace.

Higher density infill projects often face opposition from residents in neighboring areas who may have the Not In My Backyard (NIMBY) attitude. They have every right to refuse pain so newcomers can benefit. Special attention must be given to the impact on parking, traffic, and schools. Developers must convince current residents near a proposed project that lower car ownership and less vehicles will result from the design of the project, and the same goes for proposed greenfield projects that are opposed by surrounding sprawl residents.

HEALTHY PLACES reduce *perceived density*. What matters is what people find visually pleasing and attractive to live within. When you encounter the word density relative to housing do not jump to any conclusions. Put numbers aside. Seeing is believing. And do not believe right-wing density-drivel. Sprawl shill-meister Wendell Cox and junior shill Joshua Utt wrote in a June 2004 Heritage Foundation report that smart growth "would force people to live at higher densities" and "severely limit, or even prohibit, further suburbanization." "Force" and "prohibit" are signs of intellectual terrorism aimed at frightening Americans about smart growth. These paranoid zealots seem unable to accept higher density *suburban* HEALTHY PLACES, *freely* chosen and enjoyed, and *freely* built by profit-seeking developers. Cox calls smart growth a "naïve civic religion." He worships the car-culture.

HIGHER RESIDENTIAL DENSITY REDUCES CAR USE.

The "2001 Mobility" report from the World Business Council for Sustainable Development made these observations: "the provision of road infrastructure can accelerate the outward relocation of households and businesses. Within a few years of being opened, it is not unusual for these roads to carry traffic levels that…were not forecast to occur until after 20 or more years of service. …building infrastructure to get rid of all congestion is not a solution. …when people leave their homes they isolate themselves in cars. This can lead to a loss of sense of community and social cohesion. …there is a distinct, if inchoate sense that the increased use of cars over longer commutes has led to a more harried, less friendly society." Business interests, not environmentalists, reached these conclusions.

Think transportation. Do you see the advantages of reducing the distances between the locations you need to get to, so that you make shorter and fewer automobile trips? Do you want to replace automobile trips with walking to local, convenient destinations? Would more convenient access to safe and reliable public transportation be attractive? More and more people are answering yes to these questions.

Higher residential density is profoundly important for reducing automobile use. With higher-density housing, stores serving neighborhood residents can succeed, allowing residents to walk to buy groceries or to the dry cleaner. Mileage reduction can happen even if people still commute to work by car, because so many auto trips – 85 percent – are for other purposes. Vehicle ownership decreases with increasing residential density, reaching one car per household when density rises to 20 to 30 units per acre. In general, apartment residents average 1.0 motor vehicle per household, while owner-occupied houses average 2.1. One study found that in a neighborhood with 15 homes per acre, one-third fewer auto trips occur per household compared to sprawl.

Another study found that, after controlling for income levels, annual vehicle miles traveled (VMT) in households in traditional higher density neighborhoods was nearly 50 percent lower than in more recent, sprawl developments. Considerable data show that reaching densities of over 10 units per acre – as in HEALTHY PLACES – can reduce annual VMTs by 10,000 to 30,000 for households, or even more. Below this density level in sprawl, vehicle use rises extremely sharply. In sprawl-intense regions VMT can hit 100,000 or more miles annually.

Vancouver, British Columbia, has undergone remarkable success and population growth because of its high quality of place. Its high residential density is balanced by pedestrian-friendly streets and a quality transit system. Between 1994 and 1999 vehicle trips decreased by 12 percent while walking increased by more than 50 percent, confirming the principle that when residents are given solid alternatives they cut car use. The city resisted building a freeway system and, instead, emphasized its transit system and mixed-use, walkable neighborhoods.

Higher densities are crucial for public transit. Densities higher than about 10 to 15 units per acre are needed to support public transit of some kind, with buses requiring less density than rail options. But such developments may not be mixed-use and heavy car use may be necessary for non-commute transportation needs. Well designed transit-oriented developments or transit villages are catching on. They increase transit use, reduce driving 20 to 40 percent, reduce residential parking spaces 20 percent, and increase affordable housing.

One thing is crystal clear. Many people want to live in higher density neighborhoods. Consider the successful "Digital Harbor" revitalization in once industrial areas around Baltimore's inner harbor. Award winning developer Struever Brothers Eccles and Rouse has turned once empty factory buildings into offices, apartments, and sometimes retail areas. The old blue collar residential area of Canton has come alive again after years of neglect. Home sales doubled from 1996 to 1999 and prices jumped 70 percent, but remained relatively low with an average price just over $100,000. While Baltimore's population dropped 20 percent from 1980 to 2000, Canton's increased 36 percent. All this happened despite a high density approaching 20 homes per acre. They are relatively small attached row houses, mostly without garages or lawns. Why so much demand? Bill Struever explained: "Young people love being in these wonderful old buildings in a neighborhood where they don't have to drive to get to work." And they can also walk to the harbor, shops, restaurants and night spots. They don't need cars.

Higher densities generally mean lower land and other costs per home that make it easier for developers to include some affordable housing in projects. Affordable housing with easy access to public transit is especially needed for low to moderate income people, including public sector employees and many elderly residents. Sprawl shills blame smart growth for insufficient affordable housing. This is completely illogical. The shortage would not exist if 50 years of sprawl had provided enough affordable housing. Moreover, sprawl advocates generally do not support public transit which spurs affordable housing.

Higher residential density is an opportunity to drive less, a lot less.

LARGE-LOT SPRAWL FRAGMENTS GREENSPACE.

"Sprawl is a major concern because it is consumptive of all the things we have the least of in the West: water, tax money, clean air, and other environmental resources," said former Colorado Governor Dick Lamm. It is especially bad because so much Western sprawl is large lot sprawl. Carbon County, Wyoming, in early 2003 required *a square-mile, or 640 acres* for the minimum lot size on open range. Other local governments require 3 to 50 acres. "Farmettes" or "ranchettes" ruin country vistas and often destroy productive rural land uses such as farming or timbering (see Figure 3-2). This figure shows disorganized sprawl. Rampant rural sprawl is widespread in the most beautiful wilderness and forested areas.

Local governments often require large lots because they think it will stop sprawl and preserve open land, and because they think fewer homes and people will reduce spending on new government services. The strategy should never be equated with smart growth. Large-lot zoning does not "save" open space; it squanders and privatizes it. New Jersey home builders have complained about large-lot zoning by municipalities, often 10 acres for a single home, but in 2004 William Dressel of the League of Municipalities said: "They [builders] brought this on themselves because, as a powerful lobby, they opposed every tool we advanced for 30 years. ...I think the citizenry is concerned that we are paving the whole state and must put some controls on sprawl."

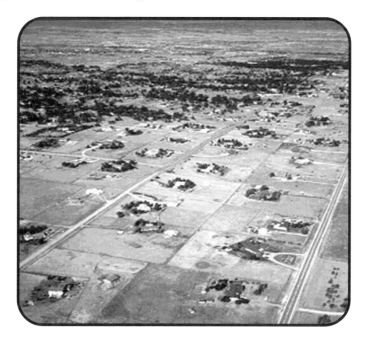

Figure 3-2. Very low density sprawl with custom built homes on large lots.

Once, people built modest rural homes on large lots and perhaps did a little farming and had some animals. Now, large-lot sprawl promotes the construction of mansions and destroys natural habitats and biodiversity. True, there is a lot of open, greenspace between the widely scattered houses, but it is *private fragmented* greenspace, not *public* park, forest or wilderness areas for all people to enjoy. The most valued greenspace is accessible by the general public, even if only as occasional visitors. Public greenspace most merits conservation and protection. Large-lot development is not regimented but it is a disorganized form of sprawl. It is the epitome of conspicuous, gluttonous land consumption. Some call it "snob sprawl" or "Gucci sprawl." Ordinary sprawl developers often "leap-frog" these areas, pushing subdivisions still further out.

Large-lot land owners usually expect public services, despite large distances from towns or cities and from other homes, even though in some areas homes are often used for short periods during the year as second homes. There are over 9 million second homes nationally, and the market is sizzling. In Colorado's four-county ski country, second homes drive the economy more than tourism, and have crowded out affordable housing for local workers. Because Colorado state law exempts properties of 35 acres or more from subdivision regulations, large lot sprawl has gobbled up more than 2 million rural acres, over three times the 625,000 acres for all of Colorado's cities, towns and suburbs where most people live. These lots are too small to ranch and too large to mow. They have put some half million residents in wildfire danger areas. True, such development creates low school costs, but other costs are high, such as for roads and emergency services. Colorado counties spend $1.65 in services for every tax dollar received from ranchettes, according to a Colorado State University agriculture specialist. In Larimer County a resident complained that the county only graded his road once a year, but all property taxes on the road provided was $800 annually, compared to the $7,000 cost for one-time road maintenance.

For those with $3 million to spend on a lot, Gray Head in Telluride, Colorado, exemplifies a ritzy sprawl development eating up once pristine wilderness. The 885-acre project offers 35-acre home sites on a former sheep ranch. The rugged terrain features 200-foot rock spires, trout streams and waterfalls, and it is home to herds of deer and elk. The area is eight miles from Telluride, where multimillion dollar homes cover mountain sides. A local civic leader bemoaned "With every new subdivision, there's less open land."

Eleven percent of all prime ranchland in the Rocky Mountain West is threatened by large-acre sprawl development with "prairie palaces." Montana State University researchers found that rural sprawl, such as ranchettes in the Yellowstone National Park, is driving some species toward local extinction. And work at Colorado State University found the lowest biodiversity in rural sprawl areas as compared to ranchlands and protected lands.

Large sprawl footprints stomp rural areas and squash their history. Some developers justify their rural sprawl projects by clustering the homes somewhat and preserving relatively large amounts of land.

However, such "conservation" developments are often not mixed-use. They are sprawl un-places with major impacts on rural landscapes and biodiversity. Private "dream" houses in once pristine and beautiful natural settings destroy *public* scenic beauty and recreational opportunities, everything from hiking to hunting. After the houses come strip malls. Soon, after farms and ranches disappear, tourism drops. Jim Reidhead, director of Larimer County's Rural Land Use Center, got it right: "People say they want to move into rural areas. What they want to do is superimpose an urban lifestyle on rural America." And Mary Ann Fidler of Samsula, Florida, a farm resident and sprawl fighter said, new sprawl residents "don't want the dust, the smell – they don't want the animals mooing at night."

Pity long-term rural residents. Many owners of large rural tracts who once made money from working their land eagerly wait for sprawl developers offering a financial windfall. Mike Willis with South Carolina's Department of Natural Resources described this greed: "The younger generation is learning it can sell the property and, in lots of cases, become instant millionaires. We have a generation that thinks water comes from a faucet, food comes from Harris Teeter and clothes come from a mall. People don't realize what is being lost when we destroy the land." Farmers who resist become isolated and they or their heirs eventually capitulate. Residential landowners with just a few acres who chose rural seclusion or were born into it suffer invasive sprawl, strip malls and rising taxes. *Sprawl kills rural lifestyles.* Some relocate to regain privacy in more distant rural areas, hoping to escape the mad march of sprawl. Charles Pattison of 1000 Friends of Florida commented on this: "People can't live in the community where they grew up and have to move away, or they have to live farther away and drive more, creating more traffic congestion."

At the expanding edge of sprawl one family's freedom to choose sprawl robs another family's freedom to enjoy a rural lifestyle. One family finds privacy; another loses rural seclusion. One family gets a big house; another loses scenic vistas. One farmer hits the jackpot by selling out to a sprawl developer; another farmer faces encircling sprawl residents angry about bad smells of livestock and fertilizer. Chase Schneider farms in Loudoun County, Virginia, and is surrounded by sprawl; "I know kind of how the Indians felt now," he said. One family gets bright streets and mall parking lots; another family loses the blanket of night darkness and star watching, the wondrous connection with the rest of the universe. Martha Pagliotti and her husband felt chased from their home of 33 years near Arvada, Colorado. Sprawl blocked their view of mountains and prevented star gazing at night. She commented "They've let this state be beyond ruined." One family accepts automobile dependency; another family can no longer safely walk or ride horses on rural roads now jammed with heavy traffic. Kelly Jacklin of Provo, Utah, owns 15 horses and has felt the impact of sprawl development: "We used to ride along the roads, but now there is no shoulder, and because of the traffic it is just crazy and dangerous." The final insult from rural sprawl is that it is forcing the closing of "trailer parks" offering low cost housing to low income people who then have difficulty finding affordable housing.

Remember the words of Joni Mitchell, "they paved paradise and put up a parking lot." Sprawl killing unique natural beauty and rural culture is a national tragedy.

MONSTER HOMES SERVE PRIVACY CRAVINGS.

Barbara Walsh once had a wonderful woodland view from the back of her house in North Castle, New York, but then a developer tore down a small cottage, wiped out dozens of mature trees and built a 6,000-square-foot house. "They're just plopping this McMansion in there and it's absolutely dwarfing the rest of the homes," she said.

After the cinematic invasion of the body-snatchers comes the real invasion of the neighborhood-snatchers. It is attack by the sprawl culture. People may rightfully expect their home to be their castle, but building castles is quite a different matter. Private space is the addiction of the rich, who take all they can get from land pushers.

The ultra-rich have set the pace for ultra-excess in the sprawl culture. Bill Gates has a mega-mansion outside Seattle with some 65,000 square feet. Television producer Aaron Spelling's Hollywood home has 35,000 square feet; Oprah Winfrey's house has 23,000 square feet. One billionaire is thinking of building a house in Washington, D.C. with over 100,000 square feet. In gated Jumbolair Aviation Estates in Ocala, Florida, actor John Travolta has a 21,000-square-foot home, and spaces for his Boeing 707 and Gultstream II jets next to his house.

Across the nation "ordinary" rich people are building monster homes, called "starter castles," "McMansions," and "trophy houses," the ultimate conspicuous consumption. Owners of monster homes often spend hundreds of thousands of dollars to demolish an older house, sometimes two. They often remove old trees. That is why these huge new million-dollar homes are also called "scrape-offs," "teardowns," and "pop-ups." In 2002, about 25,000 single family houses were built on lots after older homes were bulldozed, and this trend is rapidly escalating. In 1998, to get more privacy, Apple Computer's Steve Jobs tore down a one-story bungalow on an adjacent lot and planted a fruit orchard. In Winter Park, Florida, a perfectly fine 20-year 3,000-square-foot lakeside home was torn down so that a 5,000-square-foot house could be built. This would not be happening if there was abundant land.

Mega home space is more for indulgence than large families. Often just two people live in these mega-homes and sometimes just one person rattles around in the *internal sprawl space*. Many hooked-on-space people want to live in older communities, often because they want to avoid long car commutes to and from work (see Figure 3-3). In their midst bulky 5,000 to 10,000-square-foot homes are out of scale and dominate the local viewscape. Often they have an architectural style quite different than that prevalent in the neighborhood. They destroy the historic character and charm of older neighborhoods. These newcomers bring sprawl values with them, and do not care about "blending in." Their monster homes make the older nearby homes look like dog houses. Their selfish action negates neighborliness. The "eyesores-for-profit strategy" of uncaring developers and home builders serves self-centered consumers. An official of Toll Brothers, a large builder of these houses, said: "We sell what nobody needs." All too often an initial invasion ignites a trend. Older and smaller affordable homes disappear.

Infill monster homes are often so large that they occupy most of their lots, leaving extremely little open space around them. Adjacent homes can lose sunlight and views of sunsets and greenspace. The giant houses usually are set close to the street and have three or more car garages with large, wide driveways. They make streets less pedestrian-friendly. To add insult to injury, local property taxes can increase because of monster houses. More is not better when a cluster of monster houses are crowded together. The land looks oppressed by the monsters atop them. Such places are often gated and walled, but their obtrusiveness insults surrounding neighbors. Infill monster houses are not consistent with smart growth, or a smart way to revitalize older areas; they are too few in number to curb suburban sprawl.

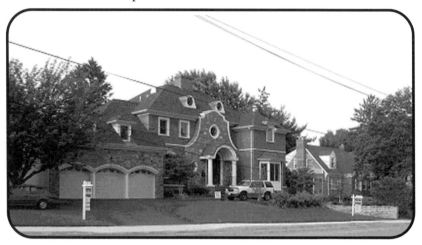

Figure 3-3. Infill McMansion dwarfs older, original home next to it.

Angry local residents usually protest, if they become aware that one or more monster homes are planned for their neighborhood. In a San Francisco neighborhood graced with historic Victorian homes and unique turn-of-the-century bungalows, residents fought replacing a 700-square-foot cottage with a 6,000-square-foot monster house five stories high, which would use up the entire lot. A resident said "Your home is your refuge. And the street outside is the living room of the neighborhood. Both are worth fighting for." Exactly right. But in the end, few local zoning laws prohibit monster homes. This is slowly changing. Denver changed its ordinance to require new homes leave at least 40 percent of the lot open; house height and shape can also be regulated.

The analog of the monster house is the Sport Utility Vehicle. Make no mistake about it. The SUV is the bastard offspring of the sprawl culture. Automakers' market research found that SUV buyers are more likely to be self-centered, self-absorbed, and unneighborly. They are less social than most Americans. They seem ideal for the sprawl culture. And forget the nonsense about the greater safety of SUVs that is often cited as the main justification for buying SUVs. The occupant death rate is higher in SUVs than in cars, and they cause more deaths in other vehicles in crashes. The mentality and values driving people to monster houses are also driving Americans to SUVs. Think of SUVs as "Sprawl Un-place Vehicles."

Not surprisingly, peoples' lifestyles also affect their pets, with about 50 percent of pets being overweight. Cats and dogs are moving around less and eating more than they should. In some McMansions with elevators, low level "paw-buttons" are placed conveniently for pets. They may even have their own rooms.

MIXED-USE PARKING AREAS SERVE MULTIPLE USES.

Paved deserts are everywhere. Nearly two-thirds of all the land that is covered by the built environment is for paving over land to create the "habitat for cars," including highways, streets, parking spaces, parking lots, garages, driveways, gas stations, auto dealerships, and other surfaces serving vehicles of all kinds. In downtown Atlanta, 60 percent of the surface area is for parking.

On a per person basis, no mode of transportation requires more physical space than motor vehicles. An incredible amount of land is used for parking. In Houston, there are 30 parking spaces per resident. Far out suburban sprawl areas may be worse. Typically, office workers who commute by car require at least 20 percent more space for their cars than the size of their office area. An eight-story office building could require a 10-story parking garage for all employees.

Automobile addiction is enabled by the government and private sector providing free parking. People resent paying for parking, whether it is street meters or garages. About 80 percent of commuters and an even greater fraction of shoppers enjoy free parking. Of course, no parking is really free. Wherever parking is provided, some entity has had to pay for the land and the construction of the parking spaces or facility. Surface parking spaces cost about $2,000 apiece; spaces in a garage cost $10,000 to $15,000, and ones below ground can cost $20,000 or more each. These costs are embedded in the cost of doing business and this affects consumers and workers. Not only is there no free ride, there is no free parking.

Seemingly "free" and abundant parking actually increases vehicle trips, which increases traffic congestion. Every parking space is a traffic generator. When parking is made more difficult or costly, people reduce their trips to those destinations. Limiting parking can stimulate ride-sharing, van pools, bicycling, use of public transit, and walking. Making parking easy does just the opposite. Incentives reduce vehicle trips. Silicon Valley companies that gave their employees passes for free transit use found that parking demand dropped by about 19 percent. An engineering firm in Bellevue, Washington, offered $40 per month to those who walked, bicycled, carpooled or took transit to work. Single drivers dropped 39 percent, revealing the truth about the "slave-hate relationship" Americans have with their cars.

Having less parking area is good for the environment, because impervious surfaces, like asphalt and concrete, increase water runoff that causes water pollution in streams, rivers, wetlands, and coastal waters. Excessive runoff prevents downward migration of water with contaminants, such as automobile oil, and the natural cleansing that takes place over time in subsoils. High runoff in highly developed areas also contributes to flash flooding in local streams and rivers.

Government agencies impose many requirements on developers and builders for minimum amounts of parking that vary according to the type of building. In most jurisdictions, there is no maximum for the total amount of parking provided, so developers who think that lots of parking sells put more of it in projects. For office buildings a common "standard" requires at least 5 spaces for each 1,000 square feet. Each parking space requires a total of about 300 square feet. So that means the parking area is 50 percent more than the office space! All such standards or zoning requirements are based on traditional heavy reliance on cars.

There are better ways to think. Portland, Oregon, has encouraged and strongly supported public transit. One study there found that because of its light rail system downtown, six 42-story parking structures did not have to be built. The closer an office building is to a public transit, the less parking is allowed. In one case, a new office development on a transit mall was allowed 84 percent less parking spaces. One developer built an office building without any parking spaces.

There are similar parking standards or requirements for shopping places, residential buildings, and schools. For retail shopping, many places require 5 spaces per 1,000 square feet. The essence of sprawl is that different types of buildings are widely separated, so that parking is needed for each of them, even though the parking areas may be empty much of the time. Shopping malls have vast expanses of parking lots that are underused most of the time; they are built to serve needs during the winter holiday season. In most places, special government approval is needed to supply *less* than the standard amount of parking, which takes time and money. Traffic engineers advocate for parking capacity which prompted architect and former planning commissioner Martin Dreiling to comment: "We need a holy war versus traffic engineers. A lot of great projects are killed by traffic engineers."

In mixed-use communities parking areas can serve multiple users. For example, parking for office workers can serve customers of shops, restaurants and movie theaters in the evening, as can school parking. Some parking lots can serve as areas for farmers and flea markets on weekends. Because of short distances between spots, one-stop parking saves time and fuel, and also cuts stress. People can go shopping, have a dinner and go to a movie or a public meeting in a civic building, and park only once within walking distance of everything.

Another approach in urban mixed-use places is using vertical, structured parking, with retail space on the ground level, sometimes with residential units on the top levels and stores on the ground level, and often with a façade that hides the fact that the building is a parking facility. This reduces land use for parking, helps keep the different types of community buildings close together, and offers an attractive viewscape. Another technique is to "wrap" garages with liner buildings containing, for example, loft apartments over retail shops. Garages can become nearly invisible. The City Lights project in Orange County, California, has 792 apartments in a square doughnut building; in the center "hole" is a parking garage with pedestrian bridges to all four levels of the apartment building and in all four directions. Overall density is 50 units per acre.

Fewer parking spaces are needed when buildings of any type are located close to public transit. An enormous resurgence in housing construction in Los Angeles proper and not its many suburbs has been aided by the city dropping its requirement for builders of apartments and lofts to provide parking spaces. Commercial areas and strip malls have been transformed into relatively high density housing in mixed-use neighborhoods.

Government agencies sometimes over-build transit parking lots on the assumption that many people will drive to the station. Some portions can be used for mixed-use development to increase the number of people living close to the station. It is smarter to make it easier for people to *live* close to transit. At the Ohlone-Chynoweth light rail station in San Jose, California, only 30 percent of the 1,140 original parking spaces were used. Now it has only 240 parking spaces, 330 units of affordable housing, a retail plaza, a child-care facility, and a community recreation center.

Another innovation offers good and bad news. In fully automated and computerized garages people leave their cars at the entrance, which are moved on pallets. Parking space density is high. One such garage in Hoboken, New Jersey, provides 324 spaces compared to only 95 spaces possible with a conventional ramped garage. Construction costs are about twice that for a conventional above ground garage, but comparable to below ground garage costs. Using this technology in urban cores to replace surface lots and ramped garages is more efficient land use. But using it just to provide more spaces promotes vehicle use.

This much is certain. When you look around and easily see large parking lots and commercial garages, it is a "carscape," a sure sign that you are not in a HEALTHY PLACE. In a HEALTHY PLACE "park" has so much more value as a noun than as a verb.

HEALTHY PLACES OFFER SECURITY AND SAFETY.

Sprawl shills link higher density living with unsafe conditions, but residents in higher density HEALTHY PLACES say otherwise. A three-year resident of King Farm in Rockville, Maryland said her favorite thing to do in the community was: "Walk the neighborhood. We really like the fact that so many people walk around day and night and one can feel safe in the community. We have really enjoyed our porch and looking at the changes in the neighborhood."

"We all enjoy our privacy, but everyone feels safer and more secure here knowing their neighbors, especially the families with children," said a resident of East Lake Commons, an excellent HEALTHY PLACE outside Atlanta with a racially diverse and eclectic mix of singles, young couples, small families, empty nesters and retirees from across the economic spectrum. Another resident said "Visitors to the community are visible to the residents. That is real security and real privacy."

Greater webs of citizen surveillance have become more important as funding of police departments has been squeezed. Driving around spread-out suburban areas with mostly deserted streets is very inefficient for police patrols, and many such areas never see any police presence. In sprawl, the emphasis is on home security systems and gated restricted access places.

The closer physical proximity of homes in HEALTHY PLACES makes suspicious behavior more easily observed. Exactly what was taken for granted in old-time neighborhoods in both cities and small towns, *more "eyes on the street" and more concern about neighbors.* In HEALTHY PLACES people know their neighbors, not just next door, but broadly in the community. Mixed-uses within the community promote more outdoor human presence throughout the day. People use greenspaces for recreational activities. Residents working from their live-work units spend time outdoors. As do elderly people and retirees. Local libraries and post offices bring people out. Diverse households, occupations and interests promote the presence of residents throughout the day. Streets where kids play, neighbors talk, and people walk produce more "feet on the street" to recognize strangers and inappropriate behavior.

Diversity of housing in HEALTHY PLACES raises an issue about rental apartments and safety. Apartments provide higher density housing and are critical for affordable housing, without which many service workers cannot live reasonably close to their jobs. About one-third of U.S. households are in renter occupied housing, much of it in apartments, while two-thirds are in owner occupied housing, most of it in single family houses. Contrary to some views, apartment residents are more socially engaged, equally involved in community groups, similarly attached to their communities and interested in local politics, as compared to house owners, according to research at the University of Chicago. On a per home basis, there is little evidence that the rate of police activity is higher in apartment communities than in single-family residences. Research at the University California, Los Angeles found transit stations do not cause increases in crime, which is important because of multifamily housing in such areas.

In sum, there is nothing intrinsically unsafe about higher density. What matters is great mixed-use community design and residents who literally look out for each other.

EMPLOYEES WANT TO WORK NEAR HOME.

Winston Tabb drove between his home in Reston, Virginia, and his job in Washington, D.C., for 30 years, a 60-mile round trip that took him "two hours at least, on a good day." Then he took a job in Baltimore, chose a home within a walk of 10 to 15 minutes, and boasted: "I like the freedom of it. I like the exercise. I like the quickness. I like meeting people. I'm passionate about it." He sounds like a walkaholic.

In the wake of September 11, 2001, living in a true community near work has received more attention. The terrorist attack on New York City's World Trade Center reminded many people and companies of the advantages of decentralizing and distributing offices. Small and medium size employment centers within HEALTHY PLACES offer benefits to workers and their employers. The workers are able to live near their work and reduce automobile use, and the companies face less risk from disruption of business and have a higher performing workforce.

The 2001 American Housing Survey by the Census Bureau found that, among people who moved the previous year, the chief reason cited for picking a new neighborhood was convenience to the job. About 31 percent said it was a factor, compared to 24 percent a decade earlier. This is consistent with the fact that in the 1990s the increase in the average time to get to work was 4.5 times greater than the increase for the 1980s.

Developers of HEALTHY PLACES are learning that employers increasingly recognize that suburban employees want to work in a mixed-use place rather than a typical office park or downtown. The many opportunities to go out on foot to local stores and eateries, the local green infrastructure, and perhaps even their homes, are highly valued. This makes office space in HEALTHY PLACES attractive business opportunities for developers. Many HEALTHY PLACES have included significant employment centers, almost always as offices. While local retail establishments, restaurants, and professional offices provide some jobs, they are typically small numbers compared to the number of residents. Here are some HEALTHY PLACES with impressive employment opportunities.

Post Riverside in Atlanta, Georgia, has over 537 apartments with 334 more planned, and at one end of the town square a nine-story office building that has about 750 workers.

Abacoa in Jupiter, Florida, has over 6,000 apartments and single-family homes and a large amount of office space, retail establishments, and a university campus that altogether provide over 7,000 jobs.

Maple Lawn, Maryland, is planned for about 1,600 homes and 4,000 residents and as many as 5,000 workers in offices.

Nocatee in Florida, will have a population over 30,000 and over 7,000 jobs in offices, retail and light industry.

Coffee Creek Center in Chesterton, Indiana, is planned for 1,200 residences and commercial space offering over 3,000 jobs, close to the expected number of residents.

Mission Bay in San Francisco, an urban infill development, will have over 15,000 residents and over 30,000 jobs.

King Farm in Maryland will have close to 10,000 residents and office buildings with over 10,000 jobs.

The Lowry community, built on a former Air Force base in Denver, Colorado, will have some 11,000 jobs and over 12,000 residents at build-out.

Mountain House, a new town under construction 60 miles from San Francisco, California, is planned for 44,000 residents in 12 villages and 21,000 jobs.

Before sprawl, many Americans walked home for lunch with their family, and then walked back to work. HEALTHY PLACES offer the chance to rediscover that old-world convenience.

SHOPS BELONG IN A COMMUNITY.

"It's great to be able to go shopping and get my coffee without dealing with the traffic," said Mike Muscutt, a resident of Creekbridge in Salinas, California.

In 1960 there was just 7 square feet of retail space per person, now it is 38 square feet, 400 percent more. From 1986 to 2003 the U.S. population increased 20 percent, but the number of shopping centers and malls increased 63 percent. Yes, more data of the absurd. The unrepentant conversion of rural land into commercial sprawl development is what Andy Serwer in *Fortune* magazine called "the insane proliferation of retailing." Keep sprawling, keep building roads, keep building more malls, keep spending more time shopping. Good for business, bad for people.

What consumers really want is not more retail, but more *convenient* retail – a good mix of retail stores and eating places they can get to without driving. Few people get what they want. Only 26 percent of all homes in the nation are near stores, and for new single family homes, only 12 percent are near shopping. In high-sprawl Atlanta, less than 10 percent are near shopping, while in older, dense Chicago over 30 percent are close to shopping.

Businesses come and go as market preferences change, but all require a sufficient customer base. For infill HEALTHY PLACES in cities and suburban areas, retail stores benefit from the nearby population. But in totally new greenfield communities retail may require more time to take hold. Build-out can take many years. In the early years a low number of residents can make retailing infeasible. One particular challenge has been grocery stores. It helps to have employment centers that provide a larger customer base than just relying on the immediate residents.

The small town flavor of HEALTHY PLACES requires smaller scale stores and restaurants, hopefully with local owners and workers who live in the community. Customers can be on a first name basis with store owners, sales people, and service providers. Shops and restaurants can be unique to the location, rather than chain and franchised operations that are found everywhere and do not contribute to local character and personality.

Despite the challenges, integrating retail into communities is done, as shown by these examples:

> Haile Plantation near Gainesville, Florida, is more than 20 years old and a true mixed-use community with a vibrant Village Center. With some 55 businesses, it provides just about everything any resident could desire, including medical services, restaurants, a supermarket, a bank, a post office, boutiques, a dry cleaner, a veterinarian, and many shops in a pleasing, walkable setting.

> The Post Riverside community in Atlanta has a bank, a dry cleaner, restaurant, deli shop, a dentist, an insurance agent, a travel agency, and a hairdresser.

> In Fairview Village near Portland, Oregon there is a Target store,

restaurants, a coffee shop, brew pub, bakery, post office, public library, and more.

The Russett community in Maryland has a supermarket right outside that people can walk to, as well as other stores.

Harbor Town in Memphis, Tennessee, offers its residents a grocery store, coffee shop, day spa, restaurants, a video rental store, a hairdresser, and a gift and garden shop.

Soon after the first residents moved into The Village of Providence in Huntsville, Alabama, they could go to three restaurants in the town center that will have a variety of shops, doctors, lawyers, and banks.

The developer of River Ranch in Lafayette, Louisiana, provided a local grocery store early in the build-out of the excellent mixed-use community. The store is in the Town Square, where there is also a restaurant, a home accessories store, a planned 55-room boutique hotel and an Eckerd's drug store that will be built.

The developer of Daniel Island in Charleston, South Carolina, got the Publix grocery chain to build a store when only 1,200 of the eventual 7,000 home sites were developed. The company was guaranteed that it would be the only grocery store in the community. With about a quarter of homes built, the downtown area satisfied most routine needs.

Early on, the developer of Middleton Hills in the Madison, Wisconsin, area decided that instead of spending money on advertising it was better to build a neighborhood center building; a quarter of the space was used for community mailboxes, common meeting space and the Prairie Café and Bakery, with the remainder for office space.

Who could be against close-by town centers? Sprawl shill-meister Randal O'Toole found a way. "Because it's walkable doesn't mean people will walk. People will drive for most of their travel," he said. Obsessive belief in cars and dismissal of Americans' free choice of walking over driving are sure signs of a fanatic. He also said "I'd say don't do mixed-use developments unless there's a market for them." Well, there *is* a market for them. When shills ignore markets that favor smart growth, they disparage developers of HEALTHY PLACES.

Shops in HEALTHY PLACES are an important thread of the community's social fabric. Chatting with neighbors in shops and while walking to and from them is special. Never underestimate the power of small talk to spur neighborliness. And rid yourself of any notion that malls are some modern version of community or town centers. Researchers have observed that shoppers in malls have a distinct slow mall walk and glazed eyes. Malls shape behavior, as children become "mall rats," compulsive consumers, and automobile addicts. In shopping malls and big box stores, people are not learning what is on the minds of their *neighbors*, nor conversing about *their* community. Strangers pass by strangers or sit near strangers in food courts, then get in their separate cars and fight traffic congestion to get back to their sprawl cocoons. All they share is *consumption*, which for too many Americans makes life worth living.

Legally, malls are private places, not public or civic gathering places, and not true town centers. The courts, including the United States Supreme Court, have consistently ruled that people do not have the same civil rights in a mall that they have in a village square or neighborhood street. You do not have the same free speech guarantees that apply in true public spaces. Many malls ban pamphleteering and other types of political activity. Malls regulate access and activity and control behavior, because they have the right to. Their aim is not promoting social discourse and community spirit. It is only to promote spending money.

In bygone days shopping enhanced community life. It can happen again, if residents shop locally and spend time walking and having opportunities to talk to neighbors. As a resident of King Farm in Maryland, Tiffany Berman said, "This is the first time we've ever been able to walk to a Safeway. We really don't use the car at all in the neighborhood. It's a really unusual place."

LIFESTYLE CENTERS OFFER A FAUX ESCAPE FROM BLANDBURBS.

Developers know how to subvert good ideas. Traditional shopping malls are facing tough times; an estimated 21 percent of over 2,000 malls are dead or dying and hundreds of empty malls dot the sprawl landscape. So developers have latched onto the mixed-use concept and consumers' desire for something more interesting. *Rather than support* HEALTHY PLACES *instead of blandburbs, the strategy is to keep Americans locked in sprawl and let them out to spend money in "lifestyle centers."* Lifestyle centers have exploded from virtually none a few years ago to over 60 now. But they are only superficially consistent with smart growth and New Urbanism.

These places are open-air arrays of a relatively large number of stores and eateries in a very attractive setting. There usually is a faux "main street" to simulate a downtown district or town center rather than a mall. "Village" and "town center" are often part of name. Legacy Village is outside Cleveland, Ohio, but it is neither a legacy nor a village. The goal is to create a compact, walkable and visually pleasing place. They usually have nothing but upscale chain stores and restaurants just like malls, rather than locally owned and distinctive stores or restaurants. Often there are a small number of housing units above some of the retail places and perhaps townhomes around the commercial area. But success depends on being a "destination," and nearly all customers arrive by car. Parking garages are usually tucked away behind shops. There may be a movie theater, outdoor stage, and other entertainment amenities to help create a pleasurable "experience" akin to leisure and entertainment rather than to mall shopping.

A decade ago it was found that 46 percent of women shopped as a psychological "pick-me-up" when they were feeling low, compared to just 21 percent now. As one architect-design firm advised: "People crave rich experience. It's a well-documented desire that testifies to a broader search for meaning that transcends material goods. …create places and offerings that activate the senses – live music, fresh air, wood you can knock on, looking across the table and having a real conversation." Other analyses have focused on the consumer "boredom factor," especially boredom with conventional sprawl malls.

A 2003 survey found that two-thirds of shoppers preferred lifestyle centers – manipulated satisfaction in manufactured cityscapes. The average shopper spends twice as much as one in an indoor mall, and 92 percent of visitors spend money, compared to just 50 percent for indoor malls. The Grove in Los Angeles, completed in 2002, had 18 million visitors in 2003, 5 million more than Disneyland.

Lifestyle centers aid the sprawl status quo. After credit cards are put away, lifestyle centers are just a faux, temporary escape from blandburbs. Be a good American, jump in your car, cope with traffic, shop and dine in a cute Disney-like place, and hit the road again to go home with still more stuff and a stuffed stomach. Such is the real trivial pursuit game.

SCHOOLS SHOULD SERVE ALL RESIDENTS.

Throughout most of history children walked to school. It is impossible to have a real neighborhood and community without schools.

Fairview Village has an elementary school and a preschool. It also has special footpaths for children so that they can safely walk to school without crossing busy streets. The Hidden Springs Community in Boise, Idaho has a new, small public charter elementary school for a little over 200 students, and a preschool. At Horizon West in Florida, with villages around a town center, all homes are required to be within walking distance of an elementary school. Hometown NRH, near Forth Worth, Texas, will have 700 homes and an innovative elementary school built close to a city recreation center, performing arts center and city library; it has a forested environmental learning area. Community and library rooms are upfront to serve adults after hours. Hometown's developer said that "The speed of life is based on how fast a child can walk to a park or school, not how fast a car can sprint to the Wal-Mart." When located within walking distances of residences more participation of parents in school activities is likely. When located within communities, school children also enhance the success of local businesses.

Large isolated schools serve sprawl subdivisions and like them lack place personality. Sprawl could not have succeeded unless local governments had built new, big-box schools that resemble shopping malls with large parking lots. School sprawl consumes large amounts of land and adds to traffic congestion and unsafe roads. The Souderton Area School District in Montgomery County, Pennsylvania, wanted to purchase 158 acres of farmland for $8.74 million – that's $55,300 per farm acre – for a new high school. The county planning commission opposed the site, because it would spur sprawl development and force most students to get there by bus or private car. Local activist Pam Learned said it "would undo 10 years of work to combat sprawl."

                                    SPRAWL KILLS +

Large sprawl schools explain the decrease in elementary and secondary schools from 200,000 in 1940 to 62,000 in 1990, despite a 70 percent rise in population. The average size of an elementary school more than tripled from 155 students in pre-sprawl 1950 to 473 in 2000. Super-size schools for sedentary super-size children are shameful. What matters most is educational quality. Years of research on education has revealed that smaller schools produce an array of benefits over large schools:

+ Improved academic achievement, as shown by grades, test scores, subject-area achievement and assessment of higher-order thinking skills.
+ Reduced rates of truancy, classroom disruption, vandalism, theft, violent crime, substance abuse, antisocial behavior, and gang participation.
+ Better student-teacher relationships and more personalized educational experiences.
+ Improved school safety and security.
+ Greater student participation in school-sponsored activities.

Michael Klonsky of the University of Illinois in Chicago summed things up: "In a big school you can't do the things that good research shows are needed: personalization; building a professional community among the educators; make the curriculum relevant to the lives of the students and the teachers; making the school safe. These big schools have 10 to 20 times the level of serious violent incidents as smaller schools." From 1998 to 2003 the Bill and Melinda Gates Foundation gave over $1 billion for small schools in New York, Boston, Chicago, Milwaukee and other cities. This reflects a wider view. A survey found that 66 percent of parents and 79 percent of teachers believed that smaller high schools provided a strong sense of belonging and community among students as compared to 4 percent and 1 percent, respectively, for larger high schools, with the remainder seeing no difference.

Rough guidelines for an appropriate size of smaller schools include no more than 300 to 400 students for elementary schools, and between 600 and 900 students for high schools. It should also be recognized that many HEALTHY PLACES projects help revitalize urban and suburban areas, and for these projects the use and reuse of older and often historic school buildings in surrounding areas is very appropriate.

Disappointment with large schools in sprawl areas has caused many parents to switch to home schooling, which is growing rapidly. In the United States there are now between 1.5 million and 2 million home-schooled students in grades K-12. Home-schooled children routinely show higher educational achievement than those in public schools.

Of course, in many newer rapidly growing suburban areas local government does not have the revenues to build new schools or expand older ones. The irony is that moving to sprawl suburbs often puts children in highly overcrowded schools or trailers used to handle the overflow. Or maybe busing is an issue. Traverse City, Michigan, built a new high school on a sprawl site outside city limits and soon after the school district could not afford to provide transportation for students, who could not walk or bike to the far off location; for two years most parents and students had to use their own cars. This situation worsens as residents in many places rebel against raising taxes and developers use their political influence to prevent government from levying impact fees to cover new school construction.

Schools should be easy to get to by walking. Parents should recognize that when their children walk or bike to school they are less likely to become overweight. Sadly, only one in eight children walks or bikes to school. Many schools do not require daily physical education classes; which among high school students dropped from 42 percent in 1991 to 25 percent in 1995, according to the Surgeon General. California testing of nearly one million fifth, seventh and ninth graders found higher academic achievement for physically fit students. A 2003 national survey of adults by the National Association for Sport and Physical Education found that 95 percent of parents think that regular, daily physical activity helps children do better academically. But most parents do little to make their children active. In the last 20 years the number of overweight children between ages 6 and 19 has soared, tripling to nearly one of every three kids.

When sprawl exploded after World War II, schools changed. Not only did they become physically isolated and separated from homes and real neighborhoods. Schools became large, single-focused "factories" where students were the "product." They lost their function as centers of their communities. Schools should serve all residents. To its credit, the U.S. Department of Education, in its 2000 report "Schools as Centers of Community: A Citizens' Guide For Planning and Design," said: "A successful school can strengthen a community's sense of identity, coherence and consensus. Like a new vision of the old town square, it can serve as a community hub and a place where students and others can learn about collaboration and the common good." Schools with multiple uses improve learning and academic performance, and also build social capital in communities.

Smaller neighborhood and community schools can provide places for many types of civic activities, some during the day such as a health clinic and some when classes are not in session. In the evenings and on weekends a school can be a place for adult education and recreation, and for community theater. It can serve as a town hall and neighborhood center. *The important principle is that schools and other civic buildings should have multiple uses, and serve as community meeting and gathering places.* With multiple uses, childless households will benefit from schools and support them.

Consider this case. After twice rejecting a bond issue for a new high school, voters passed a $25 million initiative, because community based planning produced a design to serve the entire community. Gaylord High School serves senior citizens, provides a daycare center, is a performing arts venue, offers community health care clinics and higher education classes, makes recreation space available, and even houses weddings. Facilities are used day and night, year round. The school is now a catalyst for more interactions among residents.

Parents often justify living in sprawl suburbs because of better schools. Yet the mega-schools addict their kids to automobiles and sedentariness. It takes courage for any politician to stop promoting sprawl by building new mega-schools. South Carolina Governor Mark Sanford said the following in his 2003 state-of-the-state address:

> Our current policies encourage the construction of massive, isolated schools that are inaccessible to the communities they serve. Rather than walking or biking to their neighborhood school, many students spend more time stuck on buses than they do with their families. …In addition to depriving many students of a quality education, these remotely sited mega schools also accelerate developmental sprawl into our rural areas - and what comes with it - increased car trips, lengthened bus routes, and a disappearing countryside.

In July 2003 South Carolina eliminated minimum acreage requirements for schools and allowed waivers in school square footage.

COMMUNITIES NEED ARTS AND CULTURE.

"Arts and culture is the genesis of the revitalization of communities,"
said Pittsburg, Pennsylvania Mayor Tom Murphy.

Arts and culture are a substantial part of the American economy and
the leisure landscape. The nation is home to some 22,000 non-profit arts,
culture, and humanities organizations that have about $37 billion in
annual revenues. In 1998, Americans spent over $9 billion on admissions
to performing arts events alone. This was $2.6 billion more than spent on
admissions to motion pictures and $1.8 billion more than spent on
attending sports events. There are 1,200 art museums nationwide. Growth
in the arts in recent years has been impressive. But scale and growth statistics do not tell the whole story.

Something has changed in recent decades, along with the spread of
sprawl. Sprawl has separated individuals from cultural activities, events
and venues. It coincides with a shift from personal participation to spec-
tator and consumer status. While attendance at all sorts of commercial
and non-profit venues has been increasing, the number of citizens *producing and participating in* arts and culture has been declining.
Americans are playing musical instruments only half as much today as
they did in the mid-1970s and the fraction of households where someone
plays an instrument has dropped from 51 percent to 38 percent in that
same period. A 1997 survey found that 35 percent of Americans had visited an art museum in the past year, 25 percent had attended a musical, and
16 percent had attended a classical music performance. Conversely, less
than 3 percent had acted in a publicly performed play, 10 percent had performed in a choir or chorus, and 11 percent had played music, even if
playing alone.

In past decades the arts were based more on volunteers than larger
scale commercial productions. Towns had their own playhouse, music
hall and singing groups. There was a stronger connection between art
spaces and public spaces at the community level. *The shift from a nation
of arts participants to arts spectators matches the decline in social capital*

and the increasing dominance of sprawl. Time-poor sprawl residents have less time and energy for participation. Not only are people separated from public spaces, but sprawl un-places do not stress public art and participatory community activities. And strip malls and massive shopping centers are not known for their arts and culture amenities.

Concurrently, technology also played an increasing role in making spectators out of people. Remember, sprawl and television grew up at the same time. The lure of 500-channel cable television, Internet options, computer games, home videos, and many forms of take-it-with-you music devices, has further reduced the once-prevalent experience of families and neighbors *watching and performing together.* Technology-based individualization of arts and culture does not contribute to social capital and gives considerable control of content to commercial providers. Isolation-enhancing products for individuals do not contribute to social interaction, neighborliness and community spirit. Less performing also means less physical activity.

Real communities serve the arts and culture needs of diverse residents. Civic engagement activities, like community meetings and voting, are often seen as "civic vegetables," good but not fun, but shared arts and culture activities are more like "civic desserts." Art-rich and culture-rich communities include: open-air amphitheaters; public art spaces for permanent sculptures, murals, exhibits and artistic fountains; plazas and other public spaces serving as venues for small performances, festivals and farmers markets; and neighborhood schools serving as homes for community theater and other arts groups.

Close-by arts and culture give a HEALTHY PLACE personality and character, because they:

+ Nurture social capital by facilitating interactions among spectators, performers, and producers.
+ Enhance and beautify public spaces to make walking and biking more interesting.
+ Help communities celebrate the heritage of their residents and the location.
+ Connect people to their common humanity, despite cultural and economic differences.

Here are some HEALTHY PLACES that offer residents arts and culture amenities:

> + The City Heights Urban Village urban infill project in San Diego, California, has works of six artists representing the culturally diverse community interspersed around several civic buildings. The 38-acre community also includes a performance center.
> + Cherry Hill Village with some 2,000 homes planned is in the fastest-growing area outside Detroit, Michigan. The Village Square area will include a performing arts center.
> + The mixed-use Willingboro Town Center in New Jersey will include an amphitheater overlooking a computerized 16-jet fountain.
> + In Highlands Garden Village in Denver, Colorado, a historic theater is being renovated to serve as a performing arts center.

Mizner Park in Boca Raton, Florida, is a showcase infill project on 28.7 acres; it includes 272 apartments and townhouses, some above storefronts for which people pay 20 percent more than for an ocean view, and considerable office and retail space. Four multistory parking garages are placed at each corner of the site. Residential density is five times higher than the rest of the city. The public plaza and grounds are beautifully landscaped with decorative walkways, benches, and fountains that entice pedestrians to stroll throughout the site. An amphitheater offers free concerts and other events. The Boca Raton Museum of Art hosts many community events. The Centre for the Arts is to feature a new state-of-the-art amphitheater seating 5,000 people, and a 1,800 seat acoustically superior concert hall.

One innovative developer set up a legal framework so that one-half percent of all lot and home sales, forever, go to a community fund to support civic, arts and culture activities. Once people escape sprawl and become time-rich, they will want more arts and culture venues close-by in their community, especially ones they can walk to.

AFTER LEVITTOWN CAME COMMODITY SPRAWL.

In 1947 sprawl was born in the form of Levittown on Long Island, New York. Most of the ideas were actually formulated in the 1930s, but not used on a large scale until Levittown. From 1947 to 1951, 17,447 low cost, small

750-square-foot houses were built and sold initially to World War II veterans and their families (see Figure 3-4). Just 750 square feet! Levittown homes would fit on the driveways of many recent large sprawl homes. Buyers could choose a porch or a car port. At one point over 80,000 people lived there. About 53,000 people reside there now.

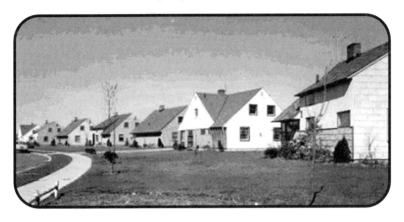

Figure 3-4. Levittown in its early phase, circa 1950.

The initial selling price was $7,990 for inside lots – just $67,109 in 2004 dollars, showing how cheap the homes were. By the end of the 1990s, the houses were selling for $162,600 on average, and sometimes over $200,000, although most had been significantly improved over the years. Levittown provided home ownership on an unprecedented scale, following nearly twenty years of little development and home construction, which created a severe housing shortage. With Levittown, the building industry changed from a piecemeal, custom-built business into a mass production, assembly-line operation. Levittown was immediately a huge success. Make no mistake about it. It *was* a great place to live.

Step back in time. There are lessons to be learned about how we got to sprawl supremacy, and the road not taken to mixed-use places. When World War II ended successfully, the United States faced these major, even desperate challenges for the economy:

+ The public feared the return of pre-war economic depression.
+ Millions of men and women left the armed services, and factory jobs were threatened as companies needed time to switch to consumer products.

+ There was enormous pent up consumer demand for housing.

+ Many people had relatively large amounts of cash from wartime work and businesses and because of a scarcity of consumer goods during the war.

+ There were a lot of postponed marriages and child bearing.

Moving from a war-time to peace-time economy needed help. The federal government responded with the GI Bill to steer ex-soldiers into education, the Interstate Highway System to provide construction jobs and increase demand for automobiles, and incentives for enormous amounts of housing to provide jobs and increase consumer spending. The growth of roads, automobiles, and suburban housing seeded sprawl, as landscape and culture. High volume, mass production of homes made perfect sense. And the automotive industry had considerable capacity that no longer was needed for military production; it was ready to make huge numbers of cars.

In the post-war years, the population was much smaller than now and it was reasonable to think that the nation had unlimited land resources. The 1947 population was about half of today's, and the fraction of people living in suburbs was about one-third of today's. Nor was there much of an environmental consciousness. It would be another two decades before that crystallized. Major cities had become congested and crowded during the war effort, and suffered from a lack of infrastructure investment in the pre-war depression and war years. When the war ended, Americans yearned for open space and rapidly available affordable housing. The American dream of the single-family house in suburbia was born.

Back then, sprawl *was* a smart solution for the nation. So many Americans had suffered and scrimped before and during World War II. The "Greatest Generation" deserved the good life as soon as possible. At first, many jobs in cities served suburbanites. But in the 1980s and 1990s, jobs and shopping shifted to suburbs, edge cities, and the exurbia beyond suburbia.

There are valuable lessons from Levittown; some pertain to sprawl and some to HEALTHY PLACES. The Levittown sprawl template:

Farmland was purchased incrementally. Land owners waited until their turn came and then they made a killing.

There was virtually no emphasis on individuality of houses; the cookie-cutter approach succeeded.

The federal government ensured success by making available about $20 billion – a staggering amount of money in the late 1940s. These funds were for up-front, government-guaranteed financing for risk-free mortgages. Veterans could buy homes with no money down.

Local government changed the building code to allow use of cement slabs instead of a basement.

Social exclusion and outright segregation prevailed. (But exclusion of African-Americans was largely true before Levittown. The Federal Housing Administration preferred "homogeneous" neighborhoods. Though the written policy was removed after a 1948 Supreme Court ruling declaring racial covenants unenforceable, exclusion remained.) Levittown was consistently described as monolithic: all residents were white, young and married with at least two children. Even now, African-Americans account for only 6 percent of residents.

Spiraling taxes have plagued the area over the decades, because of little commercial development. A big cost for taxpayers was schools. Originally, septic systems were used to avoid the costs of sewer infrastructure, which later had to be built at taxpayer expense.

Our current dominant automobile addiction shows itself by most Levittown residents still driving to those local village greens still thriving.

Levittown lessons for HEALTHY PLACES:

Design promoted community, and included small pocket parks and village greens as public spaces. The village greens included small stores and were within walking distance of homes, as were ball fields and community swimming pools. Over time, however, many of the stores failed because of the rapid emergence of strip malls and shopping centers on a major turnpike close to the development.

Social capital was high, as evidenced by some 200 community groups in the early years. Solid friendships were common with many lasting for 40 and 50 years, or more. A spirit of neighborliness was helped by the ban on fences around homes to create more open greenspaces, and a relatively high density of closely spaced, small homes. On the occasion of the 50th anniversary of Levittown a former long-time resident said: "One thing about Levittown is neighbors take care of each other. I moved to New Jersey, and in my neighborhood, I know maybe three people." The strong social spirit still exists.

Streets were important public spaces and had sidewalks and a lot of landscaping. The kitchen and living room in homes faced the street, with a large picture window, so mothers could watch their kids playing in the street. Winding lanes were used to slow traffic. But street connectivity was poor, causing people to walk long distances.

Some of the success was linked to access to public transportation. Many early residents did not have cars but used the Long Island Rail Road to commute to New York City; in 1954 half the residents commuted to New York City.

The developers knew how and why to use public involvement to get what they wanted from local government. Some 800 people attended a hearing on the proposal to remove the requirement for basements. Future residents feared not getting the housing they wanted if the developer did not get what it wanted.

The worst aspects of Levittown have defined nearly all sprawl housing, and the best aspects were lost as greed in the present displaced design for the future. The original focus on public spaces to promote community was lost while the lack of social diversity remained. For too long the black and white reality was cities for the poor and minorities versus suburbia for middle class whites. Zoning laws for suburbs made anything other than single land use development illegal. The pattern of buying up farmland remained a staple of sprawl development. The lack of jobs and shopping within suburbs explained escalating taxes, and this remains a problem, as does the shifting of infrastructure costs to taxpayers. *The sprawl culture was born in suburbia just as the baby boomers were.*

Even before Levittown there was support for sprawl, notably Frank Lloyd Wright who, as a famous architect, influenced people's views on the built environment. In his 1945 book *When Democracy Builds,* he preached elevating the private home above the public realm, the isolation hallmark of sprawl. Head for the open frontier in the most rural areas, and leave your neighbors behind, he advised Americans. He said "Avoid the suburb... Go way out into the country." He believed "human satisfactions" were destroyed by dense population. His ideal was one person per acre. Actually, what Wright was promoting and doing himself was more akin to building McMansions on huge lots of rural land, than to Levittown-type subdivisions. He bought 800 acres some 26 miles outside Phoenix for his second home. Much of current sprawl is closer to Wright's vision than to Levittown.

Levittown suited average Americans. It was much denser than Wright's ideal, because it was close in time and distance to the original walkable, mixed-use cities and old pre-war suburbs, and because of the huge demand for homes. After Levittown, developers stopped designing communities and just built sprawl subdivisions. William Levitt's business legacy was simple, get help from government; the sprawl industry became adept at that.

Here is another sprawl history footnote. The first free-standing, enclosed suburban mall in the early 1950s was originally envisioned by its designer Victor Gruen as the center of a new mixed-use "downtown." He planned apartment buildings, houses, schools, a medical center, a park and a lake. But only the Southdale Mall outside Minneapolis was built. Decades later Gruen criticized malls because of "the ugliness and discomfort of the land-wasting seas of parking" surrounding them. Levitt and Gruen had unintentionally created monsters whose profit-driven offspring would devour America's land and shred its social fabric.

At the height of post-Levittown suburban development, one of the nation's distinguished thinkers and authors, William H. Whyte, coined the term urban sprawl in the January 1958 issue of *Fortune* magazine. His words still ring true: "In the next three or four years, Americans will have a chance to decide how decent a place this country will be to live in, and for generations to come. Already, huge patches of once green countryside have been turned into vast smog-filled deserts that are neither city, suburb, nor country and each day – at a rate of some 3,000 acres a day – more country is being bulldozed over. ...the subdivisions of one city are beginning to meet up with the subdivisions of another." The more correct term now is "suburban" sprawl because most sprawl spreads out from existing suburbs not city boundaries and "rural sprawl" is more straightforward than "exurban sprawl."

Lewis Mumford warned in his 1960 book *Landscape and Townscape* "the continued growth of loose suburban areas will undermine our historic cities and deface the natural landscape." Later, Whyte said in his 1968 book *The Last Landscape*: "For years we wasted land with impunity, now we no longer can." Unfortunately, we could and did. Americans have not heeded Mumford's and Whyte's warnings given in sprawl's early days. Sprawl still consumes land with impunity despite its clear and present harm. More people feeling the pain will help us beat sprawl.

SPRAWL CHANGED CULTURE.

Consider the second half of the 20th century following World War II. The U.S. became the driving force for the global economy and emerged as the only world superpower, and on and on. Yet one largely unnoticed change was the unraveling of America's social fabric. No newspaper headlines declared the loss in social capital, even though it was a jolting change from the spirit and community that prevailed during and immediately after World War II. But today few people know firsthand what existed back then, and what was lost. About 80 percent of the present built environment was constructed since World War II, during the golden age of sprawl that changed our culture as much as it changed our landscape.

There was a time, when walking or shopping or sitting on a park bench, people could easily "make conversation" with other residents of any age or sex. It was a friendlier culture. For decades, nobody asked: Is losing physical and human connectedness really "progress"? Is a higher economic standard of living – really a "standard of having" – worth a lower quality of life? Does prizing private space but not the public realm enhance our democracy? Saying "no" to these questions is seeing what sprawl hath wrought.

Sprawl's impact on health was also unseen. High levels of cigarette smoking, exposure to unregulated toxic substances (such as asbestos in workplaces and lead in homes), and far less advanced medical science and technology offset the advantages of the old-style built environment that existed prior to World War II. Sprawl and its major impacts, especially sedentariness, offset the health benefits achieved by so many behavioral, regulatory and medical advances of recent decades.

Now, expensive medical "solutions" should be replaced by prevention through a built environment designed for active living. Americans have too much faith in the quality of health care. A landmark study published in the *New England Journal of Medicine* in June 2003 said that Americans only have a slightly better than a 50-50 chance of receiving optimal care in either a doctor's office or hospital, for either preventive care or treatment for acute and chronic conditions. Dr. Donald M. Berwick observed "If auto repair defect rates were the same as this, we wouldn't be alive today." Studies have found that even for their obese patients, physicians advise only one-third to exercise and less than half are told to lose weight.

A day after this story broke, an article in the *British Medical Journal* made the case for people taking a daily "polypill," a single daily pill to prevent heart disease and stroke. Robert O. Bonow, president of the American Heart Association declared: "This is exactly the wrong message to be sending. To suggest that you can continue to gain weight and smoke and not exercise and do that because now we have a magic pill – that is exactly the wrong message." Exactly right.

Imagine a couple in a sales office of a sprawl subdivision; they look overweight and in the women's handbag is the latest hit diet book. They ask whether the place promotes walking and a healthy lifestyle. The sales agent smiles, pulls out a copy of an article about the polypill and tells them "not to worry." An expensive magic pill versus the no-cost magic of physical activity, blandburbs versus HEALTHY PLACES, these are today's choices.

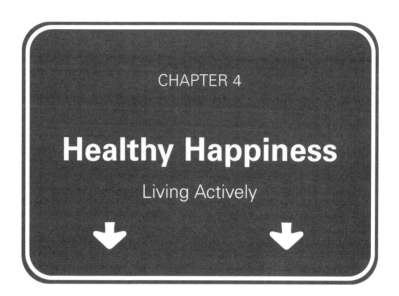

CHAPTER 4

Healthy Happiness

Living Actively

Sprawl kills.

Selecting a community to live in really is a matter of life and death.

Everyone agonizes over a new home decision and tries to balance a complex set of perceived benefits and tradeoffs that cannot be entirely quantified. But the one benefit that has not ordinarily been included is personal health, as if that has nothing to do with selecting a place to live in. It does.

In recent years, many books have been written about suburban sprawl, automobile dependency, and alternative lifestyles. Most authors try to encourage citizen outrage, social movements, and public policy changes, or a better understanding of American history and social trends. I had a different goal. How people can make better housing decisions to achieve a higher quality of life on their terms, not those of the housing industry and corporate America. Housing choice determines whether entrenched unhealthy habits can change for the better, and whether good habits will be sustained.

You come first. If your housing decision also makes the world a little better, fine. Sprawl does not make the world better. Sprawl living gulps down natural resources, and worldwide emulation of the American sprawl culture will eventually lead to resource wars. Self-interest beats altruism and sacrifice as effective motivation to make better housing and transportation decisions. In HEALTHY PLACES, replacing vehicle use with walking makes you healthier and cuts petroleum use and air pollution, a true win-win action. Large scale environmental improvements require actions by enormous numbers of people, companies, and governments. But you cannot control what large numbers of other people do. It is interesting that the direct and indirect costs to the nation of physical inactivity totals more than $150 billion annually. You cannot deliver that result. You can improve *your* health and reduce *your* health care expenses.

On the more negative side of the distinction between personal and cumulative benefits is the argument that many sprawl supporters make. They discount the importance of building HEALTHY PLACES, because yearly new housing construction represents a tiny fraction of existing housing stock, about 1 percent. So, they argue, why spend so much time trying to make it easier to build HEALTHY PLACES to appeal to relatively few people? From a national perspective, in terms of a cumulative benefit, it seems statistically insignificant. Not so, however, when you look at it from a personal perspective. A HEALTHY PLACE may be the best way to help you live healthier and longer.

This chapter presents the health benefits of HEALTHY PLACES. It may seem over-dramatic to say that sprawl kills, but where one chooses to live really is a matter of life and death. In 1975, about 75 percent of Americans agreed that they were in good physical condition. By the late 1990s, that fraction had dropped to 55 percent. It will keep dropping unless more people choose living in a walkable, old-fashioned neighborhood. The built environment needs to be seen like diet and foods, something you choose.

The smart growth movement holds up a psychological mirror for Americans to see a reflection of the cultural conspiracy of sprawl suffering. "Social phantasy system" is a concept of psychologist R. D. Laing, who believed that people develop "pseudo-sanity" to cope with "pseudo-realities." It is a virulent form of defensive self-delusion that aids survival, but reduces critical, objective thinking necessary to see the downside of a lifestyle. Living inside the sprawl lifestyle seems natural and normal. From outside it looks synthetic and irrational. Believers in true community, neighborliness, and active living see a sprawl social phantasy system with people afflicted with pseudo-sanity and saddled with pseudo-realities, because they believe in a fake American dream.

Famed psychologist Erich Fromm saw something similar when he wrote long ago about "socially patterned defects" that enable people to adjust to a system that from a humanistic perspective is "fundamentally at odds with our basic existential and human needs." Fromm pointed out that destructive impulses can be rationalized and "a whole social group share in the rationalization and thus make it appear to be 'realistic' to the members of such a group." The sprawl world dehumanizes its inhabitants. It destroys the environment, social capital, healthy active living, and free time. Yet it is rationalized as perfectly normal by consumers more focused on privacy and materialism. Half a century of sprawl dominion has created a cultural norm – that living in blandburbs is realistic, reasonable, and rational. In truth, it is a sick and destructive lifestyle. Brooding blandburb residents suffering from sprawl "dis-ease" look into the smart growth mirror and ponder "Is there something better?" There is.

SEDENTARINESS CAUSES OVERWEIGHT AND OBESITY.

Former Surgeon General David Satcher said: "I found the fountain of youth and it is physical activity." According to the current Surgeon General, Richard H. Carmona, Americans "are eating too much and moving too little." And in March 2004 Health and Human Services Secretary Tommy G. Thompson said: "To know that poor eating habits and inactivity are on the verge of surpassing tobacco use as the leading cause of preventable death in America should motivate all Americans to take action to protect their health." Take action. Seek a HEALTHY PLACE.

Retirees Penny and Jim Hessell took action; they became one of the first residents in Windsor Park, a 20-acre new community with 88 homes in Fruita, Colorado, which has a network of walking and biking trails, ponds, and parks. Jim said "We were looking for this perfect place. We found the communities we were getting involved in were so sedentary; nobody wanted to get out of their house and do anything." An advertisement for Brambleton, a large 2,000-acre mixed-use community for 6,240 homes in Loudoun County, Virginia, used a picture of a bicycle rider in a greenspace with this caption "Can Brambleton Help You Lose 10 Pounds?" More ad copy boasted of "parks, miles of exercise trails, tennis, swimming, sport courts and 15 playing fields." Developers can market active living and Americans can take action to protect their health.

A visitor from another planet could be fooled about Americans. Besides all the thin beautiful people on television and in the movies, visible everywhere are people addicted to fitness: obsessive runners speeding through neighborhoods, 500,000 people running in marathons, hordes of cyclists spandexed for multi-mile treks, 50,000 hyperfit people punishing themselves in triathlons, and a multitude of sweating regulars in gyms and health clubs.

Millions of these people are the exceptions that prove the more general truth. Most Americans do not embrace or maintain physical activity. All the fit male and female bodies seen in advertisements, commercials, and entertainment venues define and sell an idolized America that the vast majority of us will never experience, no matter how hard we try, no matter how much money we spend, no matter what we eat. Many know this. Many blame their genes. Others fault their economic circumstances and lack of time. Many keep chasing body-perfection. Many others give up. Hardly anyone thinks about the importance of where they live.

Here is the real America. Some 70 percent of adults are not regularly physically active, according to a 2002 report by the Centers for Disease Control and Prevention, including 30 percent who are not active at all. Inactivity increases with age, exactly when regular physical activity provides the greatest benefits. Inactivity is generally higher for minorities, lower income groups, the less educated, and women. Active living is hardly sought. HEALTHY PLACES are hardly known.

The general recommendation for health-promoting physical activity is 30 minutes a day of moderate type activity, although smaller chunks of activity throughout the day are beneficial, and greater total time is even more beneficial. A moderate amount of physical activity uses approximately 150 Calories of energy per day, or 1,000 Calories per week. A range of activities is shown below, with times compared to brisk walking.

LESS VIGOROUS, MORE TIME. MORE VIGOROUS, LESS TIME.
+ Washing and waxing a car for 45-60 minutes
+ Washing windows or floors for 45-60 minutes
+ Playing volleyball for 45 minutes

- Gardening for 30-45 minutes
- Bicycling 5 miles in 30 minutes
- Dancing fast for 30 minutes
- Pushing a stroller 1 1/2 miles in 30 minutes
- Raking leaves for 30 minutes
- **Walking 2 miles in 30 minutes (15 min/mile)**
- Swimming laps for 20 minutes
- Playing basketball for 15-20 minutes
- Bicycling 4 miles in 15 minutes
- Jumping rope for 15 minutes
- Running 1 1/2 miles in 15 minutes (10 min/mile)
- Shoveling snow for 15 minutes
- Stair walking for 15 minutes

On average, being obese means losing seven years of your life, and three years if you are just overweight. Among real Americans, 31 percent are obese, and 35 percent are overweight, according to 2002 data from the Centers for Disease Control and Prevention. It boggles the mind that two-thirds of Americans are overweight or obese! Sometimes both categories are grouped together and called overweight. The percent overweight increased more than 50 percent from 1990. In sprawl-ravaged Georgia the increase was over 100 percent. Nationally, obesity doubled from 1970 to 2000. Even worse news is the growth in severe obesity, meaning at least 100 pounds overweight and near certainty of severe medical problems. From 1990 to 2003 severely or morbidly obese Americans escalated from about 4 million or 3 percent of adults to 7.5 million or about 5 percent of adults, according to the American Obesity Association. All this happened despite more attention given to food and diet, food labeling, and exercise, and also when perfect bodies are shown to us on literally everything we look at, *except each other.*

In the real America there were about 103,000 stomach surgeries for weight reduction in 2003 at a cost of $3 billion, with some 300 dying, over 20,000 requiring repeat procedures, and about 30,000 developing serious side effects. Some 150,000 surgeries are expected in 2004 — a 50 percent increase in one year! Physicians have reported that some people are eating more to qualify for the surgery. Add to these some 400,000 yearly liposuctions to remove fat. But Washington University researchers found that fat removal through liposuction does not reduce risks of heart disease and diabetes. All this medical spending fattens health insurance costs and increases the Gross National Product, where "gross" reflects the ugly side of the real America. The light at the end of the blandburb tunnel is the ceiling light you see as they roll you into surgery.

This much is certain: *Insufficient physical activity relative to food intake explains being overweight or obese.* The medical community increasingly recognizes that regular, moderate physical activity is generally more effective than dieting to control weight. A desire for old-fashioned walkable neighborhoods is more than nostalgia. Choosing the right built environment to support physical activity can be as significant as not smoking cigarettes. It is just as important as good diet and nutrition, and likely more important for most people.

Physical activity is crucial to closing the excess energy (calories) gap. People need to burn more of the calories they are eating. The overweight epidemic is not caused by genetic factors, because genetic makeup in the overall population has not changed over recent decades when overweight and obesity have skyrocketed. In theory, the chief cause of the overweight and obesity epidemic could be gluttony or sloth – too much eating or too little physical activity. In practice, blandburbs support both sins. For every 60 minutes of driving the risk of being obese increased 6 percent, according to a survey of 10,878 Atlanta area residents. Blandburb residents don't stand a chance. As University of Colorado Professor James O. Hill said: "We drive to everything. We've created the perfect environment for creating obesity."

University of Tennessee researchers confirmed the importance of physical activity in preventing overweight and obesity. In an Old Order Amish farming community, where only pre-electrical and pre-motorized technologies are used, and consisting of 96 men and women, ages 18 to 75, daily physical activity was measured by pedometers. Men logged 18,000 steps and women 14,000 steps per day, compared to a healthy level of 10,000 steps a day, which few Americans achieve. The obesity rate was only 4 percent; a little more than a tenth of the U.S. rate. The overweight fraction was 26 percent, close to 80 percent of the U.S. rate. But their diet is far from being weight-conscious; it is high in calories, fat and refined sugar, but snacking between meals is rare. In more sedentary Amish communities, however, where people work in tourist shops and make furniture, the rates of overweight and obesity are similar to the larger population. The conclusion is clear, extensive physical activity can offset an "unhealthy" diet.

Duke University researchers demonstrated the effectiveness of physical activity without dieting or changing eating habits. Over eight months, 120 overweight or mildly obese adult men and women, ages 40 to 65, were instructed not to diet. A control group did not exercise, others walked briskly for 30 minutes a day or 11 miles weekly, and others jogged 17 miles weekly on average. The non-active group gained an average of 2.5 pounds. Of the walkers, 73 percent maintained their weight or lost a few pounds. The joggers lost an average of 8 pounds. Dr. Chris Slentz said "This study revealed a clear dose-response effect between the amount of exercise and decreases in measurements of central [mid-section] obesity and total body fat mass, reversing the effects seen in the inactive group. The close relationship between central body fat and cardiovascular disease, diabetes and hypertension lends further importance to this finding."

Another a study of nearly 5,000 healthy, employed adults over the age of 20 found that those who were physically active five or more times a week were 50 percent less likely to be obese, regardless of the level of physical activity in their work. A study of over 15,000 Europeans found that both decreased physical activity and increased hours spent sitting down during leisure time increased obesity by over 50 percent. Physical activity matters.

Obesity can increase the risk of adult-onset diabetes by as much as 34 fold, and diabetes is a major risk factor for amputations, blindness, kidney failure, and heart disease. Over half of adult diabetics are obese. One study found that people who were obese were more than twice as likely to develop cancer of the larynx, almost three times more likely to develop cancer of the small intestine and 1.4 times as likely to develop lymphoma. Excess weight has also been found to contribute to cancers of the kidney, breast and uterus, colon and rectum, esophagus and gall bladder, cervix and ovaries, pancreas, liver, and, in men, stomach and prostate. The American Cancer Society says that one-third of all cancer deaths are due to poor nutrition, obesity and physical inactivity, which substantially affect developing cancer in the first place.

"Obesity Raising Disability Rates" was *The New York Times* headline. Data for 1984 to 2000 from some 36,000 households for people between the ages of 18 and 69 revealed that disabilities associated with diabetes and musculoskeletal problems increased dramatically over that period for people less than 60 years old. Above that age there was a decrease over that period. Obesity in the younger people was deemed the main reason for rising disability rates.

Obese people have more than three times the risk of their stitched breastbone rupturing after open heart surgery, increasing the risk of death. The solution is to use extra-strength stitching. To manage severe obesity new super-size stretchers can handle up to 650-pounders. New wider ambulances have special hydraulic lifts, shock absorbers, and winch-and-pulley systems to pull heavy loads into the ambulance. Triple-wide coffins can handle a 700 pound corpse. In the real America techno-logical accommodation comes to the rescue.

Arguably, too much attention has focused on the gluttony side of the equation. Dieting has not worked in the long run for most people. A report published by the President's Council on Physical Fitness and Sports said: "Physical inactivity is certainly a major, if not the primary, cause of obesi-ty in the United States today." Sloth is more complex, related to the design of the built environment and the use of sedentary-enhancing technolo-gies, such as television, escalators and elevators. The ugly truth is that fighting the sedentary lifestyle in blandburbs is very difficult, and car-dependent, stressful sprawl living encourages bad eating habits.

When you put down this book remember this. Being overweight or obesity is *a cause* of disease rather than a disease itself; sedentariness is *a cause* of being overweight or obese, and a poorly designed built environ-ment is *a cause* of sedentariness. How much of a cause in each link in the chain of logic depends on personal circumstances. Food, weight loss, and pharmaceutical business interests back making overweight and obesity a disease, which would reduce personal responsibility and create a victim mentality. Sadly, in July 2004, the Bush Administration opened the obesi-ty-as-disease door for the Medicare program. Writing in *The Washington Post*, nurse practitioner Carolyn McCarthy observed: "But adults are responsible for their adult choices; if they claim to be victims of obesity, they must name themselves as their victimizer." And parents who do not ensure the right choices for and by their children victimize them. Allen Steadham, head of the International Size Acceptance Association, said: "Obesity is not a disease. All this does is open the door for the diet and bariatric surgery industries to make a potentially tremendous profit." Through taxes and insurance rates, those who are fit will subsidize the obese.

How do Americans see the overweight issue? A 2004 Time/ABC News

Poll found that 58 percent of Americans would like to lose weight, but only 26 percent exercise at least three times a week, despite the fact that 86 percent believe not getting enough physical exercise is an important cause of obesity. Forty-four percent say it's hard to walk anywhere. An Associated Press poll found that 75 percent of overweight Americans blamed themselves and 8 percent blamed their families. Here is an example of a healthy attitude: "When the weather is good I am deliberately inefficient, and I will make many runs downtown," so said Alice McLerran of Bellport, Long Island who walks instead of driving.

SPRAWL HARMS KIDS.

"City officials allow developers to build the same dysfunctional sprawl pattern suburb over and over. …It's not surprising that many kids become addicted to games or television or drugs. They need an escape from the lethal combination of monotony, conformity and the confusion of personal value with material status," so observed University of Texas Professor Dean Terry.

The national epidemic of overweight and obesity is deadly to children. America's children are like the canary in the coal mine, sending us a clear warning. As U.S. Surgeon General Richard Carmona said: "As we look to the future and where childhood obesity will be in 20 years…it is every bit as threatening to us as is the terrorist threat we face today. It is the threat from within."

Duke University researchers created a Child Well-Being Index that measured various factors in several domains from 1975 to 2002. They reported that "the modern day epidemic" of obesity was the single biggest health problem for children ages 1 to 19 and drove health well-being down 15 percent below 1975 levels. The social relationship domain was also below 1975 levels and the emotional/spiritual domain was below levels since the late 1980s. Between 1975 and 2002, the overall index had risen an unimpressive 5 percent.

It boggles the mind that 10 percent of kids entering kindergarten are already obese! More data of the absurd. The prevalence of overweight in children from 6 to 18 years old was 6 percent in 1976-1980, 11 percent in 1988-1994, and 15 percent in 1999-2000. From 1971 to 1999, the prevalence of obese children and adolescents more than doubled. Now, 24 percent of young people between 2 to 17 years old are obese. Arkansas tests all school children and found that 22 percent were obese and 18 percent overweight. From 1996 to 2001, 2 million adolescents became obese and an additional 1.5 million remained obese as they matured into adulthood. Over 80 percent of obese adolescents become obese adults. For adolescents who are just overweight, between 70 and 80 percent will become obese adults. Race matters. In 1999-2000, 24 percent of black, non-Hispanic girls and 29 percent of Mexican-American boys were overweight. In 2002 the National Heart, Lung and Blood Institute reported that by age 18, 31 percent of white girls were living sedentary lives, compared to 56 percent of black girls. CDC data for 2002 showed that 31 percent of white women aged 20 and older were obese, compared to 49 percent for black women.

As early as third grade, some children are being diagnosed with hypertension and type 2 diabetes, both formerly associated with adults. Between 1982 and 1994 there was a 10-fold increase in type 2 diabetes among children. All this explains why the Centers for Disease Control and Prevention committed nearly $200 million in 2002 for an advertising campaign to get children more physically active. But will it work on children stuck in sprawl?

Adults' sprawl lifestyles affect children. When both parents are obese, the probability of a child being obese is between 60 and 80 percent, compared to just 9 percent when both parents are lean. Pregnant women obese in their first trimester have children who by age 2 are twice as likely to be obese, and by age 4 are 2.3 times as likely. A 2004 University of Iowa study of parents and their children found that over about 20 years, the annual rate of weight gain increased by 150 percent for children age 15 to 18, clear evidence of lifestyle changes, not genetics. A study found that 75 percent of parents of overweight children did not realize their kid's problem. And pediatricians at Children's Hospital of Pittsburg did not note that children were overweight in two-thirds of office visits by obese children.

Children's behavior has degenerated. Children spend about 75 percent of their waking hours being physically *inactive.* In the early 1970s, 80 percent of children played sports every day, but now only 20 percent do. In 2001, children aged 5 to 15 years walked or biked to or from school less than 15 percent of the time, a remarkable decrease from 48 percent in 1969. The Centers for Disease Control and Prevention found that in 1999, among children living less than one mile from school, only 31 percent of trips were made by walking, a remarkable decrease from close to 90 per-cent in 1969. Surveys by the National Sporting Goods Association found that children ages 7 to 17 riding a bicycle six or more times a year dropped 18 percent from 1991 to 2002. Where did all the time go? A Kaiser Family Foundation study found that children under 6 spend as much time in front of screens as they do playing outside. The average child now watch-es 5.5 hours a day of electronic entertainments other than television. Another study found that obesity was 38 percent higher in children watch-ing television more than three hours of television a day; a different study of young children found that the risk of obesity doubled per hour spent playing video games and nearly tripled per hour of watching television.

Childhood development of brain chemistry and capabilities, both intellectual and emotional, are affected by the built environment. Kids become "wired" for sprawl isolation and automobile addiction. The Commission on Children at Risk formed by Dartmouth Medical School and others was composed of physicians, neuroscientists and social scien-tists. "Hardwired to Connect" released in 2003 said that humans have a "biologically primed need to connect to others." The instinctual desire for connections has a biological basis. Social environments and built envi-ronments that promote connections positively "affect gene transcription and the development of brain chemistry." Conversely, social disconnec-tion and low social capital impair brain development. An analysis of 269 studies from the 1950s onward found that steady increases in self-report-ed anxiety and depression among children have resulted from the decline of social connectedness. This matches the growth of blandburbs over the past 50 years.

Twenty-one percent of children ages 9 to 17 have a diagnosable mental disorder or addiction. From 1987 to 1996 there was a 300 percent increase in the use of psychiatric drugs by children. The suicide rate among college students has tripled in the past 35 years.

To sum up, children are increasingly physically inactive, and physical-ly and mentally unhealthy, and the vast majority of them live in sprawl-space. *Getting educated in super-size sprawl schools, eating super-size fast-food meals, and becoming super-size themselves, children dream of the day when they can get their own super-size SUV and a super-size monster house.* Children must learn that a healthy body is easier to attain and keep than a perfect body. Smart parents benefit their children by living in a community that promotes active living and where blandness does not foster boredom, because bored sedentary kids self-medicate by eating or worse behaviors.

PHYSICAL ACTIVITY MAKES YOU HEALTHY.

What a frightening forecast by the Centers for Disease Control and Prevention: One-third of all the people born in 2000 will get type 2 diabetes if current sedentary trends continue.

In mainstream America the sedentary lifestyle prevails, a lifestyle linked to cardiovascular disease, diabetes, hypertension, osteoporosis, arthritis, asthma, some cancers, depression, and anxiety. The President's Council on Physical Fitness and Sports said: "A major cause of death in the U.S. is sedentary living." Moreover, "over 30 percent of the deaths for coronary heart disease, type 2 diabetes and colon cancer would be prevented by moderate-intensity physical activity." Other work has shown that being physically active on a regular basis can reduce by 50 percent the risk of getting coronary heart disease, obesity, diabetes, stroke, and colorectal cancer.

Information keeps expanding on the many health effects of physical activity and inactivity, *independent of other factors*. General statements about health benefits of physical activity may convince you, but specific evidence is even more compelling. Capsule summaries of research findings are given below. The point is not remembering all the facts and figures. Let the information flow over you and take you to the truth of active living.

GENERAL AND MULTIPLE HEALTH EFFECTS:
A Stanford University study of over 6,200 older men, tracked for an average of six years, found that physical inactivity is a better predictor of death that other risk factors, such as smoking, hypertension and heart disease. This held for both healthy men and those with known health risks. The risk of death in the fittest people was about half that of the least fit. The message for physicians was that physical activity merits as much attention as smoking and high blood pressure.

A number of studies have found an inverse relationship between mortality and level of physical activity, including one that found men who engaged in moderate physical activity had a mortality risk just 73 percent of that for the least active men. Another study of older men found that the mortality rate was cut in half for those walking two miles a day.

A study of adults over 40 years old having at least two chronic diseases found that those who exercised at least 30 minutes a week had half the risk of death than those exercising less than that.

A review of the scientific literature concluded that being active for 30 minutes most days of the week was associated with a 20 to 30 percent reduction in all-cause mortality in younger and older men and women.

A CDC study of 2,896 adults with diabetes found that those who walked two hours a week had a 39 percent lower all-cause mortality rate and a 34 percent lower cardiovascular disease mortality rate. This was independent of all other significant factors, like sex, age, weight, and smoking. Those who walked 3 to 4 hours a week had a 54 percent lower all-cause mortality rate, and 53 percent lower rate from cardiovascular disease.

Many studies confirm that regular, moderate physical activity correlates with better functioning of the immune system, which means less vulnerability to viruses that cause sore throats, colds and other respiratory infections. A study of 160 overweight and obese women found that those who walked briskly for 45 minutes a day five days of the week had half the days of sickness as those who remained sedentary.

Members of a California runners club over the age of 50 who ran for about four hours weekly reduced their likelihood of disability later in life, in comparison to a control group who ran an average of 20 minutes weekly and who had a death rate three times higher than the first group, according to the 13-year follow-up study.

The World Health Organization concluded that exercising in three

10-minute sessions is as effective as a 30-minute workout. Accumulating 30 minutes of moderate-intensity physical activity throughout the day reduces the risk of developing coronary heart disease by 50 percent, the risk of developing adult diabetes by 50 percent, and the risk of developing hypertension by 30 percent.

A study found that people who regularly commute by bicycle have a 40 percent reduction in mortality compared to people who do not cycle to work.

A study of 7,553 predominantly white women aged 65 and older found that the risk of death, heart disease, and cancer was reduced in the six years following the initial six years of the study, during which the women had physical activity equivalent to walking a mile every day. The lower mortality rate was similar to that of women who were already active when the study began. Interestingly, for women who were active but became sedentary the mortality rate was similar to that of women who were sedentary all along. This result showed that physical activity benefits cannot be "banked;" you must maintain physical activity.

According to several papers published in the Journal of the American Medical Association, people who are physically inactive are at a two- to three-fold higher risk of premature death, as compared to physically active people.

The Washington Department of Health reported that in 1998 the lack of regular physical activity caused an estimated 12 percent of all heart disease, 12 percent of all cases of high blood pressure, 15 percent of all cases of colon cancer, 27 percent of all diabetes, and 20 percent of all osteoporotic falls with fractures. These were responsible for an estimated 1,272 deaths and 5,768 hospitalizations.

HEART DISEASE AND STROKE:
A CDC study found that being sedentary was the most common modifiable risk factor for coronary heart disease. It was present in 58 percent of cases, compared to cigarette smoking in 25 percent, obesity in 22 percent, and hypertension in 17 percent, showing that

physical activity is more important than these other well-known risk factors.

Research at Brigham and Women's Hospital on women middle-aged or older found that brisk walking for about 2.5 hours a week cut the risk of heart disease and stroke by about one-third. About 74,000 women between ages 50 and 79 were tracked for six years.

A study of 17,000 Harvard alumni found that sedentary men were 64 percent more likely to have a heart attack than those who exercised enough to expend 2,000 calories per week, including walking 20 miles a week.

Men in the lowest 20 percent of physical fitness have two to three times the risk of dying overall, and three to five times the risk of dying of cardiovascular disease, compared with men who are fitter.

The risk of stroke was reduced 30 percent and the risk of heart disease was reduced 40 percent by walking briskly two to three hours weekly.

A Harvard University study found that men who ran for an hour or more weekly cut their risk of heart disease by 42 percent, compare to non-runners; walking briskly for more than 30 minutes daily gave an 18 percent reduction; training with weights for 30 minutes or more per week reduced the risk of heart disease by 23 percent.

Duke University researchers found that exercise accounted for more and larger HDL particles (good cholesterol) and fewer LDL particles (bad cholesterol).

Lawrence Berkeley National Laboratory found that jogging or running increases good cholesterol in women and men. This translated, for women, to a 29 percent reduction in the risk of heart disease for running 40 or more miles a week, and 45 percent lower death rate from cardiovascular disease.

A study found that how long a person exercises – not its intensity –

is more potent in reducing the bad forms of cholesterol, but not to how much weight is lost. The cholesterol-improving effect of walking a mile is the same as running a mile.

Research discovered a new way that exercise protects against heart disease. Exercise mimics the anti-inflammatory action of certain drugs through elevated blood flow. A number of studies have correlated physical activity with lower levels of C-reactive protein and, therefore, lower risk of heart disease and type 2 diabetes.

A study of 201 generally sedentary and overweight women, who had their daily calorie intake reduced from 2,200 to 1,500 calories, improved their heart health whether their daily exercise regime was 30 or 60 minutes of moderate or vigorous activities. This was in addition to significant weight loses.

TYPE 2 DIABETES:
A Harvard School of Public Health study of over 68,000 healthy women, age 36 to 55 years, for six years found that each hour a day of brisk walking was associated with a 34 percent reduction in diabetes; and 43 percent of new cases could be prevented with an active lifestyle of 30 minutes a day of brisk walking and less than 10 hours a week of television watching. This lifestyle would also prevent 30 percent of obesity cases.

A Harvard study of nearly 40,000 men, age 40 to 75, for ten years found that those walking 20 minutes on most days reduced the risk of diabetes 20 percent, those doing 30 minutes cut the risk by 30 percent, and those that were even more active cut the risk by 50 percent; watching television more than 40 hours weekly tripled the risk of getting diabetes.

Walking was found to predict diabetes in a National Institutes of Health study. Women who briskly walked the most had just 58 percent of the risk, compared to sedentary women, taking into account age and hypertension. Even moderately paced walking produced a significant risk reduction.

A Harvard study gave an exercise test to over 8,600 men. They were divided into three groups. After six years the men in the low fitness group had nearly four times the risk of diabetes as compared to those in the high fitness category, regardless of their weight.

A Cooper Clinic study of men with diabetes found that low fitness and sedentariness greatly increased the risk of all-cause mortality, independent of other factors.

CANCER:

Walking or other more vigorous forms of exercise, for seven or more hours a week, reduced breast cancer as compared to those who exercised one hour or less, according to a study of 122,000 nurses age 30 to 55 and tracked over a 16 year period. A comparable study found a similar benefit in women aged 25 to 42.

A study of 75,000 women age 50 to 79 found that women who currently walked briskly, or exercised differently but at a similar intensity, for 1.25 to 2.5 hours weekly were 18 percent less likely to develop breast cancer than sedentary women.

For women without a family history of breast cancer, a study of over 1,100 women found that women who consistently exercised had a 35 percent lower risk of getting breast carcinoma in situ, as compared to women who did not exercise at all.

A study of 1,008 Ashkenazi Jewish women with breast cancer found that women who inherit mutations of the BRCA1 or BRCA2 gene have a 55 percent risk by age 60 and 82 percent risk by age 80 of developing breast cancer, but its onset was delayed by sensible eating and exercise, such as dancing, team sports or walking, during adolescence.

The risk of colon cancer and polyps was cut in half by engaging in moderate daily exercise, according to a study of 22,000 men age 40 to 84.

OSTEOPOROSIS:

A study of 1,000 women and 700 men found that walking protects the bone density of hips and has a protective effect on the bone mass density of the spine.

MENTAL HEALTH AND OTHER IMPACTS:
CDC found that people who exercised had 1.3 fewer days a month feeling sad, blue or depressed; the average for all adults was 3 days.

Older women who walked regularly had less memory loss and other declines in mental function as compared to less active women.
A brisk 30-minute walk three times a week was found as effective as antidepressant medication in reducing the symptoms of major depression in middle-aged and elderly people.

A study of 1,700 men aged 40 to 70 found that regular physical activity reduces the risk of erectile dysfunction.

A University of Wisconsin study of women over the age of 60 living independently and in assisted-care facilities found that women were more likely to give themselves high ratings for overall quality of life and physical health if they were more physically active. The conclusion was that older adults hurt their health more by not exercising than by exercising.

University researchers found that exercise protects the brain against aging.

"Women over 70 who walked at least six hours weekly had the mental sharpness of someone three years younger. Men over 70 who walked two miles daily had half the risk of dementia of those who walked a quarter mile daily."

Regular physical activity can prevent or help various leg problems, such as blood pooling, varicose veins, and restless legs syndrome. Physical activity addresses disturbed sleep patterns.

You may feel numbed by so much data. Here is the main lesson: There is remarkable evidence already, with more coming all the time, for the health benefits of active living and the price paid for a sedentary lifestyle. You can count on benefits once you do 30 minutes of moderate physical activity on most days. Remember, even greater benefits come from 60 minutes a day, which has been recommended by the Institute of Medicine for preventing weight gain and achieving maximum health benefits. The American Heart Association recommends 60 minutes of moderate to vigorous physical activity every day for children and adolescents. For the maximum health risk reduction physical activity should improve cardiorespiratory fitness as usually measured by oxygen needs during a treadmill test. But there are still important benefits from moderate activity.

You probably have not heard about "metabolic syndrome," a cluster of closely associated medical conditions. It is seen as a lifestyle condition strongly linked to physical inactivity and excessive body weight. If you have it, you are two to three times more likely to die prematurely from a heart attack or stroke, often preceded by diabetes. The syndrome is diagnosed when a person has at least three of these five conditions (in order of decreasing importance): high triglycerides, high blood pressure, insulin resistance, low HDL or good cholesterol, and excess abdominal fat shown by high waist circumference. However, about 20 percent of people with the syndrome have a normal weight, and some obese people do not get the syndrome.

The Centers for Disease Control and Prevention estimated that more than 20 percent of adult Americans have it. It affects up to 40 percent of people over 40, causing some physicians to speak of an impending epidemic among aging baby boomers. Cardiologist Paul Howard warned "This is the epidemic of the 21st century." Syndrome prevalence has soared some 60 percent in the past decade. Even more disturbing, research found that 12.5 percent of children between the ages of 8 and 17 had the syndrome, after 3,200 students had been studied. A Yale University study found that half of severely obese children and adolescents and 39 percent of the moderately obese had metabolic syndrome. The syndrome explains increases in diabetes among children.

A study reported in 2004 of 1,881 diabetes-free men and women found that 28 percent of the men and 22 percent of the women had metabolic syndrome; men had a 78 percent greater risk of stroke and the women had more than double the risk. The syndrome accounts for about 20 percent of all strokes in the general population, and 40 percent in Hispanics.

An important finding came from a study of 780 women with blocked arteries over a three year period. Of these, 58 percent had metabolic syndrome and 76 percent were overweight or obese. Being overweight or obese *did not* correlate with a greater risk of complications or death from heart disease, but those having metabolic syndrome had about twice the risk.

The good news is that research on men found that exercising more than three hours weekly cut the risk of developing the syndrome by half. That is why treatment of the disease emphasizes increasing regular physical activity. As reported in late 2003, research on 5,115 men and women ages 18 to 30, and followed for 15 years, found that poor physical fitness, as shown by treadmill testing, correlated with a six-fold higher probability of developing metabolic syndrome, diabetes and hypertension. The big conclusions were that "the development of risk factors for heart disease and stroke isn't just the natural result of aging," and that people "can protect themselves against those risks by maintaining their physical fitness," according to Dr. Mercedes Camethon of Northwestern University.

Does thin equal fit? Does fat mean unfit? In truth, you do not have to be thin to be healthy. You can be heavy and healthy, if you are not sedentary, which is very important for those people genetically predisposed to be overweight. Dwell on this fact for a moment. People who are officially overweight or obese but who are physically active have death rates comparable to thin and average-weight people who are also physically active. A study by the Cooper Institute for Aerobics Research of some 25,000 men over eight years found that unfit lean men were nearly twice as likely to die as the fit, including obese fit. Another study of nearly 10,000 women found that physical activity resulted in a 43 to 52 percent reduced risk of death, regardless of overweight or obesity. In other words, obesity does not necessarily increase mortality risk. Along the same line, Dr. William E. Kraus at Duke University Medical Center said that his research on the effects of exercise showed "that you don't have to lose weight to improve your cholesterol profile."

Many physicians now believe that being sedentary is unhealthier than being overweight, and that regardless of your weight you will benefit from increased regular physical activity. Rather than focus solely on dieting, more people should put equal or greater emphasis on physical activity. Rather than trying to get fat people to become thin, why not help them become healthier? Steven Blair, with the Cooper Institute said: "Being active and fit is good for you whether you're young or old, man or woman, tall or short, skinny or fat." He also said that if Americans walked briskly for 30 minutes a day "the public-health battle would be won." Of course, no matter what your level of physical activity, good nutrition and weight control is smart.

In early 2003 the American Heart Association released its "Guide for Improving Cardiovascular Health at the Community Level." This was quite significant because previously the paradigm for physicians was to treat individuals at high risk. It was a radical shift to recognize that population-wide interventions were necessary and appropriate. It recognized the importance of deleterious lifestyles and behaviors as causes of heart disease and stroke. One of the key behaviors targeted was a "sedentary lifestyle characterized by less than 30 minutes of moderate-intensity physical activity per day." A key recommendation was: "Every community should commit to providing safe and convenient means for walking and bicycling as a means of transportation and recreation." In other words, active living design is a medical solution.

A few months later the American Heart Association released a Scientific Statement "Exercise and Physical Activity in the Prevention and Treatment of Atherosclerotic Cardiovascular Disease." This was a strong message to physicians about the preventive and curative benefits of aerobic physical activity. Healthcare providers were advised to "support the implementation and maintenance of exercise programs for their patients across the lifespan."

Physical activity is also good for corporate America and the national economy. A study by General Electric found that employees who exercised were absent from work 45 percent fewer days annually than those who did not. Reducing the time and stress for commuting to work increases worker productivity. A new trend is "healthy architecture" where the design of office buildings and campuses require employees to walk more. For example, a new Sprint campus has parking lots that are intentionally a five-minute walk away from buildings. What about the health insurance industry?

A major health plan company in Minnesota surveyed about 5,700 of its members aged 40 and over, and verified the importance of regular physical activity. For every additional day per week with physical activity medical care costs decreased by 4.7 percent, regardless of age, sex, race or the presence of diabetes and heart disease. Benefits were seen in only 18 months. In similar work on sedentary adults over age 50, those who increased their physical activity to 90 minutes per week reduced their medical costs by \$2,200 per year. Obese members of the Kaiser Permanente HMO have health care costs 44 percent higher than those with healthy weights. Obviously, all parties paying for health care would benefit by supporting efforts to increase physical activity. With consumers paying more of their medical costs, even with health insurance, they have an economic incentive to be physically active.

Believe this: *Physical inactivity is unnatural.* If physical inactivity was "normal" it would not cause so many health problems. True, we no longer gather our own food and fuel, and most of us do not do manual labor, but we still need to be active. Humans are genetically wired or programmed to be physically active and to consume food to survive. The programming to eat still works all too well, especially with abundant and relatively cheap food. But the built environment and a myriad of products, technologies and services choke our biological need to be physically active. Lost is the natural balance between the two genetic programs. With so much gluttony and sloth the sprawl lifestyle is not just unhealthy, it is sinful. A HEALTHY PLACE helps you restore the natural balance between consuming and burning calories.

PRE-SPRAWL COMMUNITY DESIGNS ARE HEALTHIER.

Two San Diego neighborhoods were compared. One was an older one with high walkability and the other one had low walkability. The actual time spent being physically active was measured; the average was 207 minutes per week in the high area versus 147 minutes in the low area. That extra 60 minutes might help explain why only 35 percent of the people were overweight in the high area, compared to a more normal 60 percent in the low area. The high area had higher residential density, more mixed-use, and safer streets with greater connectivity and aesthetics.

The right community design undeniably supports walking and other outdoors physical activity. But virtually all mass-produced suburbs built in the past 50 years are not walkable, mixed-use places, and at least 60 percent of Americans live in such automobile dependent suburbs. This is up from just 15 percent in 1940, showing the fundamental change between pre- and post-World War II lifestyles. In the 75 largest metropolitan areas, 75 percent of people now live in such blandburbs. From 2000 to 2025 it is likely that near 90 percent of new housing will be in sprawl un-places, if past trends continue.

Much research has shown that when community design makes it easy, enjoyable, and safe to walk or bike, then people will walk and bike more. Street connectivity is a key factor. Cul-de-sac streets in blandburbs mean that for some visible destination "you can't get there from here." In neighborhoods with relatively small, square, and connected blocks, residents walk up to three times more than in places with non-connecting, cul-de-sac streets. Having access to public transit means that up to twice as many people walk or bicycle, as compared to sprawl, automobile-dependent places where street safety is a major issue.

"The Metropolis Plan" released in early 2003 to guide growth in the greater Chicago metropolitan area through 2030 had a goal of building more walkable communities and business districts to improve public health. The data showed that through various land use, housing, and community design measures the share of trips made by walking and biking could increase from about 10 to 16 percent. This 60 percent increase would be accompanied by a 40 percent decrease in the average time spent in vehicles, a 65 percent decrease in the average time spent in traffic congestion, and a 60 percent reduction in open land consumed for new development with 30 years of population growth. Also, the number of new households within walking distance of greenspace would nearly double. Community design matters.

Here is some proof for this. The American Society of Civil Engineers found that residents in more walkable, mixed-use neighborhoods would drive 43 percent fewer miles as compared to typical sprawl subdivisions. For 12 neighborhoods in the Puget Sound area, pedestrian traffic was three times greater in the walkable areas as compared to suburban sprawl areas. In Portland, Oregon at least 20 percent more trips were made by transit, walking or biking in areas of 5 or more homes per acre, as compared to areas with an average of one home or less per acre. For Canadian neighborhoods in an urban center (more than 900,000 residents), a small urban center (less than 50,000 residents), and a suburb near the urban center, there were four times as many non-motorized trips in the most walkable areas, compared to the least walkable ones. Because of abundant bike lanes and paths in Davis, California, bike trips now account for more than 25 percent of all trips, compared to less than 2 percent nationally. Data from 2001 showed that 21 percent of Americans age 65 and older do not drive and only 7 percent of these walk on a given day in sprawl areas compared to 33 percent in denser areas. Another study found that 43 percent of people with safe places to walk within 10 minutes of home had healthy regular physical activity, compared to 27 percent not near such places. Community design matters.

A 2003 review of available evidence for functional walking concluded that residents in highly walkable communities had twice as many walking trips per week compared to those in low walkability areas. Mixed land use provided nearby destinations to walk to, and good street design helped. One or two extra walking trips a week can burn off enough calories to drop nearly 2 pounds a year, which is the average amount that adults tend to gain annually.

Pre-sprawl neighborhoods are like time capsules. They support once prevalent physical activity because they are more likely to have sidewalks, denser interconnected networks of streets, and a mix of business and residences. Older places support the healthier "old fashioned" lifestyle – the walk and talk, rather than the ride and hide style. *But everyone cannot live in old places, even with infill projects in older suburbs and cities, so new places must be designed like the old ones.*

Here are data that support the benefits of older communities: Analysis of 1980 data for sprawl areas built since the early 1950s and HEALTHY PLACES built before World War II around San Francisco found that car usage was 32 percent higher in the sprawl areas and walking was 50 percent higher in the HEALTHY PLACES. In the Puget Sound area there was a 62 percent decrease in the number of walking and bicycling trips in developments built after 1977, as compared to places built before 1947. Similarly, research at the National Institutes of Health on a nationally representative sample of adults found that living in urban and suburban homes built before 1974 had a 40 percent higher level of walking one or more miles twenty or more times per month as compared to those who lived in homes built in or after 1974.

A South Carolina study found that students were four times more likely to walk to schools built before 1983 than to those built afterwards, which were more likely to be in sprawlspace. The 2003 EPA study "Travel and Environmental Implications of School Siting," compared two Gainesville, Florida high schools. At the one in the city 15 percent of students walked or biked and 85 percent used cars; at the one on the edge of the city all students used cars and the trips were twice as long.

Here are research results directly connecting walkable areas with overweight and obesity.

The *Atlanta Constitution* surveyed its readers; 72 percent did not believe that where you live affects your weight. But a study for Atlanta found that the total fraction of overweight and obese white males in walkable, mixed-use areas was two-thirds that for residents in low walkable neighborhoods. In areas with two or fewer homes per acre, 68 percent of white males were overweight, compared to 50 percent in areas with more than 8 homes per acre. The figures for white females were 32 and 22 percent. For obesity in white males, the figures were 23 and 13 percent. In terms of mixed-use, 20 percent of residents in the least mixed-use neighborhoods were obese, compared to 15 percent in the most mixed-use.

Boston University researcher Russ Lopez used 2000 Census tract data in 330 metropolitan areas and CDC data on 104,000 adults. Increases in a sprawl index increased risk for being overweight and obese. For example, the risk for obesity in Atlanta region residents would be reduced by about 17 percent, if Atlanta (sprawl index = 80.65) had the sprawl level of Boston (46.57). Insightfully, Lopez explained: "When people have less time, they have less time to be physically active and cook. People have been moving to the suburbs for healthier lives, but Americans should rethink this."

Another study used national data on community design and health. It examined information on over 200,000 people living in 448 counties and found that more walkable counties with the least degree of sprawl correlated with greater amounts of walking, lower levels of overweight and obesity, and less prevalence of high blood pressure.

In late 2002, the Task Force on Community Preventive Services appointed by the Director of the Centers for Disease Control and Prevention concluded that there was strong evidence showing that creating or improving access to places for physical activity, such as walking trails, really worked. Places that promoted physical activity actually were effective in helping people to exercise more. Typically, 25 percent more people exercised at least three times a week. Recognized benefits were weight loss or decrease in body fat.

Trust this conclusion. The right community design – old or new – promotes physical activity and better health. Of course, you must take advantage of the design. Bobby Rayburn, president of the National Association of Home Builders, thinks that sprawl is a "horrible term" and believes that the health case against sprawl is "absolutely crazy." Shill-meister Randal O'Toole agrees; he said "the nation's recent 'obesity epidemic' has nothing to do with the suburbs. It is not even certain there is such an epidemic…" Samuel R. Staley is also a shill and said: "People should have the choice to live somewhere where they can be fat." That's easily done, because the market offers so few communities that help residents be physically active and healthier.

SPRAWL DRIVERS POLLUTE THEMSELVES.

Cars have bad breath. Reducing vehicle use reduces personal exposure to air pollution from vehicles' exhaust. Vehicles take your time and money and give you toxins too. Many groups advocate reducing automobile use to reduce air pollution and global warming. But these are classic cumulative benefits that require actions by countless people to be significant on a regional, national, or global basis. Reducing *personal exposure* to air pollution is quite a different benefit.

Less time in cars and traffic congestion means breathing less air with the most concentrated levels of toxic air pollutants, such as volatile organic compounds like benzene, toluene, and xylenes. You probably will not smell exhausts, unless the vehicle ahead of you is a really old car or a diesel truck. Vehicles produce lots of stealth pollutants. Motor vehicles account for over 50 percent of the carbon monoxide, 30 percent of the nitrous oxide and 25 percent of the carbon dioxide emissions produced nationwide from all sources. Smog or ozone is a huge problem; it forms when sunlight interacts with nitrogen oxides and volatile organic compounds. Though it decreased during the 1980s, it got worse in the 1990s.

Sprawl shills like to talk about advances in engine technology, pollution control devices, and fuels that have reduced vehicle pollution emissions on a per mile basis. But these benefits are being offset by the increased number of vehicles, increased use of them, the increased size and lower fuel efficiency of them (particularly SUVs) high numbers of old vehicles, and increased road congestion and stop-and-go traffic, which causes worse pollution.

Chronic, long-term exposure to automobile pollution is a serious health threat. The issue is not whether you become exposed, but how much exposure. The American Lung Association says that vehicular air pollution causes as many as 120,000 unnecessary or premature deaths annually, and $40 to $50 billion in annual health care costs. High ozone levels caused by car emissions lead to respiratory problems, cardiovascular effects, immune system deficiencies, and higher rates of birth defects. High carbon monoxide levels in heavy congestion can restrict oxygen flow to the brains of drivers trapped in traffic, potentially impairing their performance once they hit the gas again. University of California postmortems on seemingly healthy young Los Angeles auto accident victims found that 80 percent had serious lung abnormalities, and 27 percent had severe lung lesions. By matching death rates and air pollution levels of more than 500,000 Americans in 156 metropolitan areas for over 16 years, in 2003, it was reported that because of a decrease in cigarette smoking, air pollution had become more risky to the cardiovascular system than respiratory diseases.

Where you live matters. A 2000 study of Denver children living near high-traffic roads found they had six times higher risk of developing all types of cancer, and eight times of getting leukemia. Other studies found higher levels of asthma, bronchitis and pneumonia among children near high traffic roads. A study of long-term exposure of 5,000 adults living near high traffic roads found that they were almost twice as likely to die from heart or lung disease and 40 percent more likely to die from any cause, as compared to people living in low traffic areas.

Strong evidence of unhealthy car pollution came from 17 days of the 1996 Summer Olympic Games in Atlanta. During that period there was a 22.5 percent reduction in peak weekday morning traffic, and a decrease of 27.9 percent in peak daily ozone concentrations that are linked to vehicle use. The positive result was a drop of 41.6 percent in the number of asthma emergency medical events in the Atlanta area.

Asthma in children is a growing national epidemic. In children under five years of age asthma increased 160 percent in the past 15 years. About 20 percent of children have asthma. Vehicular use is one of the most significant causes of smog pollution, which in the summer of 1997 was responsible for 6 million asthma attacks, 159,000 visits to emergency rooms to deal with asthma and 53,000 asthma-related hospitalizations. Research has also found that asthma prevalence correlates with obesity and physical inactivity, and not just indoor and outdoor air pollution. Nationally, with some 4.8 million children afflicted, asthma is the leading cause of school absenteeism attributed to chronic conditions. The disease is also linked to poorer academic performance, increased chance of not finishing high school and increased need for special education programs.

Another aspect of sprawl is a massive use of school buses; nearly 600,000 of them transport some 24 million students to school each week day. Collectively, children in the United States spend 3 billion hours on school buses each year. As sprawl subdivisions have spread out, suburban school buses have faced more traffic congestion, longer routes, and more idling which produces higher pollution levels. The national rise in asthma among children may be linked, in part, to the diesel exhaust exposure in school buses. High levels of air pollution have been measured inside school buses. Children are particularly susceptible to health effects of diesel exhaust exposure because of their narrow airways and faster metabolism and rates of breathing. Now, it turns out, nearly all bused children are exposed to significant levels of diesel exhaust, which contains a host of toxic chemicals, including several known human carcinogens and soot which causes fine particles to lodge deep in the lungs. Diesel soot has been link to missed school days, asthma hospitalizations, chronic bronchitis, pneumonia, heart disease, and premature death.

Some environmental groups stress the use of natural gas fueled school buses, but the healthier alternative is walking or biking to school. Children who walk to school are more alert and better behaved than those riding a bus, according to teachers. Even when children live relatively close to their school, they are likely to use buses, because there are no *safe* walking routes to school. Unsafe routes result from the lack of sidewalks and unsafe intersections. Some school districts actually require students to use buses, despite some living close to school or having safe routes. The option of "walking school buses," having parents escort children to ensure their safety is a better idea.

Ironically, sprawl evolved from zoning laws designed to separate people from highly polluting "smokestack" industries, such as foundries and chemical plants. But now sprawl causes people to be in close proximity to large numbers of polluting vehicles – trucks and buses as well as automobiles – despite the fact that they live in suburbs far from polluting industries. Sprawl drivers are polluters polluting themselves. Sprawl school buses are polluting children. The combination of physical inactivity because of automobile dependency and greater exposure to vehicular pollution is the sprawl-health double-whammy.

The lesson is clear. Less breathing of polluted air means less risk of respiratory diseases, heart diseases, various cancers, and premature death. But blandburb residents have few alternatives to heavy traffic on roads connecting suburban sprawl housing to jobs and everything else.

PEOPLE BECOME LIKE BLANDBURBS.

In 1950, during sprawl's initial big-bang after World War II, *The Atlantic Monthly* editors wrote "Every motorist is aware of the monotonous new communities, the clusters of little pastel houses, which have mushroomed up overnight within a thirty-mile radius of most American cities. Have they been planned with forethought or simply with a rich profit in mind?" Robert Moses answered in "Build and Be Damned." New York's "master builder" recognized the city's problems and hoped that "In the suburbs and near-by country, we still have a chance to do the right thing without stultifying compromise." The parks advocate noted "what was once a pleasant bit of nature has been ruthlessly leveled and ripped up to make a subdivider's holiday." "A community must have leadership and conscience to resist the ruthless modern developer," he advised. Few have. *The Atlantic Monthly* later called Moses the "Godfather of Sprawl" because his parkways had contributed to Long Island development, but Moses had been disappointed in the Levittown-style of suburban development. He had not anticipated induced demand for parkways conceived for weekend leisure driving, not commuting.

Lewis Mumford once quipped that our national flower is the concrete cloverleaf, and in 1953's *The Highways and the City* he observed: "In using the car to flee from the metropolis the motorist finds that he has merely transferred congestion to the highway and thereby doubled it. When he reaches his destination, in a distant suburb, he finds that the countryside he sought has disappeared: beyond him, thanks to the motorway, lies only another suburb, just as dull as his own." Motorists kept moving outward for 50 long years. Dullness won. Sprawl developers became unstoppable. Suburbs became blandburbs. Suburbanites became victims in a sprawl social phantasy system.

A healthy mental state results when people feel that they have control and mastery over their lives. But residents routinely trapped in sprawl and traffic are likely to feel helpless and victimized. They will focus more on private home and car space where they have more control, but be more alienated from the public and community realm. Could rising rates of divorce, depression, alcoholism and drug abuse be related to sprawl-caused despair? It seems plausible. Depression has been showing the largest increase. Between 1987 and 1997, the percentage of Americans being treated for depression more than tripled. Antidepressants have become the second largest class of prescription drugs at nearly 140 million prescriptions annually, one for every two Americans. One explanation is widespread anger about quality of life impacts from sprawl, like loss of free and family time and suffering in traffic, because depression is anger turned inward. It turns inward because people see no solution and their own decisions condemn them to the sprawl's pseudo-realities.

Think blandness and stress.

I have formulated a three-stage model for understanding the ill effects of the sprawl lifestyle; like all models, it simplifies reality. First, Suburban Blandness Syndrome results from the overall character of the sprawl built environment, namely its bland and boring uniformity. Second, Sprawl Stress Syndrome results from the regular stressful impacts of automobile dependency and a built environment that is psychologically oppressive. Third, Sedentary Death Syndrome covers the ultimate physiological consequences of a sedentary lifestyle over extended time. Recall that figure of 365,000 premature deaths from physical inactivity and poor diet.

Sprawl infects. In blandburbs people undergo suburbanization of the mind that makes *them* bland and boring. Instead of rejecting the sprawl environment, people adapt and unconsciously become like it. Mental energy and vitality are drained by bland, boring and barren residential and commercial surroundings, especially in the absence of regular physical activity. This is Suburban Blandness Syndrome – the silent suffering of people dulled by their dull surroundings. Think of it as the complete opposite of being energized and spiritually uplifted in the presence of great architecture or beauty. Americans have freedom in a prison of blandness. When critics condemn a film, a restaurant or just about anything they invoke blandness. *Blandness is a root cause of human disappointment, pain and suffering.* And it is preventable. The smart growth movement is also an anti-blandness movement. If blandness was a crime against humanity, sprawl developers and builders would be serving life sentences. Blandness *is* a crime, but bears no penalty in the sprawl culture. Hence, we have a blandness-for-profit sprawl economy. Banality sells because it is marketed so relentlessly.

The award-winning film *American Beauty* captured the complex feelings of isolation, ennui, depression and rebelliousness among affluent sprawl residents. As one reviewer said, the film captured the "dark underbelly of suburban madness." The film portrayed life in blandland without ever explicitly referring to sprawl, without ridiculing it. It just showed life in it, including a scene where a teenager is shocked when two friends decide to *walk* home from school. She says incredulously: "That's like almost a mile!"

The film shows sprawl's suffocating blandness eating away spirit, creating vacant minds and expressions. It is the real America where products are branded, places are blanded and minds are stranded. Pressures inside the heads of characters are disturbingly palpable. Something is killing them as reflected in the film's opening, with Lester Burnham saying "in a year I'll be dead... But in a way I'm dead already." Personal isolation is the result of withdrawal from the bland public realm, the natural environment and social networks, explaining wife Jane Burnham's life lesson: "You can't count on anyone except yourself." Combine personal isolation with bland and boring surroundings and you make boring people. In the film, teenager Ricky's cruel curse to cheerleader Angela is "you're boring and totally ordinary." It works. She is shaken by the insult.

Despite its dark themes, *American Beauty* may have been such a commercial success because people could relate to the suffering of Lester Burnham, who feels empty, exhausted and "dead already," and to his wife who is lonely and untrusting. Viewers could see the downside of sprawl living, the existential embarrassment, eroding meaning of life, self-confidence and dignity. They could feel the pain of privacy escalating to reclusive anonymity, loss of identity, social atomization and anomie. The screen characters were bored and boring; each expressing their feelings of angry rebelliousness and desire to escape. Lester escaped to marijuana, his wife to infidelity, and his daughter and boyfriend to somewhere else.

Chronic blandness produces chronic stress that leads to chronic disease. Immersion in blandness causes negative brooding and a yearning for self-transformation, individuality and distinction. Discomfit and unhappiness become chronic stress, physical and mental. Suburban Stress Syndrome is a painful mental state of automobile addiction, constant time-crunches, too little physical activity and poor nutrition. Not everyone succumbs but many do, especially children. Life can never be stress-free, but a better designed built environment can help. And that help is needed right now because more than half of U.S. adults say they experience high levels of stress on a daily basis, according to CNN. This is consistent with a study of mental illness in 14 nations in the *Journal of the American Medical Association* that found the United States has the highest level at 26.4 percent of adults, consistent with a 2004 Harris poll that found 27 percent of adults received mental health treatment in the past two years. Our sprawl-savaged society has half of adults stressed out daily, a quarter mentally ill, and two-thirds overweight or obese! Sounds like sprawl pseudo-reality that only the pseudo-sane can accept.

Privacy and materialism have not worked. Rather than turn outward to people and civic engagement to offset boredom and stress, people desperate for self-fulfillment, self-identity and meaning turn inward. Meaning is sought through piercings, tattoos, and cosmetic surgery. Rather than active living, health is sought through stomach stapling to fight obesity and psychoactive drugs. Violence is also common. Children go on tire slashing rampages and throw rocks from overpasses onto speeding cars, perhaps to show their hatred of cars and drivers.

Most extreme is killing and escape by suicide. Ironically, several months before *American Beauty* was released, the movie's darker sprawl culture messages were presaged by the Columbine High School shootings in Colorado. Amidst speculation on what factors drove the student killers to commit their crime, Christopher Caldwell added suburban layout in "Levittown to Littleton," in the *National Review*, May, 1999. He theorized that suburban children grow up in "almost hermetic seclusion – a newer and more soul-destroying condition," as compared to just the physical monotony of Levittown, considered the birthplace of sprawl. He argued that there is an "infantile seclusion" in un-places that leads to "kids building the wildest fantasies in their interminable solitude, with the help of their computers, their televisions, and their stereos." With children spending 70 percent of their trips in the back seats of vehicles, they have so much time to fantasize about a more exciting and satisfying life. But when they reach adolescence in suburban sprawl with boring lives, they seek escape from blandness.

Choosing suburban sprawl for the sake of children is incorrect thinking. Affluence aside, *all sprawl parents* need to rid themselves of the delusion that suburbs are better for their children than city schools. They are virtually the same with regard to sex, drugs, violence and delinquency, according to a 2004 report from the Manhattan Institute using data from the National Longitudinal Study of Adolescent Health. Statistics for suburban students in grades 9 through 12 are chilling (urban data in parentheses): nearly 20 (13) percent of high school seniors had driven while high on drugs and 22 (16) percent while drunk; nearly 30 (34) percent of all students had been in a serious physical fight, 22 (26) percent had stolen something from a store, 18 (16) percent had damaged other people's property in the past 12 months, 9 percent (10) had run away from home, 10 (8) percent had sold drugs, and 8 (10) percent had painted graffiti in the past 12 months. Blandland is no nirvana.

The Columbine High tragedy seemed to reflect severely disturbed teenage lives. There could come a day when the American Psychiatric Association legitimizes sprawl-induced mental illness and lawyers use it as a defense for suburban kids shooting other kids in schools or for committing vehicular homicide.

AUTOMOBILE ADDICTION IS UNHEALTHY.

Larry Klimovitz gets up at 4:20 a.m. so he can beat the heaviest traffic. "It makes the commute a lot less stressful," he said. Dee Strausser awakes at 3 a.m. because "Dealing with the traffic and then dealing with the stress of my job, I don't think I could do it." Whether their jobs are in another suburb or downtown, Americans everywhere are hitting the road earlier and earlier, trying to reduce car stress. Soon they find that hordes of other commuters are doing likewise, making it less and less effective. So they get up 15 minutes earlier, than 30 minutes, then... Day jobs are becoming night jobs. Hard to think that this makes family life better, especially if early risers cannot leave work a lot earlier, and even if they do, odds are the roads will be congested. Some people believe that Starbucks' coffee success is its high caffeine levels.

Sprawl Stress Syndrome has much to do with heavy car use and constant traffic congestion, especially on weekends. Car stress results in elevated levels of blood glucose and cholesterol, and a decline in coagulation time (cardiovascular disease factors) for times in traffic as little as 15 minutes. Prolonged commuting stress suppresses the immune function and shortens longevity. A study of 600 nurses found that those commuting by car exhibited much higher stress levels than those using mass transit when commute times were equal. Daily traffic congestion makes drivers frustrated, angry, panicky, impatient, irritated, careless, exhausted and depressed. Not exactly what is portrayed in television commercials for automobiles. Stressed-out drivers put themselves at risk when they make frantic lane changes without signaling, tailgate, use the shoulder, block other drivers from passing them, flash their head lights, run red lights and stop signs, harass bicyclists, show no deference to pedestrians, swerve outside their lanes, eat and drink and hit their horns with alacrity. Car horns have become like an animal's territorial scream or bark.

Drivers feel at risk from other drivers, as they should. Drivers are the natural enemies of other drivers. Drivers inevitably hate other drivers. Drivers are not friendly neighbors. Drivers compete with other drivers for space, speed, and time. Neighborhood walkers talk to other walkers, even if only with a friendly hello. Drivers fear other drivers, because they have weapons of destruction – their cars. Survival of the fittest principle causes alienated and angry automobile addicts to defeat car opponents. Sprawl savages.

Road rage is a symptom of frequent intense car stress. A survey found that 51 percent of Americans had another driver make an obscene gesture at them and 28 percent had another driver make a threatening move at them. A survey of Salt Lake City drivers found that 12 percent of men and 18 percent of women agreed that "At times I felt that I could gladly kill another driver." Imagine what levels might exist for cities like Atlanta and Los Angeles. Pedestrians as well as drivers tick motorists off at their peril. From 1990 to 1996, there was a 51 percent increase in the rate of events in which an angry or impatient driver tried to kill or injure another driver after a traffic dispute. In 1996, there were 10,000 reported incidents, 12,610 injuries, and 218 deaths associated with road disputes. The more you drive in heavy traffic the higher your risk of a road rage encounter.

Car stress does not end with leaving traffic. April Crispo of Deer Park, Long Island walks to nearby shops because "I don't have to be stressed with finding a parking spot." A study found that drivers take 21 percent longer to leave a parking space if another driver wants it and 33 percent longer if that driver honks. Car-space competitors treat each other badly.

Being addicted to something both harmful and plentiful is dreadful. Cars are as bad as cigarettes and alcohol in that respect. The number of family cars keeps increasing, which is why so many sprawl homes now have three-car garages that consume even more land. Sprawl home garages are getting bigger than the typical living or family room. And each vehicle puts more mileage on each year. At any given time, several family members may each be driving in their own cars, seven days a week. Each "car potato" may be stuck in traffic, but they can talk to each other on their cell phones. Car misery loves company. Sprawl residents oscillate between social isolation in their homes and vehicles. As much as sprawl stresses the natural environment, sprawl residents stress themselves with their automobile addiction. Keep in mind that sedentariness means the absence of physical activity that produces brain chemicals like serotonin that raise spirits and neuropeptides that counteract the body's stress response. For many people, depression and anxiety lead to a downward spiral into gluttony and sloth.

For sprawl living with painful car dependency also think post-traumatic stress. For many years Professor Raymond W. Novaco at the University of California, Irvine, has been studying the physical and psychological impacts of traffic gridlock. He has shown that the traffic experience reduces tolerance for frustration, reduces cognitive ability, and kills the post-commute mood at home. A negative mood can consist of tension, nervousness, impatience, and irritability. All this happens regardless of a commuter's income, age, education, or job satisfaction. This is serious sprawl lifestyle stress. Is a negative frame of mind supportive of quality family time or interest in physical activity? Not likely. Sounds more like couch potato stimulation. Traffic woes and sprawl stress may explain why, on average, adult men watch television about 29 hours a week and adult women some 34 hours a week. Internet surfing time is just as sedentary.

Here is a logical anti-sprawl idea. Pay-as-you-drive insurance (PAYD) means your mileage determines your insurance premium. Todd Litman of the Victoria Transport Policy Institute estimates that PAYD would cut driving by about 10 percent and crashes by 12 to 15 percent. Testing of this insurance method in Texas found that drivers saved an average of 25 percent, with some getting a 50 percent cut. Nationally, this approach could save Americans some $8 billion annually on insurance plus congestion-related savings of $9 billion, according to University of California, Berkeley Professor Aaron Edlin. High mileage drivers would pay more, possibly several times more, providing a disincentive for high auto use.

Face car facts. Vehicular stress is the pavlovian reaction to involuntary automobile addiction. In unhealthy un-places peoples' health worsens as they move through three stages: Suburban Blandness Syndrome, Sprawl Stress Syndrome and Sedentary Death Syndrome. First you become bored and boring, then psychologically unhinged and stressed out – both causing you to eat more than you should – and finally your bloated body fails. At the end of the suburban sedentary rainbow, you find a pot belly, not a pot of gold. Affected are millions of children and adults. To the rescue come alcohol, illegal drugs, and the pharmaceutical-physician alliance offering an expanding menu of pills for a growing GNP – our Gross National Pharmacy. After all, the sprawl culture is the culture of consumption, not prevention. For prevention, choose a HEALTHY PLACE.

CHRONIC SPRAWL STRESS CAUSES FOOD CRAVINGS.

"You have stress in life, and food is the one thing they can't take away from you," so said Marie Pomerlee, age 35, 5 feet 5, and weighing more than 300 pounds. Every evening millions of stressed-out couch potatoes get biological emails telling them to munch the worst kinds of foods. They respond involuntarily, like a shark to blood.

Sprawl stress is not just plain or acute stress that comes and goes in unusual situations, but is *chronic* stress. Chronic sprawl lifestyle stress results from a steady stream of frustrations and heartaches over long periods, like daily stress from driving in heavy traffic and never having enough time. As reported in September 2003, researchers at the University of California, San Francisco identified a biochemical feedback system that explains why people with chronic stress have a physiological motivation to eat lots of the worst kinds of food. Chronically elevated adrenal hormones create a biologically driven desire to eat high fat and carbohydrate foods, so called "comfort foods." The body's response reduces the stress-causing chemicals and you feel better. But this habitual self-medication backfires, because it leads to weight gain or obesity and an array of diseases. The situation is particularly disastrous because stress hormones like cortisol activate fat receptors in the abdomen and belly, where fat deposits accumulate. One of the researchers said that the middle-aged man or woman with a gut or pot belly has a body type that "represents the classic distribution of fat from stress." The blandburb choice is between short term stress relief or longer term disease and death. Also note that Duke University researchers have shown that the cumulative effect of repeated stress is to reduce the heart's ability to respond appropriately to the outside world.

So we come full circle as Sprawl Stress Syndrome causes the worst kind of excessive mid-section weight associated with the deadly metabolic syndrome, as described previously. This gives new meaning to "death by chocolate." Routine cravings for goodies loaded with fat and sugar are the body's way of addressing chronic sprawl stress. Exiting the road to get a fast food fat-fix answers nature's message that there is too much stress in your life. Perhaps McDonald's and other chains will claim that they are really providing a public service by providing anti-stress foods. Become stressed, find junk food, and get back on the road. Nearly 40 percent of spending on meals is for eating outside the home, which tends to be the unhealthiest type of eating. Fast food consumption has increased five-fold since 1970; in 1972 Americans spent $3 billion on fast food, which jumped to $110 billion in 2003. More sprawl, more driving, more stress, and more fast food.

Back in the home cocoon, sedentary people with Sprawl Stress Syndrome miss out on the stress-reduction benefits of regular physical activity. Watching television and computer screens and eating the worst kinds of food because of stress cravings leads to involuntary gluttony. Blame blandburb's bad geographic genes, not yours. Perversely, dieting creates more chronic stress and even more compulsion to eat comfort foods. This is why dieting by itself is notoriously ineffective but works better with physical activity. Younger people with stress may succumb to eating disorders such as anorexia and bulimia. Many consumers seek surgery to lose weight or buy exercise machines that either will not be used or will not work. Sprawl stress is good for business. And if obesity is officially declared a disease, the health care and pharmaceutical industries will have a bonanza, and health insurance costs will explode. Worse, the sprawl industry will escape responsibility for unhealthy community design.

So now you know how sprawl's two deadly sins of sloth and gluttony arise and what leads to Sedentary Death Syndrome. Mix automobile dependency and sedentariness with sprawl stress and you get chronic physical inactivity and gluttony. Sprawl is guilty beyond a reasonable doubt. Want to reduce your sedentariness, stress and unhealthy eating? Want a decent chance to win your battle of the bulge? Be active in a HEALTHY PLACE.

CONSUMERS WANT GREENSPACE.

"Nearby nature is positive even if you don't use it; if it's something you know is there, as kind of an escape, you feel better," so concluded Ohio State University Professor Jack Nasar. But seeing nature is even better. A University of Michigan study found that residents prefer a smaller home with a view of the woods over a large home with a manicured lawn. Professor Stephen Kaplan said the survey of residents in 18 subdivisions, some sprawl and some using compact design, showed "that the myth that big homes on big lots are what is most important to people and therefore everything that happens is market driven is wrong." Counting lawns as "open space" is misleading because "a lawn is not a natural feature," said Kaplan. Not all greenspace is equal.

The noted Harvard naturalist Edward O. Wilson coined the term "biophilia" to describe the innate human tendency to be drawn to nature and feel an affinity, love and craving for it. One piece of evidence for this is that more Americans attend zoos every year than attend all professional sporting events combined.

Green is the color of physical activity. Health benefits of living in HEALTHY PLACES result from lots of usable greenspace and easy access to parks and trails. "Green infrastructure" also provides public places to simply rest, feel peaceful, enjoy nature, and reduce stress. Parks of all kinds are important casual gathering places for families and residents, where conversations do not require consumption, as in a bar or restaurant. Greenspace contributes to building social capital. Parks deserve more credit for improving quality of life, improving mental and physical health, spurring community pride, creating memorable experiences, and imparting place personality.

Research has shown that contact with nature improves cognitive functions, reduces mental fatigue, reduces pain, hastens healing, and improves feelings of satisfaction and well-being. Research at Cornell University found that greenness around homes correlated with improved cognitive functioning and attention capacity in children. The greener a child's play area, the less severe their attention problem. At the University of Illinois, they found that when people living in low-income housing projects in Chicago overlooked a small slice of nature – such as a few mature trees and a patch of grass – they reported feeling significantly healthier, more productive, less aggressive, less violent, friendlier and more neighborly than residents facing alleys and concrete. They also performed better on tests of cognitive function. People were found to gather more in public spaces with trees than in ones without trees. Research at Ohio State University found that driving in scenic, nature-lined streets has a calming effect as compared to commutes on roads with fewer cars but in a sprawl area with strip malls. In a Pennsylvania hospital it was discovered that over ten years gall bladder surgery patients in rooms with tree views had shorter hospitalizations that those in rooms with wall views, as well as less need for pain medications.

On the connection between parks and health, a study of Cleveland Metroparks users age 50 and over found over two-thirds used the parks to obtain moderate or high levels of physical activity, with about half the time spent walking. These users were healthier than sedentary users and non-users; they had fewer physician visits and drank less alcohol.

The popularity of national and state parks attests to greenspace value. Sadly, Americans may have lawns, passive greenspace, but not usable greenspace. Sprawl subdivisions may be surrounded by as yet undeveloped farmland or open space, but there are usually no parks and trails immediately available for un-place residents to walk to and enjoy (see Figure 4-1).

Ironically, so many sprawl subdivisions are built on land cleared of all trees, leaving sprawl residents with few if any mature trees. Planting bushes and young trees is no substitute for tree canopy. Also, urban infill development often removes trees indiscriminately. A 2003 study by American Forests concluded that urban metropolitan areas nationwide had lost 21 percent of their tree cover in the past decade. Where there is sprawl-crazy development trees disappear. The Atlanta, Georgia region lost more than 40 percent of its heavy tree cover from 1974 to 1996; the San Diego, California metro area lost 27 percent in less than 20 years. Still more data of the absurd. Trees are important, as shown by a study that found people are more active in parks with tree-lined walking paths as compared to trails in empty open spaces.

Perversely, for millions of un-place residents, getting to a park, sports field, or trail usually means yet another car trip. *The Cincinnati Enquirer* headline in March 2004 was "Sprawl squeezes parkland." The point of the story was that booming sprawl development was gobbling up sports fields and greenspace, depriving children of exactly what they most need, physical activity playing soccer, lacrosse, baseball, softball and field hockey. This was happening not just in the greater Cincinnati area but from coast to coast.

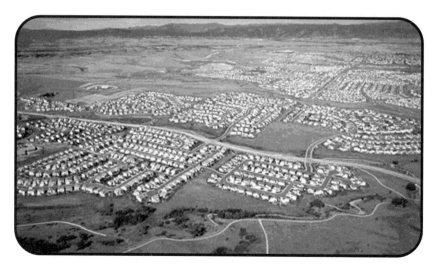

Figure 4-1. A number of sprawl subdivisions eating up open space in Colorado.

When you do get to a park, what you likely find is park parking lot congestion. People deserve parks they can walk to. More parks, not just bigger ones are the answer. Desperate for park play areas, but lacking them near their homes in sprawlspace, many parents take their children by car to playgrounds in fast-food restaurants, like McDonald's and Burger King. How clever of the fast-food industry to take even more advantage of sprawl's shortcomings.

The best HEALTHY PLACES have 20 to 50 percent of the land devoted to various kinds of greenspace, a crucial part of their public realm. Short 5 to 10 minute walks to parks and other green areas in HEALTHY PLACES are critically important. In Fall Creek, Indianapolis all residents in nearly 400 homes are within 4 blocks from a public park. In River Ranch, in Lafayette, Louisiana, there are parks and play areas within a 10-minute walk from just about every home.

Consumers know what makes their lives better. They want greenspace. A survey of Atlanta residents found that a whopping 52 percent wanted to be surrounded by woods or fields. Another survey of adults found that 95 percent said being close to a park would make them more physically active, and 48 percent said that enjoyable scenery could do the same. Once people had convenient access to trails, 55 percent increased their regular physical activity, according to another study. Consumers gladly pay more for greenspaces that contribute to quality of life and health. In Denver, 16 percent of residents in 1980 said they would pay more to live near a greenbelt or park; this tripled by 1990 to 48 percent.

Manicured lawns may be sprawl-sacred but they are inferior to public greenspaces. An enormous amount of time, money, water and chemicals are used to maintain "unnatural" lawns. Americans spend over $20 billion annually to keep their lawns green and perfect: weed-free, bug-free, and neatly cut. Add another $1.6 billion for fences around their yards. Note that a single lawnmower can spew as much air pollution in a year as driving a new car more than 80,000 miles. Large lawns can soak up more than 50,000 gallons of water annually. New homes in the Las Vegas, Nevada area cannot have grass lawns because of water concerns. Homeowners associations often mandate well-manicured grass lawns. This makes it difficult for residents to replace grass with other forms of land cover that require little maintenance and water - xeriscaping.

Are lawns worth all of this? Passive lawns offer none of the health and social benefits of community parks, greenways, forested areas, and rich natural habitats. Lawns are a sprawl culture fashion and perhaps an addiction. Worst of all, many home owners no longer get the physical activity and health benefits of mowing lawns. Once, sprawl residents were dying to escape the hard work of mowing their lawns. Now, they are dying because they are *not* mowing their lawns. Lawn service companies replace personal exertion or ride-on and self-propelled mowers minimize the effort.

Larger homes on larger lots exacerbate lawn lunacy. Suburban lawns consume 20 million acres, more land than used for any single commercial crop, including corn and wheat. That land could provide housing for more than 200 million people, with compact land use. In HEALTHY PLACES residents may still have lawns, but they will be small enough to use an old-fashioned non-motorized, push rotary lawn mower. You will work up a healthy sweat and maybe talk to a neighbor or a passerby on the sidewalk. And you will save money.

Lawns and other passive greenspaces are like gift wrapping around a package you receive from the developer of a blandburb named something like Old Oak Tree Acres, received just after you move into your big home. Inside, you find three discount coupons, one for a super-size meal at McDonald's, one for new automobile tires, and one for a riding mower. Your ample stomach tightens up as you think "Is there a message here?"

Passive greenspace or usable greenspace for active living - you should have the choice.

HIGH AUTOMOBILE RISKS IN SUBURBIA.

Cars are lethal. Over 2.5 *million* people have died violent deaths on American highways, more than four times those killed in World War I, World War II, Korea and Vietnam *combined*. The automobile easily qualifies as a product of mass destruction.

All those television commercials showing happy and successful people driving shiny new cars in beautiful places without traffic congestion divert attention away from some very ugly facts. Over 42,000 people are being killed annually in auto accidents, plus over 3 million injuries annually with costs of some $200 billion annually. That amounts to one death every 13 minutes and an injury every 11 seconds. Some 90 *million* Americans have sustained disabling injuries in auto accidents, which are the leading cause of crippling brain and spinal cord injuries.

The enormous national psychic trauma over the terrorist-caused airplane crashes and all the people killed on the ground on September 11, 2001 was well founded. But all those deaths equate to less than six weeks of auto accident deaths. The national auto accident death rate is like a large fully loaded passenger jet crashing every 3 days, week after week, year after year. Know this. Reducing your driving is one way to reduce a substantial personal risk.

With automobile dependency, living in sprawl means a higher risk of accidents. The automobile fatality rate in Atlanta in 1998 was over five times greater than in New York City, and twice as great as in Portland, Oregon. Correspondingly, the average daily per person vehicle miles traveled in 1999 was 35.3 in Atlanta versus 15.9 in New York City and 19.8 in Portland with higher levels of walking and transit use.

What makes an area safe? University of Virginia Professor William H. Lucy made national headlines when he revealed data showing that suburbs were more dangerous than cities. In fact, the lower the population density, the more dangerous they are. For example, consider Baltimore versus Queen Anne's county in Maryland. The city has a population density about 80 times greater than the suburban county, but the county has a rate of traffic fatalities about four times greater than the city. Suburban sprawl's high vehicle use correlates with high rates of fatalities in auto accidents, often in single vehicle accidents. Too much driving is on older two-lane roads that were not designed for the heavy traffic resulting from large sprawl subdivisions built in once rural areas. Sprawl stress causes people to drive too fast on them. About three-quarters of traffic fatalities occur on two-lane roads, and accidents on them are eight times greater than on Interstates.

In the real America, violent deaths in suburban car accidents are much more likely for sprawl residents than being murdered by a stranger. Traffic deaths are more than ten times the number of homicides by strangers annually in the United States. But in specific low density sprawl communities, the ratio can be more like a 100 times greater for vehicle crashes. Sprawl mothers gloating about safe suburbs should know that adolescent males in the suburbs die in auto accidents at the same rate as their counterparts die of gunshot incidents in cities. The homicide advantage for suburbs is overshadowed by a much higher rate of vehicle fatalities.

Rupert Farley, a resident in Fredericksburg, Virginia, wrote about teen-driver deaths: "The real villains are certain developers, auto dealers, road builders, and others who have lobbied so successfully for decades to force us to continue subsidizing sprawl at the expense of 'smart growth' neighborhoods. …Until we hold our lawmakers accountable and insist on smart growth legislation…the villains and their political bedmates will continue to walk away with full pockets while we continue to bury the casualties." Actually, they drive away in big SUVs. And in Kansas, because of high rates of deaths in traffic accidents on county roads, the *Winfield Daily Courier* ran an editorial that said "Unfortunately, the urban sprawl has far outpaced our capacity—and will—to accommodate it." Conversely, living in a HEALTHY PLACE reduces vehicle use and its associated risks. In fact, research using data on 448 counties found that car and pedestrian fatality rates were lower in more compact designed communities than in sprawl un-places. Blandburbs lack a "pedestrian culture."

Sprawl is pedestrian, as in dull, and pedestrian-unfriendly, as in dangerous.

Walking must be safe. In the past 25 years some 175,000 pedestrians have been killed on America's roadways. Though Americans make less than 5 percent of their trips on foot, 12 percent of all traffic fatalities are pedestrians, and some 60 percent of those deaths occur in places where no crosswalk is available. Now, about 5,000 pedestrians are killed yearly, and about half of fatal car-pedestrian accidents happen on local neighborhood streets. Sunbelt areas with high growth rates are the most dangerous for pedestrians.

Though few students walk to school, in 1999 nearly 900 children ages 14 and under were killed and 25,000 injured in pedestrian accidents with vehicles. Each year about 175 children are killed by vehicles in between school and home. There is also bad news at the other end of the age spectrum. The highest rate of pedestrian fatalities is for Americans age 70 and over. Walkers are dashing to death trying to move through gaps in traffic on streets designed for fast cars, not slow pedestrians. Pedestrians cannot compete with heavy vehicle traffic and frustrated, harried drivers. Automobile apartheid puts pedestrians at a disadvantage. Transportation engineers and departments serve drivers, not walkers or bikers. What they do for drivers makes it more dangerous for those not driving cars.

Consider this insanity. In early 2003 Georgia's Department of Transportation disclosed it was against having trees between sidewalks and streets, because sidewalks are "auto recovery zones." Sidewalks are to help inattentive, incompetent or intoxicated drivers regain control of their vehicles when they veer off roads. Trees might cause injuries to drivers. The Department believed the odds were low that cars would hit pedestrians. It discounted how value tree-shaded streets increase walkability, how trees provide more safety to pedestrians and are good for the environment. The Commissioner said: "the protection of intermittent foot traffic should not come at the expense of a motorist's life." Apparently, air bags and seat belts are not good enough. What better proof of automobile apartheid than this cockeyed reasoning.

Atlanta's pedestrian fatality rate *increased* 13 percent from 1994 to 1998, while the national rate *decreased* by 9.6 percent. Atlanta's 1998 rate was over twice that in Portland, Oregon, New York City, and Philadelphia, perhaps because Atlanta drivers see fewer pedestrians. Automobile apartheid also has a social justice dimension. The Atlanta rate was 4 per 100,000 for African-Americans, 10 for Hispanics and less than 2 for Caucasians.

Here is more car madness. The traffic studies chief of Prince George's County, Maryland said: "The street should be strictly for cars." Surely it is time to reclaim our streets for our children and for us. Adults have cherished childhood memories about playing in neighborhood streets. Now it is becoming illegal for kids to play in streets, illustrating automobile apartheid's stranglehold on American society. Nearly all prohibitions against street playing are in sprawl suburbs. Streets must be reclaimed for playing. Slowing down cars should be the priority.

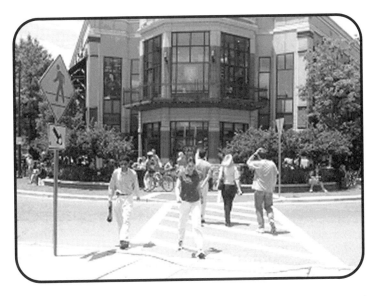

Figure 4-2. A well designed and marked street crossing gives pedestrians a feeling of safety.

Research at the University of California, Irvine found that around schools with safer walking environments, meaning fewer and slower vehicles, the number of pedestrians was about 5 to 10 times higher than around schools with less safe vehicle traffic, showing that people know and prefer safer street environments.

Consider that 25 percent of all trips are less than one mile in the current sprawl-dominant built environment, but that 75 percent of these are by automobile. This 75 percent defines an enormous opportunity for walking and biking, not for recreation, but to serve some mobility need to reach a nearby destination. The fraction of adults who walked to work decreased by 26 percent between 1990 and 2000, just ten years! More data of the absurd. At the same time the fraction of obese or overweight adults jumped more than 60 percent. Living in HEALTHY PLACES means having safe routes to walk or bike for a high fraction of short distance trips. Pedestrian safety is addressed through traffic calming measures and better street design, as discussed in Chapter 6, which help people to be physically active (see Figure 4-2).

Imagine walking more, a lot more.

THE SEGWAY IS UNNEEDED TECHNOLOGY.

Stay alert on sidewalks. A dangerous vehicle may be rolling toward you, the one shown in photographs of President George W. Bush tumbling head-first in June 2003. The Commander-in-Chief forgot to turn the foolproof machine on.

Riders stand between the two wheels and grip the handle. The motorized scooter contraption rolls along at several times the speed of walking. But where do you roll along? Sidewalks, say the Segway company, not even bike lanes, perhaps because there are not enough bike lanes. So, with a maximum speed of 12.5 miles per hours and a weight of 80 pounds, it is too slow to compete (and lose) against heavier and faster automobiles, but it is fast enough to compete (and win) against pedestrians. The Segway is marketed as a "segue" between a walking person and a car. Like sedentary Americans really need yet another unhealthy technological innovation.

Statements by Dean Kamen, the inventor of the device, show the goal of making walking obsolete: "When you stand on this machine it kind of walks for you." Better yet, a walk that "used to take you half an hour will take you 7, 8, 9 minutes." At one point he said the product "is an improvement on walking," and another time called it "the biggest improvement on walking since the sandal." Company officials said: "We designed the Segway HT to belong on the sidewalk amongst other pedestrians." *Other* pedestrians! The company had the audacity to call users "empowered pedestrians." Let's call this product the "Sedway" to remind us that it promotes sedentariness; if it reduces walking it will not be unforeseen or unintended.

What should rankle people is the considerable money spent lobbying state governments that have made it legal to use the Sedway on sidewalks, despite it being a motor vehicle. The Sedway is a public safety threat because it can crash into pedestrians and cause serious injuries. The amount of energy expended in a crash would be some 25 times greater than being struck by another walker. San Francisco had the good sense to ban Sedways from city sidewalks, one of the few governments to do so. But in November 2003 a 3-year-old girl was run down and injured by a Sedway on a San Francisco sidewalk, and the culprit sped away. Hitting blind walkers is an issue. "We're not disappointed it hasn't caught on," said Melanie Brunson, head of the American Council of the Blind. The Sedway has been banned from Disneyland, Disney World, California Adventure, and Sea World Orlando.

God help us if the Sedway lobby joins up with the sprawl lobby. Keep your three car garages for your SUVs and still have room for a Sedway. Own a McMansion? Hop on your Sedway to move around your cavernous indoor sprawl space. Sound absurd? Dean Kamen does this in his 32,000 square-foot mansion where he also has a Hummer, a Porsche, and two helicopters, one of which he uses to commute to work. He also has a pulley system that can bring a bottle of wine from the kitchen to the bedroom. Talk about sedentary-enhancing technology.

Here are some comments on this innovation:

Bill Wilkinson, of the Pedestrian and Bicycle Information Center: "This isn't competition for the sidewalks; this is an invasion."

Zac Wald, of California Walks: "Segway has put the pedestrian on the defensive. Many advocates see the Segway as the SUV of the sidewalks."

Matt Smith wrote "Showing Segway the Highway" in *SF Weekly*: "Buckets of lard. Fat, rosy cheeks. Ample alabaster bellies. Arms that flap, legs that waddle, bodies by the million shaking like bowls of jelly. In these terms, I believe, the Segway is a national threat at least as grave as Iraq. It's a high-technology lard-making device introduced at a moment when America is suffocating from obesity. Calculated in potential casualties on the field, the Segway is the ultimate American doomsday machine."

For active living, the Sedway is a step in the wrong direction. The Sedway is a solution looking for a problem. In public talks Kamen has said "We have a culture that's obsessed with nonsense." And some of it is high-tech.

SPRAWL RESIDENTS FACE RISKS INSIDE THEIR HOMES.

"If you bought a $500,000 home in the county and fire and emergency response time was double or triple what it was supposed to be, wouldn't you want to know that?" asked Donna Hathaway Beck, a resident in Prince George's County, Maryland. Sprawl development was ahead of basic county services. Twenty-one developments had been approved even though ambulances or paramedics could not meet emergency response time standards. She noted that developers "are walking away with millions in their pockets, while we're playing bingo to buy fire trucks."

Think danger – it is another dimension to the sprawl-health nexus. Consider this scenario: You made it home, after another long, tough commute and a particularly rough day at work. You are cocooned in your spacious sprawl home. But you are alone. You grab a bag of snack comfort food, hit the couch and click the TV remote. Then you feel ill. The needle on the Sedentary Death Syndrome dial is in the red zone. The signs of a possible heart attack are clear. You realize that emergency help is needed. You call 911 on your GPS enabled cell phone.

You wait.

And you wait.

If you are in a new sprawl subdivision, you may be waiting longer than you hoped, because the nearest facility with emergency service may be far way, and dangerous unpaved or poorly paved roads with heavy traffic can greatly slow down emergency vehicles.

Research by Northern Illinois University on response times for emergency medical services (EMS) found that both average and median times are significantly longer for new sprawl developments, as compared to older communities, either older, close-in suburbs or cities. The recommended EMS maximum response time is 4 to 6 minutes. But the average time for the new sprawl subdivision was 9.6 minutes. According to the American Heart Association, after a heart attack, every minute that goes by without restoring the normal heartbeat reduces chances of survival by

10 percent. Those extra minutes could reduce the chance of survival by some 50 percent. Call it the sprawl life reduction factor.

The increase of as much as 50 percent for EMS response time was also matched by as much as a 600 percent increase for police response time, and as much as a 33 percent increase in fire response time, according to the research. In sprawl-rich Colorado Springs, Colorado average police response time rose from 9 to 12 minutes from growth in the 1990s, and some types of situations were no longer responded to, as reported in 2001.

And when you find yourself alone at home when a crisis hits, you may not have a close-by, friendly neighbor to help you out – unless you live in a real community where neighbors take care of neighbors. This is even more important for people living alone, especially for older people who cannot afford constant home care or assisted living. Aging in place does not make sense in sprawl isolation.

Unchecked sprawl development in Roanoke County, Virginia prompted county fire and rescue officials to say that they would "rarely, if ever" be able to respond to emergency calls in a new project within their goal of six minutes. A local developer said "You can't answer every emergency." Imagine saying that to prospective homebuyers. Rapid growth in and around Orlando, Florida has caused increase response times from fire rescue stations; newer subdivisions can wait twice as long for firefighters to show up. Joseph Meinert, planning director for Bowie, Maryland asked: "Why would somebody buy a home in a development where the roads are inadequate, the schools are inadequate, and nobody will be able to get there in an emergency? But I guess people think that the government is looking out for that." Au contraire, if sprawl interests have corrupted government.

Some new sprawl residents receive a nasty night-time surprise, their house shakes. Loud, low flying military aircraft or thunderous explosions from firing and training ranges shake sprawlspace. Developers are not hesitating to use land dangerously near military bases and airfields. Often there is no legal requirement to disclose the proximity to such installations and the impacts on residents. There are some compatible land uses near military bases, but not residential housing and schools that put people in harm's way, particularly from airplane crashes.

Unsafe sprawl is unhealthy. Does it make sense to trade safety for private space?

SPRAWL LOCATIONS CAN BE DANGEROUS.

Living in nature is not the same thing as living *with* nature. In a Maryland suburban area 100 Canada geese were gased with carbon monoxide in a van because some residents complained about their droppings and blocking of traffic. When sprawl invades natural habitats residents also face dangerous animals, such as alligators in Florida. Citizen complaints against alligators rose from 4,914 in 1978 to 14,738 in 2001; since 1948 there have been 325 attacks on people with 13 killed. The problem is sprawl subdivisions built close to water bodies. In many other regions, black bear, coyotes, and mountain lions are roaming around homes. Does this surprise sprawl shills who say we have only developed such a tiny fraction of our land?

Sprawl kills deer when it invades their natural habitats. The major deer predator left in America is the motor vehicle. In 2002, drivers killed some 1.8 million deer. Conversely, deer kill more people in this country, about 150 in 1.5 million traffic accidents, than do all commercial airline, train and bus accidents combined in a typical year. Countless injuries to people also result from deer-car collisions, and deer cause over a billion dollars of damage to vehicles yearly.

Suburbanites may joke about rats and cockroaches in inner cities, but blandburbs pushed into natural habitats (especially forests and wetlands) and farmland are receiving their fair share of risks, including exposure to diseases transmitted to humans from animals, sometimes by way of insects, such as Lyme disease and West Nile Virus. Raccoons and other critters may have rabies.

Another threat is the "heat island effect." Blandburbs with a high fraction of paved over land, high traffic, and little greenspace are hotter than more open or rural areas. When tree-shaded surfaces in Atlanta were 85 to 90 degrees, surfaces in direct sun were 127 to 129 degrees. Prolonged periods of high temperatures can cause heat stroke and death, and they inhibit physical activity outdoors or make it risky. HEALTHY PLACES with tree-shaded narrow streets can be 10 degrees cooler in warm weather than a sprawl area. Three large trees around a house can cut air conditioning costs 20 percent or more.

Good design comes to the rescue. The developer of North Richland Hills Town Center, near Dallas, Texas, a 330-acre mixed-use community with 1,700 homes and a large office complex, wanted to promote physical activity of residents. He hired an urban micro-climatologist who came up with these heat-reducing design features: making streets narrower than usual and lining them with trees to form a shade canopy; creating three lakes and fountains to shoot up water for dispersal by winds; using light-colored flat roofs on commercial buildings; and using light-colored concrete instead of asphalt in streets. Summertime temperatures will be at least five degrees cooler than the surrounding area. The developer said: "You can create really gorgeous places, but if people aren't comfortable, you can't expect them to get out there and use it." Residents will also benefit from a 15 to 20 percent reduction in air-conditioning costs.

Sprawl developers often ignore inevitable natural hazards. Here are some examples poor location choices:

+ Houses in coastal areas face risks from hurricanes and flooding.
+ Houses on hillsides or in valleys near mountains face risks of flooding and mudslides from excessive surface water runoff because of paved-over and deforested areas.
+ Houses too close to forested areas place houses in the path of wildfires and wild animals.

Does sprawl kill? Count the ways. HEALTHY PLACES should avoid these risky situations.

THE SPRAWL INDUSTRY IS LIKE THE CIGARETTE INDUSTRY.

It probably was inevitable: a hotel for super-size people. Some savvy businessmen created a 112-room vacation beach resort, south of Cancun, Mexico, designed especially for overweight and obese people. It is a place to rejoice being big. Design amenities include: super-size doors, four-foot wide chaise lounges, wide walkways, reinforced large chairs with no arm rests, reinforced king-size beds, and large shower stalls with railings and seats, but no tubs. Four pools have wide steps instead of typical small aluminum ladders. There are no steps to climb inside the hotel. As an all-inclusive "size-friendly" hotel, food is never far away. Five restaurants serve buffets, with entrees heavy on creams and sauces, and a large selection of desserts. No single bedtime sweets on pillows – guests receive a dish with six mints. Food for thought: How long until a gated set of McMansions are built expressly for obese residents?

A lot of data have been presented in this chapter. Individual statistics are not the point. People will always argue over statistics, and especially whether a correlation between two things really proves that one causes the other. Causality is very, very difficult to prove with scientific certainty. Most things are caused by multiple factors, usually in complex ways. Scientists and lawyers can still argue whether a person's lung cancer was caused by smoking. The larger truth is that cigarette smoking is a major health risk factor for the vast majority of people, as is sprawl.

Some individuals escape the dire effects of smoking. Some people escape the many negative consequences of sprawl living. But most people will benefit from choosing a HEALTHY PLACE. The health warning on packs of cigarettes might just as well be given for blandburbs. The National Association of Home Builders said it "rejects the argument...that the choices people make about where they live can actually cause them to become obese." Like the cigarette industry, the sprawl industry denies responsibility for harming people.

The statistics presented above form a consistent pattern or "gestalt." The pattern of evidence trumps the individual figures. In legal parlance the weight or preponderance of the evidence is compelling. There is a series of sprawl-related epidemics over recent years, including these:

+ An epidemic of physical inactivity.
+ An epidemic of obesity.
+ An epidemic of diabetes.
+ An epidemic of asthma, especially in children.
+ An epidemic of metabolic syndrome.
+ An epidemic of unhealthy social isolation.
+ An epidemic of depression.

This collection of escalating negative trends or "synergism of plagues" is a "syndemic" – the sprawl syndemic that erodes quality of life. But trends are not destiny. Once understood they can trigger reactions, adjustments and changes to move back into positive territory. HEALTHY PLACES are a far better solution than expensive medical interventions and government programs to manage the *symptoms of sprawl*. If Americans can reject cigarette smoking, they can reject sprawl.

Suburbanites must overcome defensiveness and denial. It is difficult to look sprawl in the face and know it for what it is and what it does to people.

Sprawl shills reject the health impacts of sprawl. An article from the libertarian Reason Public Policy Institute was entitled "'Smart Growth Types' Dumb Rhetoric: Linking Suburbs to Obesity Just Another Silly Attempt at Social Engineering." Social engineering is a conservative metaphor for evil big government, except when it supports road building and automobile addiction. Where public health officials see a strategy to promote active living through community design, the "un-Reason" extremists see an attack on individual liberty and coercion. The right-wingers assert that "access to exercise is not the problem" but that individuals lack motivation. They see nothing in community design that is vital to physical activity, despite the massive evidence given previously.

The "suburban myth" is that *all* Americans really want – or should want – sprawl. More conscious understanding of HEALTHY PLACES' benefits – especially health benefits – can dispel this myth and de-program people. Thomas Bray is on the Board of Directors of the Property and Environment Research Center, a right-wing group concerned with property rights by defending sprawl, and a columnist for *The Detroit News*, where he said that if you assert that the public's preference for sprawl is anything other than good thinking, you must believe Americans are stupid, which they are not, or "that evil, immoral forces have conspired to deny them the choices they really want," a view he said "is simply paranoid." Sprawl shills *are* immoral forces.

As in the film *The Matrix,* our sprawl world is an elaborate deception – a social phantasy system – spun not by computers but by an army of developers, builders, and sprawl shills, the sentinels guarding the Sprawl Matrix. Americans must reject sprawl programming and regain personal control. See the truth about the Sprawl Matrix, how super-size meals and super-size homes combine into a lethal combination, how excessive calories combine with sedentariness to sicken and kill children and adults. People should live out of their homes, not just in them.

Imagine being healthier, a lot healthier.

"Here is another piece of impressive evidence of the sprawl-health connection. A 2004 Rand Corporation study of more than 8,600 adult Americans in 38 metropolitan areas reported that the rates of arthritis, asthma, high blood pressure, headache and other physical ailments increased as the degree of sprawl increased. The benefit of living in the least sprawling areas was like adding four years to people's lives. Roland Sturm connected his results with higher car use, less walking, and the resulting increase in obesity that "probably plays an important role in the health effects we observe."

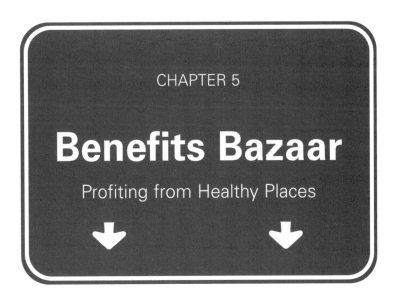

CHAPTER 5

Benefits Bazaar

Profiting from Healthy Places

Sprawl costs.

More personal benefits await those choosing a HEALTHY PLACE. In the previous chapter, the health and safety benefits of HEALTHY PLACES were presented. But considering the underdog status of HEALTHY PLACES, it is important to recognize their other benefits. Three categories are used to systematically present the other benefits: neighborliness, time, and money.

NEIGHBORLINESS. There is no more fundamental goal of HEALTHY PLACES than promoting social interactions and networks among residents. Neighborliness means friendliness, helpfulness, sociability, and cooperation. Too many Americans have already fallen victim to social isolation. They are surrounded by strangers, even after living in a place for years. After 50 years of sprawl, generations of Americans have not experienced real neighborhoods and neighborliness. Do they know the first names of the people living near them? Have they spent time socializing with them in their homes? Do they believe that their neighbors would not hesitate to help out if circumstances placed them in a bad state? Would they offer help to their neighbors? Have *you* experienced this kind of real neighborliness? Abundant privacy has not provided high quality of life and good health, but the desire for "privacy" has displaced neighborliness.

TIME. Our most precious asset is time. Time keeps coming, but like land, retrospectively time is a zero sum game. Using time one way means less of it for something else. *You cannot regain time but you can waste less of it.* Intentionally wasting time doing things that are harmful or just rob us of better, more enjoyable experiences surely is brainless. Sprawl residents waste too much time, sometimes directly and other times indirectly. A long commute is a direct waste of time, and the time after arriving home when one is exhausted is an indirect waste of time. Sprawl-wasted time is all too often seen as a rational tradeoff to obtain some other benefits. Improving quality of life and livability ultimately comes down to how much we prize our time and take charge of making the most of the time we have on Earth. To become time-rich, choose a better built environment and waste less time.

MONEY. Follow the money is great advice. After housing costs, automobiles are typically the biggest expense for people. Housing decisions determine vehicle needs and costs. Yet the interplay between the two is often ignored but is necessary for understanding the financial benefits of HEALTHY PLACES. Sprawl is often "sold" to consumers on the basis of access to low price shopping, like big box stores that tend to follow the march of sprawl into once rural areas. But is saving money on groceries and other consumer items really worth the sprawl lifestyle? Is a cheaper house in a far-away suburb really a better financial decision than a more expensive home closer to work and shopping? Not necessarily.

Together with health and safety benefits, you now have a four-part framework for thinking systematically about the benefits of a true alternative to sprawl. Use it and you will be on your way to better living.

NEIGHBORLINESS IS LEARNED BEHAVIOR.

"I moved to Plano, Texas 3 years ago not knowing a soul. My husband and I bought a house in what looked like a great cozy neighborhood. We lived there for a full 2 years. NO ONE, not one single neighbor welcomed me or even talked to us," so wrote Terri who moved from a small Oregon town. So she moved. "I now have friends and neighbors I can call on if I'm in need."

Odds are you never heard of "collective efficacy." Yet in academic circles it connotes a major paradigm change in understanding the root of crime and violence in America. Harvard Professor Felton Earls has proved that crime and violence are more correlated with collective efficacy than influences of race, income, genetics, family status and structure, and individual temperament. For high collective efficacy you need high community social cohesion and mutual trust among local neighbors. Think of collective efficacy as "effective community," where everybody looks out for everybody else. Neighbors must be willing to intervene on behalf of the common good, even intervening when seeing children of neighbors behaving badly.

University of Chicago Professor Robert Sampson explained that collective efficacy is all about "a shared vision …a fusion of a shared willingness of residents to intervene and social trust, a sense of engagement and ownership of public space." These ideas are totally consistent with HEALTHY PLACES. Conversely, collective efficacy does not ring true for blandburbs where people lead lives of harried self-absorption. For the most part, "sprawl neighborhood" is an oxymoron.

Despite sprawl, some people value a community with social trust which supports high collective efficacy. According to the Social Capital Community Benchmark Survey, in the five communities surveyed having the highest social trust, 52% of residents rated their community as an excellent place to live, the highest possible grade. In the five communities with the lowest levels of social trust, only 31% felt that way.

The causes of low collective efficacy are probably different in urban areas versus suburban ones. For example, the concentrated poverty in inner cities is absent in suburbs. But unwalkable and unsafe streets—the lack of a pedestrian culture—can be the same in neighborhoods in cities and suburbs. Walking that promotes social interactions helps develop that important shared sense of community and trust that is vital for collective efficacy. Recall the dismal data on sex, drugs, violence and delinquency for suburban adolescents given in the previous chapter. Paul A. Jargowsky of the University of Texas at Dallas made some important observations about suburban collective efficacy in 2002:

> Anonymous suburban neighborhoods in which people reside for only a short time before leapfrogging to the next development are also likely to have low levels of collective efficacy, at least relative to well-off neighborhoods from earlier times. In other words, both inner-city and suburban neighborhoods may experience higher levels of crime and violence as a result of rapid and uncontrolled suburbanization. ...The new suburbs form and are then abandoned so rapidly that many lack any sense of community. People do not know their neighbors, don't participate in the civic life of their community, and don't know the parents of their children's playmates. There is a high degree of alienation and a low level of trust. ...Premier suburbs...experience heroin epidemics and strangely elevated rates of teen suicide. ...the shallowness of human relations in cookie-cutter suburban communities is part of the explanation of the wave of school and workplace violence in recent years in seemingly unexpected places. A frequent refrain after such events is 'how could this have happened here?' Suburbanites clearly believe that residence in a prosperous suburb should insulate them from violence, but this hope has proved unfounded.

Welcome to Columbine.

To have neighborliness, residents must want it. But few people explicitly seek it. After decades of social isolation, several generations of Americans no longer remember or understand what true neighborliness is and how it improves life. Besides, if there is no real alternative to social isolation in the marketplace, then people are forced to accept it.

You don't know what you don't know.

You don't want what you don't know.

You don't seek what you don't want.

What you don't seek is competition for the ubiquitous sprawl that is still marketed as the "American dream."

It comes down to this: *You can have lawns to mow or neighbors to know.* You can click your garage opener when leaving and returning home, and stay indoors most of the time in an un-place. Or you can gain more time and have the freedom to stroll around the community, walk briskly on scenic trails, and sit on your front porch or hang out in local public places to meet and greet your neighbors who have become your friends. And you can feel comfortable in intervening if you see children in the neighborhood behaving badly.

There is cause for optimism about rediscovering neighborliness. "People value community and neighborliness. That's something that we've lost in this culture. People want it and miss it," so said the Reverend Patrick Wrisley, a satisfied resident of Celebration, Florida. As mentioned in the previous chapter, research has concluded that humans are actually biologically hardwired to want connections to other people. There is a *genetic* need for community, social interactions and caring relationships. For our own survival we need neighborliness. As the eminent psychologist Abraham Maslow said: "Humans most basic instinct is a sense of belonging." Similarly, the renowned anthropologist Margaret Mead said that people need community "for the whole flowering of the human spirit."

Too many Americans are sitting painfully on an emotional two-legged stool. There is too much dependence on family and co-workers for human connectedness, and far too little support from a broad circle of friends that includes neighbors. Healthy living means regaining a more balanced life with family and work complemented by people and activities in the community. Now, more than ever, with people changing spouses, careers and jobs more frequently, deep and enduring relationships are more difficult to form and maintain. Increasing numbers of people are living alone, because they are not getting married and for older people because their spouses have died. Good neighbors are an untapped source of friends and social networks.

Neighbors as close friends can resemble family members who have "refrigerator rights." Meaning that they can knock on the door (unlocked in an ideal neighborhood) shout hello, come into your home and feel comfortable in grabbing something out of the refrigerator, and so would you in their homes. Recall *The Honeymooners* with Jacki Gleason. Neighbors really did come over in their bathrobes to borrow something without anyone feeling uncomfortable. Children commonly thought of neighbors as aunts and uncles. Of course, you have to want such relationships and not feel that your privacy is being invaded. Too many Americans in today's "McNeighborhoods" suffer from neighbor-intolerance.

Decades of so few people living in real neighborhoods and experiencing successful neighborliness means that fewer and fewer people have learned the "skills" of being neighborly. Where has all the neighborliness gone? Developer John Ritter observed: "After World War II, the United States fell in love with cars and fell out of love with their neighbors and neighborhoods." Now, most people have a love-hate relationship with their cars. We need new learned behavior. Overcoming fear of strangers takes learning. Knowing the benefits of being neighborly takes learning. Depending on your neighbors and being dependable for them takes learning. Making conversation takes learning. Where will children learn neighborliness? Certainly not in big sprawl schools that produce people perfect for blandburbs. *The only place to learn how to be a good neighbor is a real neighborhood...a* HEALTHY PLACE. What good is a dream house if it's not in a dream neighborhood?

"NEVER SEE NEIGHBORS" is in big letters on a Texas roadside billboard. Drivers are directed to an exit where they will find the Leisure Lakes sprawl subdivision near Houston. Welcome to the "culture of privatism," where neighborliness is not even sought. "Never see neighbors," that's what smart growth is up against.

COMMUNITY DESIGN CAN IMPROVE NEIGHBORLINESS.

There's the story of a suburban sprawl resident who invited a neighbor over for dinner, and the neighbor said "Oh, that's sweet, dear, but we're not that kind of neighbor." Sprawl has taken the civil out of civilization by taking the neighbor out of neighborhood.

Like some failed experiment, 50 years of sprawl proves that the exact design of the built environment harms society. But one of the biggest names in sociology and intellectual circles, Harvard Professor Nathan Glazer, said this in a 1965 article in *The New York Times Magazine*: "We must expunge the idea that the physical form of our neighborhood has any social consequences whatsoever." No difference between living in sprawl subdivisions and true communities? Glazer was totally wrong. We have geographical neighborhoods, not social neighborhoods. Nowadays, neighborliness only exists in old and new places with the correctly designed built environment.

Washington Post columnist E. J. Dionne Jr. wrote eloquently about the community of Rockaway in Queens, New York City, where much of his family lives. It was occasioned by a terrible airplane crash on November 12, 2001, which killed all the people in the plane and some on the ground when part of the neighborhood went up in flames. One of his points was this: "To call this neighborhood old-fashioned is both true and misleading. True because the prevailing values really are old-fashioned. Misleading, because everyone is acutely aware that it takes hard work and careful adjustment to keep old values alive in the year 2001." And every year it seems to become more difficult. Rockaway is a fairly high density, walkable community of modest homes. It is old. When people become sick neighbors quickly provide food, baby sitters, and other assistance. Neighborliness has been passed down from generation to generation in a built environment that supports it. Residents benefit from neighborliness in good times and bad times. HEALTHY PLACES mean building old-fashioned neighborhoods, where residents naturally talk with each other all the time. But neighborliness is thwarted when only slightly more than a quarter of teenagers expect to live in their communities as adults.

Completed in 1982, Village Homes in Davis, California is one of the oldest HEALTHY PLACES in the nation. High social capital has been verified. On average, residents know 42 people in their neighborhood, compared to 17 in sprawl suburbs, and identify four of their best friends in the community, compared to 0.4 for sprawl un-places. They spend 3.5 hours a week with friends in the neighborhood, compared to 0.9 hours in a conventional suburb, and 80 percent participate in community activities. Also, the crime rate in Village Homes is only 10 percent of the Davis average.

People living in HEALTHY PLACES often comment about the community neighborliness feature and benefit. A consistent pattern of heartfelt views shows that the design features of HEALTHY PLACES are not abstract theories of architects and designers. They were normal in pre-sprawl America. Listen to real people living in real neighborhoods:

A resident in the high density King Farm community in Maryland said: "This is a way to be more connected to people than living in a mini-castle on a two-acre lot."

"It just feels like a neighborhood. You get out, you feel safe, you talk to people. It's just so pleasant," said an occupant of Birkdale Village in North Carolina.

A resident of Civano in the Tucson area of Arizona proudly noted: "I know more people here in two years than I knew in 20 years where I lived previously."

In Pittsburgh, Pennsylvania a resident proclaimed: "The Crawford Square area is a tight-knit community. Everyone is vested in the community and wants to be here. It feels like home. There are all kinds of people here. This is not some exclusive, gated community."

"Suburbia is death for single people. It's so depressing. I grew up in suburbia and I always felt I was displaced. Here I can mingle with people. The cross-section [of people] is so impressive. My neighbors are close to me. I love it; I feel connected," said a homeowner in I'On in South Carolina.

According to a resident in Prairie Crossing, Minnesota: "There are a lot of common pathways around the nearby pond where you meet people. Sometimes, we'll come home from work and sit on our front porch. We've met a lot of our neighbors that way."

In Harbor Town in Memphis, Tennessee, a resident captured the essence of collective efficacy: "Your neighbors are more like second parents to the kids." He estimated that he knew 50 of his neighbors, in contrast to the handful he knew in previous places. Another resident said: "It goes back to the times when people had neighbors that really cared about each other. It has a wonderful family feel – like being on vacation."

A 67-year old resident of East Lake Commons, near Atlanta recaptured what was once prized: "This place is like the neighborhood I grew up in where everybody knew everybody, and kids couldn't get away with much because Mrs. So and So around the corner would call your mother."

A homeowner in River Ranch in Louisiana said: "The community has social functions that all of a sudden happen. People gather in the street to talk. Someone else will come up and all of a sudden, everyone is sitting around and conversing about life in general."

The Ritz Towers in Boston is a two-tower, high rise, mixed-use complex with 300 condos, a hotel, health club, movie theater, dry cleaner, day care and is close to Boston Common, a marvelous urban greenspace, and restaurants and shopping. A resident said "I have more of a sense of community than I did all those [30] years in the suburbs."

A resident of Baxter Village in South Carolina said: "Knowing who your neighbors are, and being able to walk out in the community is terrific. Just the comfort and security that this area gives. Not because it's gated, but because people care about you just because you live here."

Louis Alexander of Farmingdale, Long Island walks regularly to the downtown area and said "The benefit is you see more people and stop and talk."

Such testimonials are empirical evidence that good design really works. Eventually academic research will verify it. Do not wait for data, seek experience.

In its "Best Places to Live" article in 2002, *Washingtonian* magazine opened with: "Where are the really good places to call home? They are communities with a feeling of togetherness and a sense of identity. They are places where neighbors do more than wave from their driveways." And make no mistake about it. Developers of HEALTHY PLACES are marketing the neighborliness their designs support. Here are some claims from developer's Internet sites.

"You wave at the neighbors walking past; you know every one of them by name. Take a leisurely walk to the Town Center, just for the sheer pleasure of meeting your friends there. This is Huntfield [in West Virginia]."

"There was a time when privacy and neighborliness could exist side by side, when neighbors visited with one another from the front porch, when the place where you lived was more than just a house, that time has come again, in The Village of WestClay [in Indiana]."

"Knowing the names of the children on your street. Chatting with neighbors on an evening stroll. Helping prepare for a popular community activity. These types of events create strong connections – 'social capital.' ...In Harmony, [in Florida] neighbors will be encouraged to come together and take an active role in defining the nature of their community."

"Our community plan encourages the building of relationships. The country town ambience of the Villages of Urbana [in Maryland] fosters neighborliness and a strong sense of community. Enjoy a traditional American way of life that creates fond memories for a lifetime."

"The plan of [Serenbe in Georgia] makes it a routine part of your day to run into interesting people, to have conversations that spark your imagination and develop relationships with people you might not otherwise know. ...You may discover it's much easier to find time for friends when you don't have to fight traffic to see them."

Step into the past – through community design – to have a better future.

SOCIAL ISOLATION CAUSES ILLNESS.

A nine-year study by the California Department of Health Services on nearly 7,000 women and men found that those who lacked social and community connections were 1.9 to 3.1 times more likely to die during the nine-year follow-up period. Social isolation was associated with a higher risk of dying from coronary heart disease, stroke, cancer, respiratory diseases, gastrointestinal diseases, and all other causes of death. This social connection factor was independent of and stronger than other predictors of health and longevity, including age, gender, race, socioeconomic status, smoking, overeating, physical activity, and other variables.

Few people have connected sprawl to the incredible profits of the pharmaceutical industry. Instead of having "free" time to socialize with neighbors and make a shared community better, people turn to consumption in general and pharmaceuticals in particular. People pop pills to relieve depression, anxiety, and just unhappiness and stress. In 1957, 3 percent of Americans felt lonely, which jumped to 13 percent in 2003. Talking more to neighbors and being involved with one's community may be better medicine.

One thing is certain. Social isolation or low social cohesion is a fundamental *cause* of an unhealthy condition, not a consequence of it. Low social cohesion causes people to prize walls in gated places, as compared to feelings of safety and freedom in a real community. A general research finding is that people who are socially isolated are between two and five times more likely to die from all causes, compared to individuals who have things in common except that they have close ties with family, friends, and the community. And if a person belongs to no social groups but joins one, their risk of dying over the next year is cut in half.

Professor Bruce Podobnik of Lewis and Clark College compared the Orenco Station community, a high density HEALTHY PLACE, with a typical suburban sprawl community in the same Portland, Oregon metropolitan area. He found that Orenco has a more congenial social atmosphere as indicated by high rates of perceived friendliness among neighbors, a sense of community, and participation in community groups. There was a higher level of trust, goodwill and social engagement among Orenco's residents, as compared to the sprawl un-place.

A study of a HEALTHY PLACE and a blandburb near Salt Lake City, Utah, with similar size homes and prices, found that the HEALTHY PLACE residents had a statistically significant higher rate of neighborliness in terms of knowing neighbors, borrowing from neighbors, watching neighbors' homes, willingness to improve the neighborhood, and visiting, speaking and socializing with neighbors.

A larger scale study by Professor Michael A. Krassa of the University of Illinois verified that community design supports social capital and cohesion. Street design was used to categorize 26 different neighborhoods in five cities. A tight grid street pattern defined HEALTHY PLACES, versus a lower connectivity cul-de-sac pattern blandburbs. Residents in HEALTHY PLACES:

+ Had higher numbers of interactions with neighbors and other users of public spaces, and the interactions were significantly longer, three minutes versus one minute on average. Low interaction rates correlated with a lack of sidewalks.
+ Had higher citizen engagement and activism, based on interviews with public officials.
+ More frequently mentioned their love for the area, their feelings of community, and that they had lots of good friends in the neighborhood.

+   +   +   +

+ Were more likely to love their neighborhood than the houses themselves.

+ Focused more on neighbors and networks of friends than the financial and non-human features of the neighborhood.

+ Had higher turnout for voting.

+ Had higher parental involvement with schools and school officials, according to teachers, PTA officers, and school board officials.

+ Had stronger involvement with planning, zoning and development issues associated with land use, according to developers, city planners, and zoning board officials.

Similarly, Kevin M. Leyden of West Virginia University looked at how neighborhoods affect social capital. After controlling for a number of factors, he found that people living in complete, mixed-use, pedestrian friendly neighborhoods – in the city or suburbs – had more social capital than those living in auto-dependent suburban subdivisions. When residents can interact informally with others the result is more trust, social and political engagement, and knowledge about neighbors. The annual turnover rate in HEALTHY PLACES was lower than in sprawl housing. Rather than move, residents in HEALTHY PLACES were more likely to be activists trying to protect and improve their neighborhood and community. Sprawl residents more easily substitute one house for another and use an "exit strategy" when problems arise, such as traffic congestion or school crowding. HEALTHY PLACES residents have strong ties to their neighbors and *their* community, and see moving as a less attractive option.

Researchers found that poor health correlated with states with low social capital. The chances of having poor to middling health increased by about 40 to 70 percent if people moved from a state with high social capital (such as Minnesota, Vermont and Iowa) to one with low social capital (such as Alabama, Arkansas and Louisiana). *Amazingly, one could improve one's health almost as much by moving to a high social capital state as by quitting smoking.* This research finding strongly suggests that differences among communities, rather than averages over many people in states, could produce very sharp differences in health. Indeed, some research at the community level has shown exactly this, including a community in Pennsylvania which had a very low incidence of heart disease over a long time. It was explained by extremely strong social networks that were sup-

+ 242 +   SPRAWL KILLS +

ported by design features of the old community, like front porches and walkable neighborhoods, that helped people interact all the time.

Less socially connected people generally feel worse and have lower levels of happiness. In the past several decades, life satisfaction among American adults has declined steadily, and half of it can be associated with financial worries and the other half by reductions in social capital. During recent years when social capital has been declining and sprawl mounting, the rates of depression and suicide have increased. People living alone can benefit greatly from taking advantage of neighborliness and social connectedness.

Good communities make good neighbors. Good neighbors make healthier communities.

CARS CONSUME TIME.

Jean Bennett wanted to own a house. She had to go 71 miles from her job in downtown San Diego to find one she could afford. She spends two hours driving, riding a bus and taking a train to get to her job – *each way*. "It's not so bad until Sunday night – until I start thinking about the commute again," she said. Living long distances from jobs in Southern California is common, often 100 miles one way, because sprawl developers find cheap land far from jobs.

What do people say is the number one barrier to being more physically active? Lack of time. From just 1990 to 1996 the average time an American family spent in cars every day increased 22 percent. The annual increase in time just *stuck* in traffic congestion has been running at ten times the rate of population growth! Nationally, the average driver spent 51 hours stuck in traffic in 2001, compared to 11 hours in 1982. In Los Angeles it was 90 hours in 2001. In sprawl-afflicted Atlanta, there has been over a five-fold increase in just 15 years. No wonder that Americans are time-poor. Commuting is not the sole problem; people drove 137 percent further for errands in 1995 as compared to 1969. More data of the absurd. American adults average over 70 minutes a day driving, more than twice as much as the average parent spends with their kids.

No amount of great community design will be successful in fostering regular physical activity if people do not have the time and energy to be physically active, even if they understand the benefits of active living.

Motivation is not enough. For most people, great community design is necessary but not sufficient. Time-consuming automobile dependency is the culprit. Community design must help residents reduce their car use. If not, it's not a HEALTHY PLACE. Another problem is people spending more time working to afford conspicuous consumption, even at home. The irony is that as people have become more time-poor, despite economic affluence, they have also become more desperate to save time. The sprawl culture is a hit-the-button, drive-thru, stay on-line, and remote control way of life. So much need to save time *because* so much time is wasted. Americans swallow fast-food with abandon because sprawl swallows their time.

Thad Williamson of Harvard University used data from some 30,000 interviews of people nationwide and census data to show that long commuting times correlated with reductions in number of friends, attendance at public meetings, social trust, membership in groups, personal happiness, and happiness with one's community. The report "Better Together," from a multiyear effort at Harvard University on civic engagement and social capital, concluded that "largely to make homeownership more affordable, we have chosen to pave highways and build spread-out housing developments far beyond the core cities, and in the process we have created a car-based culture that deprives us of quality time with our families and precludes the sort of casual interaction that characterizes tight-knit urban neighborhoods." Being house-rich and time-poor have curdled the American dream. Family and physical activity time is sacrificed. Blandburbanites conk out inside rather than walk outside.

Besides commuting, running errands and chauffeuring children devours time, even on weekends when people used to feel time-rich. Add the frustrating time looking for parking places. As to commuting, the greater separation between homes and jobs is shown by the amazing 200 percent increase from 1960 through 1990 for the percentage of workers with jobs outside their counties of residence. The average American driver spends over 400 hours each year in their vehicle, more than ten work weeks. It keeps going up. Wouldn't people be better off and healthier with ten more weeks of free time rather than work? Living in HEALTHY PLACES can cut that car time by very large amounts, even without eliminating commuting by car. Total car time can be cut by 50 percent or more. Live close to work and the reduction can be in the 70 to 80 percent range. Automobile addiction is not obligatory.

Excessive car use motivates time-cutting behavior. Drivers are going faster, not just 10 or 20 miles per hour over the posted limit, but 30 and 40 miles per hour over the limit. Richard Retting of the Insurance Institute for Highway Safety got it right: "We live in a hurry-up society. We've become very impatient and very much in a hurry. Many drivers seem to make up for lost time or delays they encounter in their life on the road." Drivers also are blasting through red lights and using road shoulders to escape traffic congestion.

Don't kid yourself. Drivers often talk about having "time alone to think." But this rationalization is undermined by the survival need to stay alert in heavy traffic. *Washingtonian* magazine asked about the biggest waste of time. At 36 percent, commuting was the number one time-waster by a huge margin (three times more than watching TV and surfing the Internet). Perhaps the single most sprawl commute-enhancing invention was the car cup holder. Besides drinking, drivers are on their cell phones, eating, grooming themselves, reading, emailing, and performing other tasks as they try to de-waste their excessive vehicle time. "Distracted driving" is dangerous, causing up to 30 percent of the 3 million automobile accidents a year, according to the National Highway Transportation Safety Administration. A University of North Carolina study found that drivers are distracted 16 percent of the time. Using a cell phone while driving triples the risk of dying in a car accident, and 85 percent of cell phone users talk on their phones while driving. A University of Utah study found that using a cell phone while driving was more dangerous than driving while drunk.

A man who spends four hours a day commuting roundtrip between a Virginia suburb and a job in Washington, D.C. by mostly using public transit said "I've tried driving, but you do that a few days and it just wears you out... When you get home, you're too tired to do anything anyway." A 2003 poll for the *Wall Street Journal Europe* found that the favorite leisure time activity of 80 percent of Americans is staying at home in couch potato splendor, watching television, listening to music, reading, using a computer, and presumably satiating their stress-induced craving for comfort food. And a 2002 poll on stress found that lack of time is the leading source of stress, ahead of fear of terrorism and financial worries. This is consistent with the AARP national survey responses to the question "Why do you need money?" Sensibly, some two-thirds of Americans need money to obtain medical attention and stay healthy, but a third needs money to have more free time.

Time-poor and stressed Americans are seduced by sedentary-enhanc

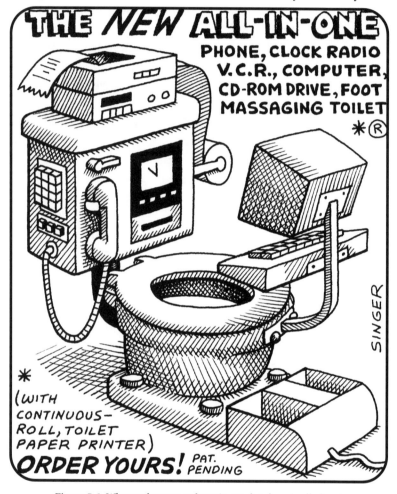

Figure 5-1. What sedentary-enhancing technology is all about.

ing technologies. Americans need to balance food consumption with more physical activity. *The sprawl-time insanity is feeling exhausted* **and** *being sedentary.* Colorado Governor Bill Owens held a press conference in 2004 to announce his intention to stop using elevators and climb stairs instead; he wanted state residents to do likewise, because obesity levels had increased for ten years. People try to recover time when total daily car time exceeds about 1.1 to 1.3 hours, which researchers think represents an ideal travel time budget. Demand increases for LSD – labor saving devices

– that eliminate countless bits of physical activity. At home, remote controls, washing machines, self-propelled vacuum cleaners and other devices (see Figure 5-1) save time and muscle use. Mayo Clinic researchers found that LSD and machine use added 10 pounds a year, unless people offset it with more activity such as walking. LSD use has risen in recent years, tracking increases in obesity.

Other than physical activity, cutting car use frees up time for family activities, education, community service, hobbies, home maintenance and remodeling, or just sleeping, because Americans are generally spending more time working than ever before. Working parents want to get home early enough to spend time with their children. For "taxi driver moms," non-commute driving consumes their time and energy. Women with school-aged children make more than five auto trips daily, requiring some 74 minutes on average. For many mothers it is much more. Shown below are the high percentages of people who agreed with this survey statement: "The current pace of development and resulting traffic congestion has resulted in my family spending more time in traffic and less time with each other." You can see that most people are making the connection between losing time in traffic and less family time, especially in the high traffic congestion Atlanta and Northern Virginia (metropolitan Washington, D.C.) areas.

Georgia	65%
Atlanta	**81%**
Maryland	73%
Virginia	63%
Northern Virginia	**84%**

So much time is spent in cars that an official of the Ford Motor Company said "The family car has become a family room on wheels. It's the hub of all the family energy and excitement." What a remarkable statement. Taken at face value, then why are people seeking larger and larger sprawl homes? Of course, the automobile industry wants Americans to see their cars as an extension of their homes. It is a marketing ploy to justify Americans spending so much time inside vehicles, and a tactic to prod consumers to spend more money on cars and their accessories.

The connection between sprawl car time and diet is grave, as in digging your own grave. Who has time to cook regularly? Sprawl living and automobile dependency contribute to terrible diets and rising rates of overweight and obese Americans. More than 40 percent of adults eat out in a restaurant on a typical day. When stressed-out parents satisfy their cravings for comfort foods they take their children along with them. Nearly one third of children aged 4 to 19 eat fast food every day; overall, one in three meals of kids is fast food. In a typical month, 90 percent of kids from 3 to 9 years old eat at a McDonald's. Few walk there. So much fast food eating and sitting in cars has devastated children.

Time matters more than ever. A survey by the Council of Governments in the very congested Washington, D.C. area found that saving time had become the number one desire of commuters, more important than convenience and saving money. So, to promote ride-sharing and use of transit they switched their television messages to "find time every day for the things that matter" and "find time for you." All this matches a survey finding that 73 percent of American workers are willing to curtail their careers to get more family time.

Cutting vehicle time is even more important for improving quality of life for children than for adults, because it can improve their entire future adult life. Giving children more "free" time helps them become more physically active. Spending time outdoors is the best indicator of physical activity for kids, which makes high quality public spaces, including safe streets very beneficial. More time with parents can prevent many developmental and behavioral problems. Kids can become healthier, smarter, have better people skills, and become more expert at whatever interests them. They can discover neighborliness and learn how to practice it. They can avoid automobile addiction.

The Center for a New American Dream sponsored a national survey of kids ages 9 to 14 in early 2003 that provided some good and bad news. On the positive side, 90 percent of kids say that friends and family are way more important than things money can buy; sixty-three percent express concern that too much advertising urges kids to buy things. On the negative side, just less than a third of kids say they spend a lot of time with their parents; 63 percent wished their mom or dad had a job that gave them more time to do fun things together; of kids' favorite activities with parents, only 11 percent chose biking and outside activity, compared to the most favorite of going to a movie at 21 percent.

"Free" time is increasingly valuable. A *Money Magazine* survey of Americans with household incomes of $75,000 or more found that 70 percent thought that their leisure time was more important than their work time. But nearly half of American workers put in more than 50 hours a week, and a quarter do not take a vacation during the year. Roper surveys found that Americans increasingly feel that they do not have enough leisure time; in 2000 49 percent felt this way. And 50 percent said they felt stress and tension on a regular basis.

Being time-poor has an economic dimension. Ironically, a core principle of developers is that "time is money," and that they must do everything possible, including influencing the political system, to avoid losing time to bring projects to completion. What is true for sprawl developers ought to be true for sprawl residents. What is saved time worth? Economists usually assume that those hours are worth what a person makes from working, but research finds that people value time wasted at up to half their wage rate. This implies, of course, that the time of higher income people is worth more than of lower income people, just in strictly economic terms. Americans should acknowledge that there is economic value in becoming time-rich. Time *is* money.

A new HEALTHY PLACE is The Village of Providence in Huntsville, Alabama, and a selling point is: "Freedom will be given to kids to walk to school or local parks, to the elderly to walk to shops and activities, and to parents to spend less time chauffeuring children around town. In short, freedom to spend their time on the more important things in life – like friends, family, and recreation." Frisco Square near Dallas, Texas, a new mixed-use community uses this marketing message: "Discover the Art of Convenience." Prospective residents are asked to "Visualize the ultimate solution for streamlining your life and maximizing your personal time." The developer said: "We want to create time for residents to enjoy the ideal environment they're living in."

Oddly, once upon a time, in a world with less efficiency and technology, people were time-rich and had time to "waste." They could "kill" time. Having nothing to do is a lost luxury, unless you are retired, unemployed or rich. Stress-free time is especially rare. In our time-poor society, time kills people, because so much of it is in vehicles rather than being physically active or with loved ones. Sedentary time kills. Sprawl commuter time kills. Sprawl stress time kills. Sprawl fast food time kills. When sprawl kills time, it kills life.

Americans need mental pop-up ads repeatedly asking: Is living the suburban, car-dependent American Dream eating up your time? Sprawl living is more a coma than a dream – a car coma – that keeps you sleep-driving through life. Research found that when gasoline prices increase people spend more time working, because they reduce leisure-time activities that sadly are car-dependent. Wake up. Live in a HEALTHY PLACE to become time-rich, before your time runs out.

HOUSING AFFORDABILITY DEPENDS ON LOCATION COSTS.

With the majority of Americans living in suburban sprawl, it is an uphill battle to persuade people that there are economic benefits from living in HEALTHY PLACES. There are myths to dispel and new ways of looking at total location costs. Time to learn that the cost of sprawl living is not as attractive as it first appears. Less obvious indirect costs are the culprit.

When most people think about the cost or affordability of housing, they usually just think about home price, purchase or rental, relative to their income. To fairly evaluate a true alternative to sprawl a different approach is needed. Housing affordability depends on community location and quality of life costs. Consider the following opportunities to increase disposable income relative to sprawl living:

+ Reduce health care costs through active living, lower vehicle use, and a higher social capital community.
+ Reduce direct and indirect transportation costs by reducing car ownership and use.
+ Reduce food costs by having more time for home cooking and less craving for comfort foods.
+ Have lower entertainment costs by participating in diverse community activities.

Reduce lawn care costs because of smaller lawns.

Such cost reductions make housing more affordable. The lower your income the more important it is to use this framework for understanding the economics of housing and community decisions.

As to health benefits, a 2000 survey of 35,000 Americans found that medical costs of inactive people averaged $2,277, compared to $1,242 – 45 percent less – for active people, where active meant at least 30 minutes of physical activity three times per week. With very high costs of health care, even if you have health insurance, take community design more seriously.

As a fraction of household income, transportation costs are usually second after housing costs, 19 percent versus 33 percent in 2001, and more than for other categories, like food and clothing combined. Transportation costs have risen faster than housing costs as a fraction of household income. Home ownership provides a long term financial reward, but cars just depreciate rapidly. In 2001 the average American household spent $7,200 yearly on buying, financing, fueling, parking, repairing, insuring, and maintaining cars and trucks. There are also taxes and tolls, and license, registration, and inspection fees. These days, in high sprawl regions, family spending on cars can top $20,000 annually from after tax, disposable income. The lower the income, the higher the fraction devoted to vehicles, reaching one-third for low incomes.

Where you live really matters. The stronger the public transit system, the less money spent on cars. A study for Chicago found that households of average income in outer-ring suburbs spend more than twice as much annually driving their cars than families living in the city along transit lines. In 2000, average annual household transportation costs for the Atlanta region were $8,513 and in the greater Houston area were $8,840, both areas known for considerable low density sprawl, compared to $6,384 in the Cleveland-Akron region and $5,800 in the Milwaukee-Racine area, both older, higher density places.

For families with three or four cars, car costs can exceed housing costs. Here are examples of sprawl sticker shock in the Atlanta region. A husband and wife carpool together and drive nearly 30 miles each way to work, and the monthly car cost is $1,230, compared to their $1,100 mortgage cost. For another couple, the husband has a 50-mile and the wife a 100-mile round trip; the monthly vehicle cost is $898 versus a mortgage cost of $858. Sprawl homes are not always what they first seem to be because of high transportation costs.

The most certain way of reducing vehicle costs is by choosing to live in a HEALTHY PLACE. The benefit can amount to many thousands of dollars a year. Car cost reduction could provide more money for housing or allow you to work less and have more time for family life and physical activities. Maryland has the "Live Near Your Work" program that offers $3,000 towards closing costs for employees who buy a home within five miles of their workplace, with a third coming from the state, a third from the employer, and a third from the local government. The Fannie Mae Corporation has two programs. Location Efficient Mortgages are available in some areas and allow people to borrow more money for a certain income, if their home location reduces transportation costs. It can easily equate to being able to buy a home worth $25,000 to $50,000 more than with a conventional mortgage. The Smart Commute Initiative rewards those living near public transportation; it can increase the maximum allowable mortgage by up to $10,000. The right wing Georgia Public Policy Foundation called this program "a feel-good and unenforceable attempt at social engineering." Why condemn voluntary use of public transit?

When considering housing affordability, stopping at home price is a mistake. Spending more money to purchase a home in a HEALTHY PLACE can make sense.

ALL TAXPAYERS SUBSIDIZE SPRAWL.

Every time you use a postage stamp you should know that sprawl has increased the cost of mail. The United States Postal Service's fiscal health has worsened as decades of spread-out sprawl required new post offices and higher cost mail delivery. Sprawl has shifted mail delivery from doorstep to curb, and finally to cost-cutting "cluster mailboxes" at central locations that sedentary sprawl residents often resent getting to. Smart design that fosters neighborliness puts cluster boxes in a public space so residents can mingle, such as near shops, a park, or inside a community building. In contrast, a home builder who fought to get single boxes for a subdivision of McMansions near Las Vegas, Nevada said: "They want their privacy. They want the exclusiveness of having their own box."

The myth is that sprawl housing generates adequate tax revenues. Do they cover the costs of providing the full range of public services and infrastructure that sprawl residents expect? No. Rampant sprawl means rising local taxes. If you hear otherwise from the sprawl industry or sprawl shills, do not believe it. Unfortunately, local governments increase tax revenues by welcoming strip malls, big box stores, and office buildings that will lure commuters (and traffic) from other areas. On a per house basis, the capital costs alone for new infrastructure can easily be in the $10,000 to $30,000 range, or even more. But virtually no government imposes high enough fees on developers to cover all these costs; often there are no fees. An Oregon study found that development fees ranged from $1,000 to $6,500 per unit, while actual public costs were $24,500 per unit. In Phoenix, the city and county subsidized new sprawl development at the rate of $12,000 per home. In Franklin, a high-growth suburb of Milwaukee, Wisconsin, when each new home cost over $10,000 for schools and services, home builders paid only $813 in impact fees. In 2004, Centex Homes agreed to pay $500 for each of the 1,300-plus homes it was building to cover some costs of new school construction; it was just 6 percent of the cost of a new elementary school. All taxpayers pay the difference.

Saving farmland from sprawl makes economic sense. Cows don't go to school, trees don't call police, and crops don't drive cars. Many studies have found that to provide public services counties spend about 20 to 30 percent more than tax revenues from housing subdivisions, but spend 50 to 70 percent less than tax revenues from farms and open space. New York farmland preservationist Pat Hancock observed: "We, as Americans, tend to use open space as if it were a disposable commodity." Bemoaning the loss of farmland to development caused him "to wonder if Dutchess County's final crop will be sprawl? Is this progress?" In Texas, *The Valley Morning Star* ran the story "Farmland gives way to urban sprawl." The 50-year old, 100 acre Texas Valley Farms was plowed under, its grapefruit and other citrus trees cleared for sprawl subdivisions. This was happening throughout the Rio Grande Valley. Farmland that sold for $1,000 to $2,000 an acre now fetched as much as $40,000 an acre for sprawl development.

As discussed in Chapter 1, the sprawl lobby spends big money to get government – taxpayers – to pay for new roads and schools in areas where new development is occurring or is targeted. They seem to be slowly losing the impact fee battle, because of financial difficulties of local governments, but they have not yet capitulated. A 2001 Florida statewide survey found that 86 percent of voters favor developers paying for new infrastructure such as roads and schools. This much is certain. *Sprawl developers benefit not so much from a free market as from a free ride, while taxpayers have increasingly expensive rides.*

In early 2004 the New Jersey Board of Public Utilities justified requiring builders to pay the full cost of gas, water and electric line extensions to new developments in rural areas by saying it "would protect the majority of New Jerseyans from subsidizing the minority that want to promote sprawl." The New Jersey Builders Association protested. In Maryland, a

Carroll County Commissioner voted in 2003 to control land development

THE SELF-FULFILLING SPRAWL NIGHTMARE or DUMB-GROWTH CYCLE:

+ Increased sprawl housing development requires more roads and water and sewer lines being built, which begets...
+ Roads widened to 'improve' traffic flow, which begets...
+ Farmland and wilderness destroyed, which begets...
+ Increased air, noise and traffic pollution, which begets...
+ The need for new schools, which begets...
+ Wider roads which increase traffic flow and attract development, which begets...
+ Police, fire and ambulance service cost increases, which begets...
+ Tax increases, which begets...
+ The feeling that a broader tax base is needed to lower taxes, which begets...
+ Increased sprawl housing development which requires more roads and water and sewer lines....

Get the picture?

because of excessive burdens on county government: "For them, it's a dollar in the pocket, and then they walk away from the project and it's somebody else's problem." Actually they drive away with big profits.

Sprawl developers fight paying impact fees, claiming higher home prices will reduce housing affordability, but there is no evidence for this and, besides, many jurisdictions exempt true affordable housing from fees. Without developers and new home buyers paying for new public infrastructure and services, spreading sprawl is like a Ponzi scheme, with today's residents paying for tomorrow's newcomers, and them paying for the next round, until taxpayers say "no" to still more sprawl growth. Developers take their profits but *all* residents pay.

Boulder, Colorado faced lower sales tax revenues because of shopping outside the city, so a developer proposed a project to house a big box store, other stores, and 100 condos, but the city would have to annex the 23 acres. Boulder residents Larry Sherwood and Janet Meyer argued: "Sprawl results when cities succumb to greed and the bait dangled by self-serving developers, rather than sticking to the plans created by their citizens in accordance with the community's values." They wanted the city to expand shopping *inside* the city. Similarly, Stephen Sommerrock in Salisbury, Maryland, where developers pay no impact fees, criticized annexation of 40 acres for a new sprawl subdivision: "We're concerned about the impact this development will have on our schools, our roads, our water and sewer services."

Americans pay a hidden "sprawl tax" to subsidize the sprawl industry. Usually property taxes increase, because they typically supply some 30 percent or more of local government revenues. Sometimes, sales and gas taxes increase. Without tax increases government revenues shift from spending in older areas to newer sprawl developments. The "dumb-growth" cycle (see Figure 5-2) answers the question that many sprawl residents ask: Why are my taxes so high? Alternatively, if public opposition limits tax increases, sprawl residents suffer from poor public services, usually overcrowded schools and dangerous rural roads. It all amounts to a lose-lose situation for existing residents, and ultimately for new sprawl residents who find out that their tax burden will be higher and public services worse than originally anticipated. When developers escape impact fees, local governments may favor sprawl subdivisions with larger, higher price homes to collect more property taxes. This means less affordable housing.

When sprawl residents push "no growth" policies, developers shift to more remote sprawl-friendly rural land where taxes are low – until government builds new infrastructure and provides public services. More distant subdivisions attract financially strapped homeowners. This cycle stimulates outward gluttonous land consumption. Richard L. Stup, a planning commissioner in sprawling Frederick County, Maryland summed it up: "We all open our arms to [newcomers], and now they want to close their arms to everybody else. People move here for lower taxes, and yet they demand the same services they had in the jurisdictions they moved from. They move here with three vehicles and make it more crowded. The people who yell the loudest are sometimes part of the problem." After spending millions of dollars on new schools some places face over-capacity because residents have moved to escape high taxes, or projected development has moved elsewhere. Infrastructure spending financed by tax-free bonds is a convoluted way of subsidizing sprawl.

Despite free land from developers, an absurdity is expensive construction of new mega-schools on cheap land where sprawl has already begun or where it will inevitably happen *because* of a new school. Often, older schools are closed, forcing students to get bused or driven to school. Considerable research has shown that renovating older schools is cheaper than new school construction and homes lose value when local schools are closed. Even with little population growth, leapfrogging sprawl results in high costs. Michigan school districts built 500 new schools from 1996 to 2003 and closed 278 older schools, even though school population grew just 4.5 percent. It cost taxpayers billions of dollars. Absurdly, school districts can often ignore local planning and growth management policies and regulations.

Also consider school busing. Over $10 billion is spent nationally by school districts to provide transportation for about 60 percent of students. Sprawl dispersion of homes means longer trips and often the need for more routes, buses, and drivers. School busing costs can increase without big increases in student population. Between 1970 and 1995 Maine school busing costs rose over six times, from $8.7 million to over $54 million, even though the number of students declined by 27,000. Similarly, in Monroe County, New York, over a ten year period school busing costs increased 100 percent, even though the number of students increased by only 8 percent.

Americans without kids in school pay a price for all the use of cars and buses for transporting children to and from school. Road congestion during morning and afternoon times associated with school transport jumps dramatically. For example, in Santa Rosa, California traffic jumps 30 percent between 7:15 a.m. and 8:15 a.m. during the school year.

In contrast to sprawl development, HEALTHY PLACES greatly reduce infrastructure costs on a per person or per dwelling unit basis, up to 50 percent in many cases. A study by the National Association of Home Builders compared conventional, low density sprawl and high density, clustered housing; it found that total site-development costs for street pavement, curbs/gutters, street trees, driveways, storm drainage, water distribution, sanitary sewer, grading, clearing land, and sidewalks were reduced by 34 percent for the cluster plan. Not counted were costs for schools and some other things. Urban and suburban infill projects can cut infrastructure costs by 90 percent.

Here is an illustration of fiscal benefits. Washington Township in central New Jersey had been a typical rural area experiencing rapid sprawl development, but then town officials pursued a smart growth strategy. The 400-acre Washington Town Center project will have over 1,000 homes. The commercial main street will include restaurants, small businesses, shops, a theater and a large retail anchor. Diverse home buyers include singles, young married couples, and empty nesters, both pre-retirees and retirees, compared to mostly couples in sprawl subdivisions, which is why the number of children is only about 20 percent of a blandburb. Less tax revenues are needed for new schools and other infrastructure, resulting in a positive tax revenue flow, and the well-designed commercial town center has preempted typical sprawl strip malls.

Here are other reports of reduced infrastructure costs through smart growth development:

For the Charlottesville, Virginia region continued sprawl development would require $1 billion for transportation infrastructure needs over some years. But building higher density places, emphasizing pedestrian-friendly design, and expanding the transit system, roadway spending would be reduced by $500 million – a 50 percent saving.

For the metropolitan Denver area, infrastructure costs over 25 years for continued sprawl development would cost $4.3 billion more than with compact smart growth.

In Collier County, Florida the Rural Lands Stewardship Program and compact development turn a projected deficit of $1.2 million per year for continued sprawl development into a surplus of $300,000 annually for the same population growth.

A traditional sprawl subdivision would mean a loss of town revenues of $40,000 annually, but the higher density Dunstan Crossing project in Scarborough, Maine would result in a net gain of $250,000 a year.

Nationally, the Brookings Institution reported in 2004 that smart growth development could reduce road building costs $110 billion, water and sewer costs $12.6 billion, and operation and maintenance costs $4 billion over 25 years.

In Canada, a plan for Ontario based on focusing growth in compact communities over 30 years would save 20 per cent in infrastructure costs.

The lesson: Smart growth means lower taxes for everyone.

HEALTHY PLACES PROVIDE GREATER FINANCIAL BENEFITS.

Homes in HEALTHY PLACES gain more value than conventional sprawl homes. A study by a builder of three HEALTHY PLACES, each at least three years old, compared them to nearby conventional subdivisions. Home appreciation in the HEALTHY PLACES was 16.7 percent, compared to 14.2 percent for the conventional places.

A University of Massachusetts study compared clustered housing to conventional sprawl areas in the same region. With clustered housing, 86 percent of the land was open space, the residential streets were narrow, and 14 of the 20 homes were two-family semi-detached dwellings, with the rest single-family detached houses. The average lot size was about one-fifth of those in the conventional area. Homes in the higher density cluster development gained more value, amounting to tens of thousands of dollars over some years. The study concluded that "the home-buyer, speaking in dollar-terms through the marketplace, appears to have demonstrated a greater desire for a home with access and proximity to permanently-protected land, than for one located on a bigger lot, but without the open-space amenity." Higher home density was offset by community green infrastructure.

Emerging Trends in Real Estate for 2002, aimed at real estate investors, made this important observation: "properties in better-planned, growth-constrained markets hold better value in downmarkets and appreciate more in upcycles. Areas with sensible zoning (integrated commercial, retail, and residential), parks, and street grids with sidewalks age better than places oriented to disconnected cul-de-sac subdivisions and shopping strips, navigable only by car."

Bottom line: Home investments do better in HEALTHY PLACES than blandburbs.

SPRAWL IS LONELY.

Get ready to shed some tears. A family moved from an urban townhouse to a million dollar 7,400-square-foot McMansion on a 10-acre mountain lot in Virginia, some 40 miles west of Washington, D.C. In three months they became disillusioned, in five months they had moved inward to a smaller home and lot. What happened? Day care was 45 minutes away. With a young child and another one on the way there was serious concern about getting emergency help. They were socially isolated; former friends did not visit. Even with two new four-wheel drive vehicles, getting anywhere could be difficult and time consuming, especially in snow. Even the rich can discover that the price of sprawl is more than the upfront dollar costs.

The health and safety benefits of living in a HEALTHY PLACE deserve high priority. But the additional benefits associated with neighborliness, time and money are likely to play a pivotal role in choosing a HEALTHY PLACE. Do not ignore them. The next chapter will help you find a community that gives you the benefits.

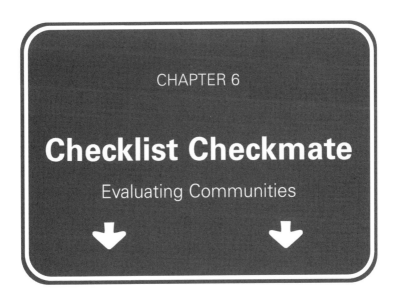

CHAPTER 6

Checklist Checkmate

Evaluating Communities

Sprawl scams.

Sprawl-speak makes it difficult to find an authentic HEALTHY PLACE.
The truth *is* out there. HEALTHY PLACES are not some theoretical ideal.
Although too few in number, they exist as models and showcases for what
is needed on a far greater scale. This chapter provides information on
many actual HEALTHY PLACES. But the landscape is also cluttered with
blandburbs that sound better than they really are. A few years ago the ten
principles of smart growth were developed and endorsed by many national and local organizations, including the National Governors Association.
They define the essence of smart growth. Here they are in succinct form:

+ Mix land uses
+ Foster "walkable" close-knit neighborhoods
+ Preserve open space, farmland, natural beauty, and critical
environmental areas

+ Create a range of housing opportunities and choices
+ Make development decisions predictable, fair and cost-effective
+ Provide a variety of transportation choices
+ Promote distinctive, attractive communities with a strong sense of place, including the rehabilitation and use of historic buildings
+ Take advantage of existing community assets
+ Encourage citizen and stakeholder participation in development decisions
+ Strengthen and encourage growth in existing communities

To help consumers, I have used these principles to create a checklist of ten questions. The checklist is a "truth detector" tool. As the excellent 2001 "South County Design Manual" from Rhode Island noted: "Like any movement designed to gather many smaller efforts into a single theme, Smart Growth has sometimes been misused by those trying to merely give sprawl a more acceptable face. ...A number of award winning 'New Urbanist' projects have been completed...that are lovely within themselves, but on the regional scale represent just another form of sprawl." Some dirty tricks are more than word games. A developer in Hudson, Ohio bought the Internet domain name www.smartgrowthhudson.com which sent people to the project's website. The developer knew that the group Smart Growth 4 Hudson opposed the project and had the site www.smartgrowthhudson.*org*.

Home builders and real estate agents push consumers to focus on private space and indoor amenities. The checklist helps you focus on the community outside. By asking the right questions and evaluating information from advertising and marketing materials, site visits, books, and Internet sites, you can decide whether a place is all that is promised and all that you want.

Ideally, a HEALTHY PLACE would satisfy all ten questions. Though excellent places may not score 100 percent, the first six questions are critically important to choosing the "real thing." Some groups claim that what they support fits the smart growth model, when actually they satisfy just a few of the principles. In using the checklist questions, think how they can relate to different phases of your life. A housing and community decision should be seen as a lot more than a financial investment to obtain shelter. It is a quality of life decision with enormous implications for long-term health and wellbeing.

TEN CHECKLIST QUESTIONS FOR EVALUATING PLACES

1. Is there a mix of housing, office space with significant employment opportunities, schools, retail shopping, outdoor recreation areas, and civic/public spaces and buildings?

2. Does the design and layout of buildings, streets, and diverse gathering places promote real neighborliness by facilitating interactions among residents?

3. Is compact design used to minimize the amount of land per dwelling unit?

4. Does the place offer greenspaces throughout the community for public and recreational uses, including continuous green pathways for biking and walking and pocket parks in neighborhoods?

5. Do streets have sidewalks and connectedness to promote easy and safe walking and multiple paths for travel through the community?

6. Are there different types of mixed-income homes, such as single-family detached, multifamily units, condos, and affordable housing?

7. Has the developer made clear how build-out over time will be faithful to the original plan and vision?

8. Does the location avoid increasing the risk or negative impacts of natural disasters?

9. Is there convenient access to public transit? For larger projects, does transit operate within the community?

10. Does the place have a consistent and distinctive style that blends in with the environmental setting and cultural features of surrounding areas?

QUALITY PUBLIC SPACES MAKE GREAT PLACES.

A non-negotiable requirement is mixed land uses. To make life easier with less car use, many needs must be fulfilled in relatively nearby locations, within about a 15 minute walk from residences. For infill projects within cities or old suburbs, amenities in the surrounding area and in close proximity should be counted. Retail shopping must be sufficient to satisfy many regular daily or weekly needs. A grocery store or supermarket, a pharmacy, a drycleaner, a bank, and one or more restaurants are what people generally would like easy access to. Residents will still go to major department stores and shopping malls for some items – but not that often. Schools, a post office, and other civic buildings should also be there, according to the population level.

Denver's former Stapleton Airport is being redeveloped as an urban infill site of about 4,700 acres with some 12,000 homes, and some 30,000 residents eventually in five communities, each with their own town center. Considerable office and industrial activity will offer 35,000 jobs. There is retail space, schools, connection to a future light rail system, and 1,100 acres (23 percent) of parks and open space. The Stapleton Strollers are a group of young, fitness-minded mothers who walk and exercise together. A Stapleton official bragged: "In this community, the basic idea is that you walk to school, walk to shopping. The car is an afterthought. ...There are parks just a couple of minutes walk from every door. What we are building here is a model community that makes human-powered transit primary, and the automobile a fallback."

PRINCIPLE: Include mixed land use

CHECKLIST QUESTION:
1. Is there a mix of housing, office space with significant employment opportunities, schools, retail shopping, outdoor recreation areas, and civic/public spaces and buildings?

HEALTHY PLACES have parks and other greenspaces throughout them. A central community square or town center with civic buildings and shops is an important feature of successful projects. *The quality of the "public realm" is just as important as the design of homes.* What is outdoors matters just as much as what is indoors.

As discussed in Chapter 3, HEALTHY PLACES face challenges in attracting retail establishments. For projects scheduled for build-out many years, can early residents wait until retail comes into their community? Some developers are successful even at early stages. At King Farm in Maryland, the village center had a Safeway, convenience store, bank, dry cleaner and other businesses, even though the development was only half built. But there was considerable population in surrounding areas.

Some factors can expedite the viability of retail, such as locating stores on the edge of the community, allowing access by outside populations. Another option is to encourage a popular store to anchor the retail street or town center, which will bring people to the area even if it is out of the way. However, various forms of "destination retail" attracting outsiders can undermine the "flavor" of a town center and cause traffic congestion. Effective retail streets have wide sidewalks, inviting people to stroll through the area, linger in it, and have a seat on sidewalk patios and benches. Streets in commercial areas should have large trees to create a positive ambience. Parallel street parking helps calm traffic and encourages customers to drive by all stores on the block.

As difficult as it is to include significant numbers of jobs within a community, many projects have accomplished the task, as presented in Chapter 3. Office space in new communities is critical for providing jobs for local residents. *Workers in communities support retail and restaurants during the day and residents support businesses at night and on weekends.* One innovation is park benches wired for laptops to allow work outdoors. This was done in Colonial Town Park, a mixed-use project outside Orlando, Florida where the number of jobs is comparable to the number of people living in the 500 new residences.

Physicians and their staffs are discovering the benefits of working near where they and their patients live. Surrounding residents get convenience that once was taken for granted before sprawl took hold. Listen to Dr. Noah Makovsky a pediatrician in Lowry, Colorado, home to 2,800 households, a commercial center, and 17-medical related places. He lives five blocks from his office and wastes no time commuting, allowing him to have more family time. He said: "My wife and I cannot see ourselves moving away from this environment. There are so many benefits that come from being surrounded by so many like-minded people who want to live, work and shop in the same place. There is no question that this move has been good for my business."

Successful mixed-use neighborhoods also require schools. For HEALTHY PLACES within older urban areas and suburbs it is appropriate to rehabilitate old schools. In new greenfield projects it is necessary to build new schools that students can walk or bicycle to. At least an elementary school is needed and, if the population is large enough, then the community should have its own middle and high schools. Children should be able to walk to school on safe streets, paths or greenways. A consumer survey found that 78 percent of people want a community where kids can walk to a smaller neighborhood school, compared to 19 percent who favor driving kids to a larger regional school.

When mixed-use really works, it makes a place special and healthy by giving it great personality and people-connectedness. *Great places are made through the quality of public spaces that lift the human spirit because they make people feel good in the presence of other people.* Some examples are shown in Figure 6-1. D. H. Lawrence captured the magic of place in his "The Spirit of Place." He wrote: "Different places on the face of the earth have different vital effluence, different vibration, different chemical exhalation, different polarity with different stars: call it what you like. But the spirit of place is a great reality."

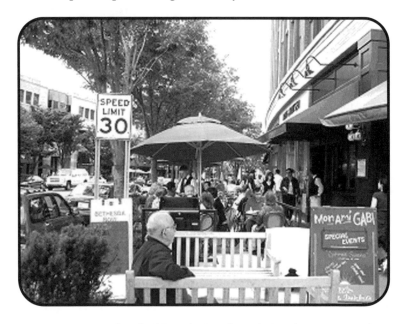

Figure 6-1. Examples of public gathering places designed to attract people.

When design of the public realm clicks, people find pleasure in the midst of other people, including: strolling on a path or through the town center, people watching at a plaza fountain, shopping in local stores, walking or biking through the community, eating at an outdoor café, watching street entertainers or an outdoor concert, or bird watching in a local greenway or park. Effective public spaces cause people of all ages to take pride in *their* community. Through shared participation and pride, individuals bond to their neighbors and community. Sprawl's social isolation breeds disrespect for neighbors and public spaces as shown by people illegally cutting down neighbor's trees or ones in public parks because they block scenic views.

Public spaces need a sense of permanence. Shops and building styles will change, but effective public spaces must endure. You want to return to them. You want them to retain whatever features you find aesthetically pleasing, fun, convenient, and safe. They are essential for positive memories of that special place. They are sacred when they nourish the mind, body and spirit. You want them protected and preserved. When are public spaces successful?

+ When they are popular routine gathering places for diverse people.
+ When neighbors interact casually and have spontaneous conversations.
+ When residents feel safe and comfortable.
+ When couples hold hands.
+ When parents walk leisurely with their children.
+ When people want to linger rather than quickly pass through.
+ When people watching is a wonderful way to pass time.

To sum up, smart growth improves the quality of housing by focusing on the non-housing land uses – the public realm – as well as the residential. Listen to these wise words of developer Vince Graham:

If as a developer you base your marketing on the idea that you are selling isolation, then every time you add something it takes away from what you're selling. But if you market community, instead of isolation, every time you add something it makes the neighborhood more complete and adds to what you're selling.

EFFECTIVE PUBLIC SPACES SUPPORT NEIGHBORLINESS.

Be careful. Sprawl developers may claim a walkable community because there are sidewalks. True walkability requires much more. Home placement, street design and green infrastructure must all work together to provide the comfort, safety, and visual attractiveness for a first rate walkable community. To promote haphazard and casual neighborly interactions in their public realm, streets must be well connected with each other, unlike the dead-end, cul-de-sac motif of sprawl un-places. Community centers, public spaces, benches on sidewalks in commercial areas and in green areas, pocket parks, and trails all contribute to effective gathering places.

> **PRINCIPLE: Foster walkable, close-knit neighborhoods**
>
> CHECKLIST QUESTION:
> 2. Does the design and layout of buildings, streets, and diverse gathering places promote real neighborliness by facilitating
> interactions among residents?

Public spaces should entice residents outdoors to spend more time walking and mingling with their neighbors. In HEALTHY PLACES, public spaces are "outdoor rooms" – extensions of homes. Aragon in Pensacola, Florida was designed to bring more people to live downtown in a waterview location. The 21-acre infill project replaced Pensacola's oldest public housing complex with 141 lots for homes and stores, and several neighborhood parks. Homes feature 19th century architecture like older neighborhoods in the city, and include porches and balconies. A neighborhood center has a grocery store. Walking paths connect to parks and Pensacola Bay. Residents can walk to the thriving business district. Architect-developer Michelle Macneil said: "We have tried to provide a variety of public amenities and spaces to give focus to the dreams of the community. One of the things we wish for is that when you provide people with good places, they will begin to see each other in daily life. We want to have opportunities that don't typically exist so that people can begin to know each other and to interact."

Worldwide, cultures have enduring public gathering places, where friends and neighbors meet and families spend time. France, Spain and South American countries have neighborhood bistros, sidewalk cafes, and boulevards for strolling. Germany has beer gardens. Japan has tea rooms and public gardens. Ireland and England have neighborhood pubs. Italy has public piazzas and sidewalk eating. Middle-east countries have bustling shopping bazaars. Starbucks seems to have learned a valuable lesson from these types of gathering places. HEALTHY PLACES have a diversity of public gathering places where residents can find people to engage in serious or frivolous conversation. Public gathering places have been called "third places," to contrast them with first place homes and second place workplaces, but they are best seen as tied with first place.

When people leave blandburb homes they usually jump in a car. Residents rarely leave their home on foot simply "to go out." In the car culture there are few unpredictable encounters with either people or places, not counting road rage incidents. HEALTHY PLACES have porches, sidewalk networks, park benches, and trails that aid unplanned encounters. Rather than watching television or surfing the Internet, residents can walk outdoors and have casual conversations with neighbors. Streets are not paved with gold, just social capital.

Front porches are more than cute. Porches and front steps should facilitate "schmoozing" with people on the street. Betsy Tarter of Baxter Village in South Carolina said: "The front porch aspect is awesome. We sit on the porch almost every evening. Neighbors sit and chit-chat. It's just great." But not all porches are well designed, especially in blandburbs masquerading as smart growth type communities. Good porches are relatively close to the ground, do not have screens, and are wide enough for people to comfortably sit on. The distance from the porch to the sidewalk must be within a "conversational" distance to facilitate talking to passersby.

Garages fronting streets do not foster neighborliness and are not pretty; their driveways interfere with walkability. Houses with prominent garages jutting out in front of them are called "snout houses." The size of two-car garages has been increasing from 20 by 20 feet to 24 by 24 feet, a 44 percent increase in land needed. Some local governments limit the space garages can take up, say no more than 50 percent of the front of a house. Sacramento, California and Portland, Oregon have taken such action. Better design puts garages behind or on the sides of houses and multiunit buildings.

Some governments also prohibit a garage being bigger than the house. The editor and publisher of *Architectural West* and a self-proclaimed "certified gas-sniffing motorhead" said "I don't know why this rule came into existence in the first place." He saw the reasonableness of providing homes with super-size garages, four-car or even ten-car garages. Housing professionals predict that over the next few decades the norm for new single family houses will become three- and four-car garages. In San Antonio, Texas the owner of a 1,200-square-foot garage – three times the size of a typical 2-car garage – uses it for three cars and many other things. He proclaimed "It's like we can't buy enough machines, and there has to be some place to put them." Sedentary-enhancing machines, like riding lawn mowers and golf carts, require super-size garages.

On average, Americans spend 90 percent of their leisure time in their homes and cars. Blandburb residents increasingly think about escape from sprawl. Some Americans do. "Ex-pats" living in Europe discover they do not need cars for a high quality of life. Europeans make about 45 percent of daily trips by walking and biking, compared to 7 percent for Americans. In Barcelona, Spain, American ex-pat Linda Steck said "We walk extensively, which is very healthy for us. I think the biggest advantage is the sense of community that walking builds. There are 1.5 million people in Barcelona and we have never gone out without seeing somebody we know. Her husband Larry Steck said "Miss owning a car? Absolutely not." Community design makes car-free living possible.

COMPACT DESIGN USES LAND EFFICIENTLY.

Compact land use is smart and sustainable land use. Compact design means minimizing the "footprint" of development on the landscape, especially for greenfield projects; it uses land efficiently, not wastefully and not arrogantly. Compact design saves greenspace, unlike sprawl footprints that defiantly keep growing (see Figure 6-2).

PRINCIPLE: Preserve open space, farmland, natural beauty, and critical environmental areas

CHECKLIST QUESTION:
3. Is compact design used to minimize the amount of land per dwelling unit?

The Baltimore Metropolitan Council found that a typical greenfield sprawl development for 1,000 homes eats up 750 acres of open space, compared to less than 300 acres for compact design development. In the metropolitan Baltimore area, in recent years, only 20 percent of new homes were built at a low density of one home per acre or less, but this share used up three-quarters of all land developed in the region.

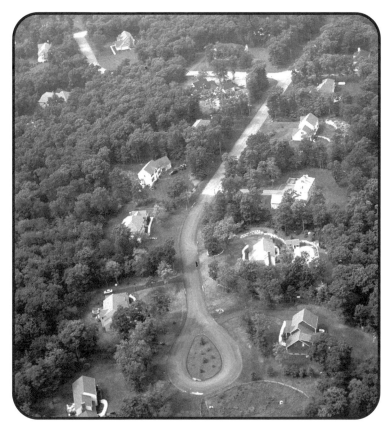

Figure 6-2. Example of inefficient, non-compact land use,
with large houses on large lots within a forested area.

In HEALTHY PLACES, lot sizes are smaller, streets are narrower, set-backs of houses are less (bringing them closer to the street), and there are fewer parking spaces in the commercial areas. Compact design reduces the amount of land needed for streets and utilities. Greenfield HEALTHY PLACES have densities of at least 8 to 10 housing units per acre, and often much higher. Infill projects will usually have 20 units per residential acre or more. Multifamily dwellings reduce land use and can raise residential densities to 30 to 50 units per acre and provide more affordable housing.

Compact land use was once normal. Consider the Minneapolis-St.

Paul, Minnesota metropolitan area. In the older core areas, in 1990 average residential density was 7.9 units per acre, compared to 4.1 in the original, inner ring suburbs, 2.8 in the newer suburbs, and only 2.1 in newly sprawling areas. The 1999 report "Two Roads Diverge: Analyzing Growth Scenarios for the Twin Cities Region," found a need for 389,000 new households from 1995 to 2020 because of a 25 percent increase in population. Smart growth would cut land use would by 65 percent and infrastructure costs by over 50 percent. Similarly, smart growth in the North Atlanta region was found to offer a 48 percent reduction in land use to handle a 24 percent increase in population.

In greenfield projects compact land use destroys less of the original natural resources, compared to paving over up to 40 percent of the land in sprawl projects. In Vermillion, North Carolina, the paved area per dwelling was 634 square feet, compared to 2,018 square feet for a conventional sprawl project designed, engineered, and permitted (but not built) for the same site. More impervious surfaces mean more harmful water runoff and less recharging of aquifers that provide drinking water in many places.

As discussed in Chapter 3, reducing parking space is important to reduce the amount of land paved over. At Coffee Creek Center in Chesterton, Indiana, reducing the number of parking spaces in the town center saved 40 acres and allowed the creation of a town green, an important public gathering place.

Using less land for *individual* homes means saving more land and greenspace for *community* use. In sprawlspace, building is "flat, not tall." With smart growth, building is still flat, but also compact, not spread out. Make no mistake, compact land use is necessary to obtain the benefits of HEALTHY PLACES.

GREENSPACE PROVIDES COMMUNITY WELL-BEING.

Natural beauty sells. The best developers know this. The more trees the better. Everything that preserves open space, farmland, natural beauty, and critical environmental areas provides benefits. Mental and physical health is improved. Economic value of homes is improved. Community life is improved. People enjoy "breathing space."

A Nebraska survey found that 80 percent of people believed it was important for a community to include walking or bicycle paths; 78 percent felt a recreation trail is a strong community asset; 47 percent use trails in their community throughout the year; and the number one reason for not exercising was lack of time.

> **PRINCIPLE: Preserve open space, farmland, natural beauty, and critical environmental areas**
>
> CHECKLIST QUESTION:
> 4. Does the place offer greenspaces throughout the community for public and recreational uses, including continuous green pathways for biking and walking and pocket parks in neighborhoods?

The best greenfield HEALTHY PLACES typically have 20 percent to 50 percent of the total land area as diverse and well-dispersed greenspaces. Interior community greenspaces should be designed for multiple uses, such as parks, sports fields, walking and biking paths, greenways, and often lakes and streams for water activities. Urban infill projects may have as little as 5-percent greenspaces. A special type of development is "conservation design," where some 50 to 70 percent of a greenfield land area is preserved as open space and there is a focus on saving or improving sensitive environmental areas.

Open space serves environmental goals by: preserving natural wildlife and native plant habitats; enhancing surface and ground water quality; providing flood control; and removing air pollution. More selfishly, open space improves community and personal well being by: providing places for physical activities; promoting community pride and civic engagement; providing gathering places; providing community identity and character; providing natural beauty and aesthetic quality; assisting in stress reduction and spiritual enrichment; and increasing property values.

Communities benefit from a balance between architects' design and layout of the built environment with landscape architects' use of the original natural setting to shape community design. For example, a site may have tree lines that define "outdoor rooms" in which development is respectfully placed. Streets can be set so that the sightlines of people driving and walking are aligned with meadows, greens, and trees. House lots can follow the pattern of hedgerows and woodlands. The designer for Tioga, near Gainesville, Florida observed continuous lines of large beautiful trees among the rest. These lines were used to lay out tree-shaded streets and an esplanade between two parallel tree lines. A new built environment inherited old natural beauty, providing residents with an exceptional sense of place.

Harmony in Florida is a premier new town. Seventy percent of the 11,000 acres will be left untouched, including two 500-acre lakes, historic oak trees, and forested wetlands. No homes will be built around the lakes. The $1 billion project will produce a community for some 18,000 residents. Along much of a large golf course there will be a linear pedestrian park, and there will be an aquatic center, playgrounds, ball fields, and pet parks. According to Harmony's website: "We think this is the way to do right by the environment and make money at the same time. ...Harmony was designed with the belief that you can't experience nature from your car. Our goal is that if you live at Harmony you will only need an automobile when you need to leave the community. And we hope that residents will be able to meet most of their needs right here."

Watershed protection is a special need nationwide, and the best designs pay attention to it. Watersheds protect our quality of life; they pay no attention to political boundaries, which is why regional planning is needed. Low Impact Development maintains or replicates the pre-development natural water environment. To minimize water runoff, the fraction of land paved over should not exceed 20 percent to 30 percent.

The Center for Urban and Regional Studies at the University of North Carolina at Chapel Hill matched 50 HEALTHY PLACES (average density of 7.18 dwellings per acre) with 50 sprawl projects (average density of 2.77 units per acre) in five states. They found that HEALTHY PLACES more effectively protect and restore sensitive areas, such as streams, stream banks, and floodplains. The results were best for greenfield projects, although even infill projects performed better than sprawl developments.

Here are examples of successful HEALTHY PLACES satisfying this question, as well as others.

EAST LAKE COMMONS NEAR ATLANTA, GEORGIA. This modest 22-acre development has 67 homes and over 45 percent open space, including a 6-acre community garden, a pond, wetlands, a stream buffer, and a woodland area with nature trails. Two "common" houses offer residents guest bedrooms for visitors, workshop spaces, a children's playroom, a teen center, and community eating facilities. Watershed protection methods are used. Residents decided to keep gravel on the interior street to cut runoff. "Green building" approaches reduce energy use. Neighboring residents were included in the site-design process, and all units in the first phase were pre-sold before construction and there is a long list of people waiting for resales.

RUSSETT IN ANNE ARUNDEL COUNTY, MARYLAND. This older, pre-smart growth HEALTHY PLACE has a design driven by concern to protect natural greenspace, including wetlands and woodlands. It has superior landscaping, many recreational areas, and 11 miles of trails through the 613 acres and 3,700 diverse homes. A resident boasted: "The design encourages walking. The kids can walk to the library or the Wal-Mart. The design tries to change the mentality of car dependence."

COFFEE CREEK CENTER IN CHESTERTON, INDIANA. This 640-acre site retains nearly a third of the land area as open space, including parks, playgrounds and nature preserves, even though all but 17 acres could have been built on. Some 2,000 residential units are planned, for a population of about 7,000. The creek runs through about 200 acres of the site. Paths in areas adjacent to homes lead into woods. The local watershed is being restored to its original condition. A 6,000 square foot open pavilion with large limestone fireplaces is adjacent to a 5-acre meadow, and an amphitheater seats 500 people alongside a cascading waterfall and 50-foot fountain. The wide housing mix includes: apartments, townhomes, and single-family homes, from small cottage homes to large estate houses. Buildings are oriented to use solar energy for day lighting and energy production through photovoltaics. The innovative Coffee Creek Congress empowers residents and community workers "to foster their vision of their community," focus on quality of life initiatives, and foster community relationships.

CIVANO IN TUCSON, ARIZONA. This 1,145-acre community has 35 percent of land dedicated to open space, mostly as natural desert wildlands, and also community orchards and trails. A key goal is to connect people to each other and to the unique Sonoran Desert. The initial neighborhood will have gathering places such as coffee shops, cafes, parks, public plazas and small commercial enterprises within the one-acre Neighborhood Center complex that is within walking distance from homes. For every acre developed, 50 desert trees and plants are salvaged for use in the community. Native, drought-tolerant plants and passive solar shading saves water. Homes feature two sets of water systems: a potable one and one for distributing reclaimed water for non-edible plant irrigation. For the initial constructed area, potable water use has been reduced by 61 percent and heating and cooling energy use by 56 percent, as compared to typical sprawl projects in the Tucson area. Passive and active solar methods are used. A design goal was reducing local vehicle miles by 40 percent.

One Civano family said this about their experience: "We have always wanted to settle down in a community where people try to live in harmony with the Sonoran Desert. When we saw the pedestrian-oriented streets lined with reclaimed mesquite trees, we knew this was the place for us. We built an adobe home with a view of the Rincon Mountains. We use more solar energy, less water, and spend more time on our front porch."

MILL CREEK IN KANE COUNTY, ILLINOIS. This 1,500-acre site will have some 2,000 homes and a mixed-use town center with two and three story buildings with retail, offices and loft apartments. The central village green contains flowers, ponds, and park benches. Clustered homes face woods, parks, open land and Mill Creek that meanders through the site. More than 43 percent of the site will remain open space, including 127 acres of preserved wetlands. Some 15 miles of hiking, biking, and jogging trails have access to a regional trail system. To protect the creek, wastewater is treated on site through an aeration lagoon on the edge of the development. Storm water is absorbed by the considerable open space, and is also treated by vegetation. Recycled water irrigates a golf course. Short driveways and narrow streets cut runoff.

ALDEA DE SANTA FE, NEAR SANTA FE, NEW MEXICO. "It's designed for people, not cars," according to Arthur Fields, one of its founders who lives there. The 345-acre project will have 476 homes of varying types, clustered together so that 60 percent of the land remains open space. A commercial plaza "will be the heart of the community" and will include a café, restaurant, community market, and support services for home-based offices.

Issaquah Highlands, outside Seattle, Washington. Five neighborhoods will have 1,400 single family houses, 1,000 condominiums, and 850 apartments for near 7,000 residents. "Green building" techniques are being used. Seventy percent of the 2,200 acres will be permanently preserved as parks, play areas, ball fields, picnic areas, forest, trails, and a natural amphitheater in an area famous for its natural beauty.

River Park, Oxnard, California. This 700-acre project will have 2,800 homes, 2.5 million square feet of commercial space, three public schools, a fire station, police center, post office, and library. One-third of the land will be kept as an extensive system of parks, open spaces, sports fields, jogging trails, and pedestrian pathways distributed throughout the community. Original mining pits were converted into water storage and recharge basins to serve as a regional water resource and to provide visual and recreational amenities for residents.

The Villages of Urbana, Maryland. This new town will have 3,500 dwellings, a commercial main street, and a 100-acre park. Several historic buildings have been restored. An early 63-year old resident said "We love this place. It's the first home we owned with a sidewalk."

Greenspace makes commercial sense for developers because it sells well. One developer in San Diego County found that he could increase house prices by 25 percent by reducing housing units by 15 percent and adding open space corridors visible from every home. Greenspaces mean more greenbacks for builders and later homeowners when they sell.

Saving wetlands matters. The Bush Administration's showed its hypocrisy when for Earth Day 2004, President George W. Bush talked about protecting 3 million acres of wetlands while visiting Rookery Bay in Collier County, Florida. Earlier, in 2003, Bruce Boler resigned his U.S. EPA position to protect wetlands in sprawling Lee and Collier Counties. He had blocked permits issued by the Army Corps of Engineers. Developers were angry. Their dirty trick was creating the Water Enhancement & Restoration Center which paid for a study that was accepted by EPA, the state, and the Corps as "sound science." Now, wetlands *cause* pollution rather than clean it; they no longer are "nature's kidneys." "It's pseudo-science with no peer review or public input," complained Ann Hauk with the Council of Civic Associations. The "junk science" enabled the Bush-appointed EPA Region 4 Administrator to stop backing Boler's efforts. If Jeb Bush's developer-corrupted Florida had no problem with a project, then George Bush's EPA would go along. Boler said "It was like the politics trumped the science." The final irony was that Boler had tried to stop the Winding Cypress sprawl project impacting nearly 200 acres of wetlands protecting Rookery Bay, the place of disgrace where President Bush received lots of press coverage. Florida got 2,300 more sprawl homes and another golf course. Did they make those more than wetlands?

Also around Earth Day 2004 the Gainesville, Florida City Commission changed its wetlands regulations to make them easier to build on. The mayor voted against it, saying the city was selling out to developers: "You are taking a wetland and saying, 'Fill it in and sell it.' …This is a sad, sad day for the city of Gainesville." In May 2004 the St. Tammany Parish Council in Louisiana granted the appeal of developers and overturned the Planning Commission rejection of a subdivision on land with 62 percent wetlands; the group Advocates for Smart Growth went to court and one of its leaders got a phone death threat he thought was connected to his opposition to the subdivision.

STREETS MUST BE INVITING TO PEOPLE.

Tenho Jackson is in his late 80s and able to walk three miles a day and sometimes twice a day in the Wyndhurst community in Lynchburg, Virginia. He can walk across the street from his continuing care facility to an eye doctor, a gift store and a coffee shop. "This is an ideal location to walk without [obstacles that] make it difficult," he said. Candy is dandy, but sidewalks are sweeter and less fattening. In blandburbs streets are for cars. In HEALTHY PLACES streets are for people. Roads are about getting there, streets are about being there – they are for enjoyable living not just cars. Automobile addicts use streets as quickly as they can. HEALTHY PLACE residents enjoy *their* streets.

Public disgust with traffic congestion has sharpened the focus on streets. A survey found that 53 percent of people consider an easy walk to stores extremely important, and 49 percent said that they prefer a less auto-oriented street pattern, with narrow streets to encourage walking. Sixty-one percent of Americans support use of state or local funds for more sidewalks, and 71 percent support mandatory sidewalks in new developments. Residents also want streets to be in good physical shape. A survey of over 2,000 people in South Carolina found that people were twice as likely to walk at least 30 minutes on most days if they thought that neighborhood sidewalks were well maintained; this was independent of gender, race, age, and education. Walkaholics become angry about cracked and pot-holed sidewalks.

PRINCIPLE: Foster walkable, close-knit neighborhoods

CHECKLIST QUESTION:
5. Do streets have sidewalks and connectedness to promote easy and safe walking and multiple paths for travel through the community?

Streets should be interesting, pretty, shaded, and connected to other streets and destinations within their neighborhood and community. Tom D'Alesandro, developer of Clarksburg in Maryland, emphasized: "You need to design with the pedestrian in mind. When you're walking, something new has to be happening about every 20-30 feet to keep your interest."

Counter-intuitively, more streets are typically found in old historic towns than in similarly sized sprawl developments, but they are narrower and the blocks shorter. Drivers in older cities and towns have lots of streets to choose from, not just a few big ones. Blandburbs have too few small streets; they rely on wide collector and arterial roads to funnel cars in and out of subdivisions, rather than dispersing traffic through several access roads, to reduce congestion (see Figure 6-3).

Below are some basic characteristics of streets that fairly serve people and cars. One thing to remember is that street environments that are interesting from inside a car are likely to be boring to pedestrians.

Conversely, streets that are interesting and safe for pedestrians will not be especially welcomed by motorists who are infrequent pedestrians.

STREET DESIGN:

Narrow streets are safer because they reduce car speed. They increase the sense of community and the feeling of neighborliness. They reduce water runoff. The consensus favors 26 feet from curb to curb. Sprawl subdivision streets are often 32 to 36 feet, which increases injury accidents about 5 times the rate for the narrower streets. Narrow streets do not interfere with fire and emergency vehicles.

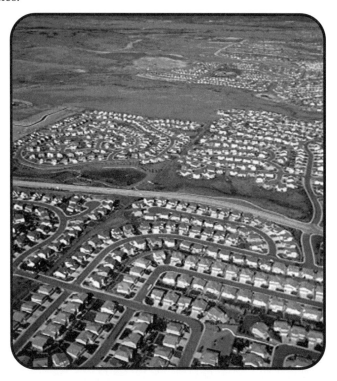

Figure 6-3. Sprawl subdivisions showing single collector streets for accessing homes with connection to an arterial road, and cul-de-sac-streets with cookie-cuter houses.

A grid pattern of short blocks with lots of intersecting streets disperse traffic, promote walking, and provide multiple, shorter routes to destinations closer to "as the crow flies" than indirect routes in sprawl mazes.

Streets and sidewalks should be connected to greenspaces and surrounding neighborhoods and destinations so that vehicle use is reduced.

Wide sidewalks make walking easy, especially for two people walking side-by-side. The minimum width is 5 feet in residential streets, and much wider in commercial streets and high traffic roads, such as from 8 to 12 feet. *A residential area without sidewalks is the hallmark of sprawl un-places.* As Margaret Mead said, "Any town that doesn't have sidewalks doesn't love its children."

A HEALTHY PLACE has well designed streets with frequent trees (see Figure 6-4 below). A "nature" strip of land between the sidewalk and the curb protects pedestrians; it must be wide enough for planting trees frequently to provide beauty and shade. Wider commercial streets can have a green median with trees and plants.

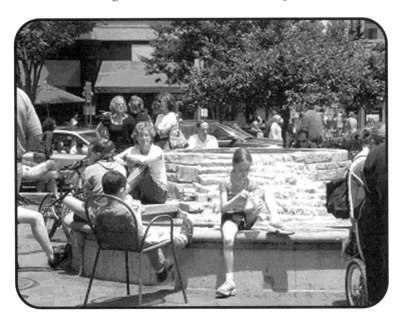

Figure 6-4. Type of street people like, with shops easily accessible, trees, benches, bike racks, outdoor eating, and trash receptacles that help keep sidewalks clean.

Ample, well-marked street crossings or crosswalks are essential for pedestrian safety.

Bike lanes are necessary to maximize safety, unless the sidewalks are very wide or there are alternative paths or greenways for bikers.

Cul-de-sacs are not smart, because they fragment the area and reduce street connectivity and walkability. (Unless there is a system of paths or trails that link residential properties together between cul-de-sacs, but this is rare.)

STREET ENVIRONMENT:
Homes should be close to the sidewalks (small setbacks) to provide "eyes on the street." There should either be no fences, or low ones, say 3-feet-high.

On-street parking slows cars and provides a buffer between sidewalk pedestrians and moving cars.

Put garages and alleys behind houses to make streets pedestrian friendly.

Excellent lighting is necessary to provide comfort and safety. Commercial streets need street "furniture," such as public art, benches, flower and shrub planters, kiosks, trash receptacles, and bike racks that do not interfere with pedestrians.

Entrances to buildings and shops should be close to sidewalks to support social interaction and "street life." But not delivery and parking lot entrances should not be close to sidewalks.

Street design that reduces traffic promotes neighborliness, social capital and physical activity. Some pioneering work by University of California, Berkeley Professor Donald Appleyard obtained concrete evidence for this connection. He studied three streets in San Francisco that looked alike but had different levels of traffic. Light Street carried 2,000 vehicles daily, Medium Street carried 8,000 vehicles, and Heavy Street carried 16,000 vehicles.

Surveys of residents revealed that those on Light Street had three more friends and twice as many acquaintances as the people on Heavy Street. Another finding was about what residents defined as their "home territory." On Light Street there was a close knit neighborhood where residents made full use of the street. For example, front steps were used for sitting and chatting, and sidewalks and the roadway itself were used by children playing. As traffic volume increased, the space people considered to be their territory shrank. People on Heavy Street had fewer friends and acquaintances because there was less immediate area in which to interact socially with neighbors; there was little feeling of community. People withdrew into their homes and avoided street activity and gardening. People even abandoned the front rooms of their homes because of traffic noise. Medium Street fell between the extremes. Residents on Medium and Heavy streets were motivated to relocate and lose long-term relationships. Appleyard concluded: "The contrast between the two streets [Heavy and Light] was striking. On the one hand alienation, on the other friendliness and involvement."

"Traffic calming" techniques alter driver behavior and make streets better for residents. Unlike traditional actions, such as traffic lights and stop signs, they are preventive and self-regulating. Narrow, well-landscaped streets with parked cars and bike lanes slow traffic. Small traffic circles or roundabouts at more heavily used intersections reduce accident rates in the range of 60 to 80 percent. The Insurance Institute for Highway Safety found that when roundabouts replaced traffic lights injury crashes dropped 75 percent and delays decreased by 20 percent. Other measures are raised center islands that narrow street width at a specific location, and raised and textured crosswalks which cut pedestrian accidents by a factor of 10.

Drivers find speed humps and bumps obnoxious but walkers should like them because they slow traffic and make streets safer. There is the story of a young child who told of his mom's dislike of a large neighborhood speed hump, but who also noted that "now she lets me walk to school." The Institute of Transportation Engineers found that on one street they reduced speed by 31 percent and traffic by 6 percent. A five-year study in Oakland, California found that children living within one block of a speed hump are 50 to 60 percent less likely to be injured by a car as compared to children whose streets lacked humps. Oakland installed 1,600 speed humps and child pedestrian deaths and injuries dropped 15 percent from 1995 to 2003.

Traffic calming to reduce auto speeds is critical. The probability of a pedestrian being killed when a vehicle is traveling at 15 mph is 3.5 percent, which increases to 37 percent if the car speed increases to just 31 mph, and to 83 percent at 44 mph. The problem is the rapidly increasing distance for stopping a car as the speed increases and the greater difficulty in seeing pedestrians. For sure, if streets are to serve people, then car speeds must be reliably reduced.

Reducing traffic volume, slowing car speeds, and reducing traffic noise improve communities by encouraging interactions among residents on the street. In one case, reducing average vehicle speeds from 25 miles per hour to 12 miles per hour on residential streets reduced noise to less than one-tenth its initial level. Reducing car speeds also increase property values. Who has thought about that? One study found that reducing traffic speeds by 5 to 10 mph increased adjacent residential property values by roughly 20 percent. A study found that reducing volumes on residential streets by several hundred cars per day increased home values by an average of 18 percent. A multi-street grid pattern with shorter blocks reduces street car volume.

A great thinker about planning and cities, Jane Jacobs, made this point: "Streets and their sidewalks, the main public places of a city, are its most vital organs." This is true for all communities. *Like wires conducting electricity, street networks can distribute social capital.* After a few months in I'On Village in South Carolina, a resident said: "Now I see the point. The homes are within talking distance of passersby and each other, which allows for more intimate conversations with your neighbors, allows you to get to know each other so much better."

LOWER COST HOMES SHOULD NOT STAND OUT.

The composition of American households has changed. Families with children should no longer dictate residential development. Now, housing is needed for diverse groups, including singles, couples without children, empty nesters, retirees, and an aging population. Less than 35 percent of the new households formed between 1995 and 2000 consisted of married couples with children. More than 40 percent were singles or unrelated people living together. Another 22 percent were single parents with children.

HEALTHY PLACES include housing for a range of income levels, preferably including affordable housing for low- and modest-income people, sometimes called workforce housing. This usually means multifamily buildings and rental units. Diverse types of housing should be in close proximity to each other, sometimes on the same block. In the best designed communities, *the lower cost homes do not visibly stand out.* They all blend harmoniously together because the quality and design of multifamily buildings is comparable to single-family houses.

PRINCIPLE: Create a range of housing opportunities and choices

CHECKLIST QUESTION:
6. Are there different types of mixed-income homes, such as single-family detached, multifamily units, condos, and affordable housing?

The Washington Post ran a front-page story with the headline "Find the Affordable Housing in This Picture." Photographs showed virtually identical houses in the 61-acre Carrington development hear Tysons Corner, Virginia with 105 homes. One was a large $840,000 detached estate house, and the contained four affordable townhomes that sold for $125,000 each. In the four-unit building, only one entrance door was visible from the street, just like the estate house. The goal? Buyers of the estate houses should not be "turned off" by the affordable housing units.

Units with ground-floor stores or offices that allow residents to walk downstairs to work are gaining popularity. Community amenities and the public realm become more valuable. In one place, live-work units contained a real-estate agent, concierge, day-care center, hair salon, a recording studio, insurance agent, and magazine publisher.

As to telecommuting or telework, modeling shows that for every 3 percent of commuters who work at home on a given day, traffic delays would drop by 10 percent. But this benefit quickly disappears if those people use their vehicles to run errands during the day, which is more likely for sprawl residents than those in HEALTHY PLACES. Moreover, telework appeals more to those living longer distances from work and clearly promotes outlying sprawl.

Why should you care about the diversity of homes in a neighborhood or community? First, if you value social and economic diversity, an inclusive rather than an exclusive community, then having a range of housing types is mandatory. There is no room for compromise.

Second, HEALTHY PLACE residents can move from one home to another *within that community* as they age, family status changes, or finances change. "Lifecycle housing" is a nice option to have. Parents or children may be able to join you. Social capital decreases when Americans anticipate moving; they do not invest time and energy in their community. When older people leave a community in which they have lived for many years, illness and death can result. Surveys have consistently found that 95 percent of older adults want to remain in their homes as they age. But in blandland, they face high costs to make their homes elder-friendly and driving can become unsafe. The "retirement community" concept is part of the sprawl culture. Louis Joyner is in his 50s, semi-retired and chose the diverse I'On community. "I couldn't even comprehend living in a situation without all ages," he said. "I am interacting with 20-year olds and 80-year olds, just by being out walking." Agnes Carr is a senior who lives in King Farm; she said "The environment is nice; it's safe, but it's not dull – you wouldn't want to be in one of those places that's all seniors." As a walkaholic, she observed "I absolutely do not see a large percentage of obese people in the street."

Third, to get the many benefits of extensive community public spaces, higher residential densities are needed, and this means having a mix of housing types, particularly multifamily units.

A major need is affordable housing for lower and moderate incomes, often defined as family incomes less than 60 percent or sometimes 80 percent of the area's median income. Teachers, police, firefighters, restaurant and retail workers should be able to live in the same community where they work. They bring an important perspective to any community that they both live and work in. These lower and moderate income people can benefit financially from reducing their dependence on cars. Many developers include affordable housing because of a government requirement or because of government subsidies. Jurisdictions often give a density bonus to a developer, allowing them to build more homes on a site than would otherwise be allowed.

Many HEALTHY PLACES have single family houses with optional accessory units or "granny flats," usually above rear garages. These are small apartments that homeowners can rent out to help cover mortgage costs. Doing so makes houses more affordable while at the same time creating affordable rental housing.

Here are some examples of first rate communities, over a broad size range, with diverse housing.

HARBOR TOWN, MEMPHIS, TENNESSEE. This early and outstanding mixed-use, pedestrian-friendly community has some 900 homes in three districts. It is a bridge away from downtown. Its mix of housing includes apartments, townhomes, and large single family houses that are distributed throughout the community and blend harmoniously together. Some apartments are above shops. Some of the townhouses are cleverly grouped together, giving the appearance of a giant mansion instead of a building with 6 or 8 separate units.

BALDWIN PARK, FLORIDA. Its 3,600 homes will include 1,300 rental apartments, 1,200 detached houses for sale, and 1,100 attached for sale units.

CRAWFORD SQUARE, PITTSBURGH, PENNSYLVANIA. This infill project on 17.5 acres is very close to downtown employment and cultural centers; it has about 500 homes, some single family detached houses for sale, townhouses for sale and rent, and apartments for rent. Half the units are subsidized affordable housing. Residents are diverse. Excellent building designs give a visual impression that all the units are high quality owner-occupied homes. There is no stigma of low-income housing. There are lots of front porches, three parks, and close-by shopping.

THE VILLAGE OF WESTCLAY, NEAR INDIANAPOLIS, INDIANA. There is a real mixture of affordable apartments, brownstones, cottages, village houses, and multi-million dollar estate houses, plus an green infrastructure including pocket parts everywhere.

THE CROSSINGS, MOUNTAIN VIEW, CALIFORNIA. Built on a former strip mall site, it has a density of 22 units per acre; there are 350 single-family houses, townhomes, row houses, and apartments. Residents can easily walk to shops, nearby offices, and the CalTrain commuter station. On the 18 acre site are parks, wide sidewalks, lush landscaping, pedestrian paths, and tree-lined streets that give a feeling of spaciousness. Bandstands and tot-lots within parks promote gatherings.

WESTMINSTER PLACE, ST. LOUIS, MISSOURI. Homes for some 1,000 people of all ages and incomes include two-story garden apartments, townhomes, single family houses, an assisted living facility for seniors, and a low-income seniors housing property. It has tree-lined sidewalks and a community pool. The community is close to nearby jobs, a bustling retail center, and a new magnet high school.

NORTHWEST CROSSING, BEND, OREGON. Housing for about 4,000 people includes townhomes, condominiums, cottages, duplexes, small apartment buildings, live/work spaces, accessory dwellings, and apartments over offices and stores in the town center. Life-cycle housing is part of the project's marketing.

STAPLETON, DENVER, COLORADO. The Workforce Housing Program will have some 10 percent of 8,000 homes as affordable housing, with a 30-year price restriction to maintain affordability. Plus 20 percent of some 4,000 rental apartments will be affordable housing. Seniors will have affordable housing in a 100-unit community for those over 55 years of age; it will be located near a 30-acre park and adjacent to a town center with stores.

CARPENTER VILLAGE, NORTH CAROLINA. In this 350-acre community, just outside Raleigh, residents can easily walk to shop, dine and run errands. On one side of the town green are 330 low-rise apartments. Branching out from the apartments are townhomes and single family houses. There are pocket parks, swimming pools, tennis courts and other recreational amenities. It is estimated that the design will reduce auto trips by 50 percent, compared to a typical sprawl development.

RIVERPARK, OXNARD, CALIFORNIA. The need for new affordable housing is a major issue in California because of its rapid population growth. In this project, affordable housing will total 27 percent, with another 4 percent set aside for very low income housing which is needed in this area for farm-workers.

HIGHLANDS GARDEN VILLAGE, DENVER, COLORADO. Diverse housing includes single-family houses with carriage homes, townhomes, artists' studios, senior housing, apartments, and cohousing (cooperative) units for a total of 290 units, with 20 percent affordable housing, on a relatively small 27-acre site that includes a network of paths, parks and gardens with space for arts and culture activities. Reduced car ownership and use is supported by nearby public transit and the availability of two Zipcars, fueled by natural gas, which can be rented by residents. The overall residential density is 20 units per acre.

Gentrification remains a tough issue for urban infill projects that from a smart growth perspective may be very good, except for displacing original lower income residents for the sake of urban revitalization. Though nearly all criticism of smart growth comes from the conservative right, the liberal left has also criticized smart growth for promoting gentrification. Tom Wetzel summed up the case in *ZNet* magazine in July 2004: "Lacking any program for democratization of land use, and no way of ensuring access of all income levels to affordable housing and urban amenities, the New Urbanist vision is in danger of being merely a façade, a set of vague slogans to legitimize the agendas of capitalist developers. Like their right-wing 'free market' opponents, New Urbanists do not challenge capitalist control of investment in the built environment. What is needed is a more bottom-up, grassroots approach that increases community participation and control over land use." Providing truly affordable housing in new development is essential and even giving priority access to original residents. A new solution is "community land trusts" that acquire land, control development and ensure long term affordability; another approach is community based planning and design as presented in Chapter 7.

Minnesota's Metropolitan Council found that 94 percent of people thought it was important to have a variety of housing types at different cost levels for people who work in a community; and 73 percent agreed that there was a need for lifecycle housing in their community. Too many projects called smart growth, New Urbanist, or Traditional Neighborhood Development lack diversity of housing types and a price range to accommodate different income levels. This omission should not be ignored.

The developers of Serenbe, outside Atlanta, Georgia, designed for 220 homes promised that the Village Coffee Shop/Bakery "will be built during the initial construction of the first residential units." The key founders, Marie and Steve Nygren, planned on moving into the development, a good sign. But in three new urban villages outside Seattle, Washington the promise of a live, work, and play community was not realized five or more years after the three developments were started. Though half completed with 12,000 residents, Issaquah Highlands, Snoqualmie Ridge and Redmond Ridge have been criticized for not delivering local shopping and jobs. Issaquah resident Maria Carlson noted "Just because a developer shows you a map with things on it, it doesn't mean those will actually occur." For the Civano project discussed above, in 2004, the nation's largest home builder Pulte Homes bought much of the land, on which three-quarters of the homes will be built. But they were not going to include the mixed-use centers in the original plan for the two neighborhoods.

> **PRINCIPLE: Make development decisions predictable, fair, and cost-effective**
>
> CHECKLIST QUESTION:
> 7. Has the developer made clear how build-out over time will be faithful to the original plan and vision?

Larger projects may require 20 or more years to fully implement. Developers should present realistic plans for construction of different phases and assurances that build-out will be consistent with the original vision. Two of the biggest and most controversial smart growth projects in the nation are planned in California. Centennial in northern Los Angeles County is planned for 23,000 homes in 12 villages on 12,000 acres, with 50 percent open space and 1.3 jobs per home. Newhall Ranch is 40 miles south of Centennial and is planned for 21,000 homes. Both would be home to more than 130,000 people. A concern for such huge projects is whether they will be built according to their original plans, and whether vehicle use will be sharply reduced because residents can stay within their neighborhoods and communities for most needs.

Regardless of initial regulatory approvals, governments provide many opportunities for departing from an original approved plan. While some housing is done early, other important mixed uses, such as office buildings, civic buildings, and retail, may not be constructed due to changed circumstances. Or a shopping mall may be built first with the promise of housing to come later. Maintaining the commitment to the original smart growth vision requires vigilance by residents. When developers live in their own community it is a good sign of long-term commitment.

Money for public services and infrastructure may not be available when needed to meet the needs of a planned build-out. With developers and builders rarely paying all such costs through impact fees, local jurisdictions often face fiscal problems. Taxpayers may vote against school bond issues and money for road expansion may not become available, for example. Developers often get land in unincorporated county areas annexed by nearby towns or cities to insure public services. Without sufficient impact fees, taxpayers in the jurisdiction get hit. The town of Smyrna in Delaware annexed 500 acres that the county and state did not want developed, prompting legislators to introduce a bill to stop such annexations. Smyna's mayor at the time was a real estate agent.

Two necessities that Americans take for granted are becoming problematic: water and energy. Consumers' faith in sprawl developers and government agencies is misplaced. Sprawl development has resulted in high rates of water and energy use. Water and energy conservation measures are important but not prevalent. A large house and lot are not much of an American dream if water and electricity are not there when the faucet is turned and the switch flipped.

Water supply has surfaced as a major issue in some Western states, especially because of the worst drought in more than 500 years. The water supply problem in California finally caused the state to pass a landmark law in 2001. It compels developers of projects with 500 or more homes to demonstrate an adequate water supply for 20 years. Major sprawl projects have already been stopped. But developers are now motivated to build projects with 499 homes or less. Water is also an issue in other states with rampant sprawl. The unrelenting growth in the Las Vegas, Nevada area has led to a $2 billion plan to build a huge system of pipelines to bring water from rural deep wells, some as far as 250 miles. Forget rural residents, the priority is maintaining sprawl growth, as the head of the regional water authority said: "The notion that we have a finite supply of water, and when that finite supply is gone you stop growing, is in the past." And who will be paying for this save-sprawl-with-pipeline strategy also being pursued in Texas, Utah and Colorado? Not developers through impact fees, but all taxpayers, unless these projects are blocked.

Electricity brownouts have plagued many places. Siting transmission towers and lines for electricity and cell phone towers pose a difficult problem. Sprawl residents do not want them in their backyards, nor wind farms with tall turbine windmills to generate non-polluting renewable energy. Increasing energy consumption because of larger homes aggravates the transmission problem. Higher residential density helps reduce energy consumption for heating and cooling, especially for multifamily and smaller units. New York State rural homes use the most energy per dwelling, while the lowest energy consuming area is high density Manhattan.

Except for fully built-out HEALTHY PLACEs, residents must stay engaged in continuous place-making. This is easier if they become more time-rich because they spend less time driving.

SMART LAND USE PREVENTS DISASTERS.

Do not depend on government to prohibit development in areas that are vulnerable to unsafe natural hazards, or the insurance industry to provide effective economic disincentives.

PRINCIPLE: Preserve open space, farmland, natural beauty, and critical environmental areas

CHECKLIST QUESTION:
8. Does the location avoid increasing the risk or negative impacts of natural disasters?

Natural hazards are *threats*; they turn into *disasters* when the built environment intersects with extreme events of nature. Preventing disasters means not placing homes and people in the path of strong natural forces, such as hurricanes, wildfires, and floods. Too much development has taken place in areas prone to natural hazards. Coastal lands are home for more than half the U.S. population, but comprise only 13 percent of the total land area. More reason to worry about sea level rise resulting from global warming. Development along the Atlantic and Gulf coasts has been remarkable, with the population increasing over 100 percent from 26 million in 1950 to 53 million in 2000. In 1998, more than 50,000 housing units were built on barrier islands from Maine to Texas, double the construction rate of 1992. Coastal population density has skyrocketed. In 1960 it was 187 people per square mile, rising to 273 in 1994, and projected to rise to 327 by 2015, according to the National Oceanic and Atmospheric Administration. The average population density for the entire nation is just 76 people per square mile.

Seaside sprawl developers turn hazards into disasters. Rows of McMansions that bully shorelines offer great views for their occupants. But shore sprawl kills scenic views for the general public, either from the land or the beach. Coastal house size keeps increasing because of a booming rental business. In North Carolina, a 10,000-square-foot house with 16 bedrooms was built as a single-family house to skirt some development limitations; it will rent for as much as $20,000 a week. Lots cost from $500,000 to $1 million in North Carolina coastal areas.

A University of North Carolina study noted: "Human activity is routinely located so that it creates a serious threat to ourselves as well as to a wide variety of natural resources and functions, many of which are beneficial to people as well as valuable in and of themselves as part of an interrelated living ecosystem." In reality, the built environment is not nearly as resilient or recuperative as the natural environment. Development inevitably exacerbates the impacts on nature and people from periodic hazardous events, and in some cases actually precipitates a disaster. For protecting public health and safety, smart land use means not locating new development in places with likely strong natural events. And engineering controls, such as levees for controlling floods or jetties to control beach erosion, often just relocate adverse impacts.

Many homeowners expect the government to always bail them out when disaster strikes. This may change. After hurricane Fran in 1996 the federal government spent $850 million in North Carolina alone. Most attempts at stemming development in hurricane-threatened coastal shore areas have failed. The 1982 Federal Coastal Barrier Resources Act, for example, withholds federal money for roads, utilities, disaster relief and flood insurance for designated environmentally fragile coastal locations not yet developed in 1982. It has not stopped developers, who go ahead, often with local and state government support. For example, in North Topsail Beach, North Carolina, in the middle of a federal zone, 960 houses and condos were built; the town paid no attention to the federal law. Its mayor is in the real estate business.

Steve Lopez wrote in the *Los Angeles Times* about the massive wildfires in Southern California in October 2003, that killed 25 people and destroyed over 3,600 homes: "we're witnessing the inevitable consequence of insane land management, and generations of public officials rolling over for developers despite past lessons. ...we wouldn't have had so many homes and lives in harm's way if planners and politicians didn't cave to developers."

According to the state forestry service some 7.2 million homes in California – more than half the state's total – are vulnerable to wildfires; the situation is similar in Washington and Oregon. In New Mexico, only 2 percent of land is vulnerable to wildfires, but it contains 80 percent of the state homes.

The massive costs to government – taxpayers – of coping with inevitable disasters mean that poorly sited housing is being subsidized. The Federal Emergency Management Agency has recognized the sprawl-hazard connection in its report "Planning for a Sustainable Future – The Link Between Hazard Mitigation and Livability":

Land development patterns over the past several decades have emphasized sprawling suburban communities and homes constructed with little or no attention paid to protection against high winds, flooding, wildfire, or other natural hazards. ...We allow some people to build in environmentally sensitive areas susceptible to natural hazards, and then we pay to help them recover when disaster strikes. This is not sound environmental or fiscal policy.

Another problem is developing land prone to flooding from heavy rains. Government permits based on average rainfall do little to protect homeowners from flooding during frequent non-average events. Pat Northey of Deltona, Florida, and a member of the County Council said in 2003: "We're opening up lots of marginal land for development. Why do we, as politicians and elected officials, every time a developer comes in with a zoning change, we grant it? We have to quit doing that." But throughout central Florida such vulnerable land is being rapidly developed.

Developers of genuine HEALTHY PLACES take better approaches, such as reducing the risk and impacts of wildfires through compact land use that avoids isolated large home sites embedded in forests; reducing the impacts of mudslides by not building on steep hillsides; not developing land near earthquake fault lines; not building in sensitive coastal areas; and not removing or leveling sand dunes that lower impacts from hurricanes. A terrific house in a well-designed community but in a dangerous location is unhealthy.

PEOPLE WANT QUALITY TRANSIT.

Anne Vu lives in a transit-oriented community in Carlsbad, California; she commutes by trains and walks almost everywhere, including to the grocery store and the beach. "We don't have to get in a car anymore. I haven't had to drive in a long time," she said. A quality "car-free" lifestyle *is* possible. Twenty percent of households in Arlington County, Virginia areas and 16 percent in several Maryland areas have no cars because they are close to Metro rail stations.

PRINCIPLE: Provide a variety of transportation choices

CHECKLIST QUESTION:
9. Is there convenient access to public transit?
For larger projects, does transit operate within the community?

"Transit-oriented developments" and "transit villages" provide easy access to public transit. The Federal Transit Administration's report "An Evaluation of the Relationships Between Transit and Urban Form," summarized abundant evidence that higher residential density and closeness to transit reduce car use substantially. A Metropolitan Transportation Commission (California) study found that in traditionally designed, higher density, mixed-use residential neighborhoods, 34 percent of daily trips were by walking and transit, compared to 11 percent in sprawl subdivisions. Other work found residents near stations are five times more likely to use transit than the average resident, and transit use drops off as distance to homes increase, which means high density is decisive. Convenience means a walk to transit within 15 minutes. Housing densities above 10 to 15 units per residential acre support transit; transit villages usually have 20 to 25 units per acre. Affordable housing in transit-friendly projects is critical to serve lower income people.

Residential property near transit has higher value. In Dallas a study found that existing property near light rail increased 25 percent over comparable property not near the rail line. In the Washington, D.C. metropolitan area, residential property near a Metro station costs $6 to $8 more per square foot than more distant properties. Home owners in transit-friendly locations will surely do well, because transit is rapidly becoming more popular and important. Mounting traffic congestion serves a useful "feedback" role. It is "driving" more and more people away from sprawl and to public transit. Public transit is up 23 percent since 1995, and is now at the highest level in 40 years. Public transportation use has been increasing at nearly twice the rate of car use in recent years. Improved and expanded transit systems, development near transit, and "Guaranteed Ride Home" programs have helped.

Despite automobile addiction, support for public transportation is strong. A 2003 national survey of adults for the American Public Transportation Association found these strong results: 81 percent agreed that increased public investment in public transportation would strengthen the economy, create jobs, reduce traffic congestion and air pollution, and save energy; 72 percent support the use of public funds for the expansion and improvement of public transportation. While strongest in urban places, this support held in suburban, small town, and rural locations.

A 2004 national survey by Associated Press found that 51 percent of respondents believed that the higher priority for government spending is expanding public transportation, versus 46 percent for building more roads. In the congested Atlanta region, a survey found that 61 percent think that the long-term solution for traffic congestion is expanding mass transit and creating communities that allow for shorter trips, compared to just 22 percent supporting new road building. Already, some 6.4 million people nationwide use public transit to commute to work.

A 2001 national survey found that the best reason for using transit was avoiding traffic and congestion (35 percent), saving money (28 percent), avoiding road rage and aggressive unsafe drivers (19 percent), and cutting commute time significantly (9 percent). These results are consistent with the survey result that 62 percent of people say that traffic congestion is worsening in their communities, and two-thirds expect it will be even worse in five years. The Associated Press poll found that about two-thirds of drivers allow more time for travel because of traffic problems. Nowadays, you must expect getting stuck in traffic.

For public transportation to succeed, it must be high quality and competitive in cost, time, convenience, and flexibility to cars. An analysis of 39 urban areas over one million in population showed that as public transit systems increased in size on a per capita basis so did their per capita use. Another study found that over half of Americans have public transit available, but less than one-third believe it is satisfactory, making it uncompetitive for a significant number of people. When given a good choice many people choose quality transit over their cars:

More than one third of the San Diego Trolley riders choose it over their automobiles.

Over 60 percent of the St. Louis MetroLink light rail system's riders formerly drove to work.

In Portland, Oregon, 75 percent of riders said they could drive but choose transit.

In Salt Lake City, 45 percent of light rail riders were new to public transit; in Denver it was 39 percent.

Public transit is more likely for infill HEALTHY PLACES in urban and older suburban areas, because the population base needed to support the system is available. Not so for HEALTHY PLACES built on the outskirts of developed areas. But HEALTHY PLACES are more likely than blandburbs to have people who know each other and use van- and car-pool arrangements. For large HEALTHY PLACES, with thousands of residents and major employment centers, internal transit is feasible, such as buses or trams.

A successful transit-oriented development is Orenco Station in the

Portland, Oregon metro area; it has nearly 2,000 homes and a density of about 14 units per acre. Residents can reach town center shops and services within a 5 to 15-minute walk. A light rail station is just minutes away. More than half the residents use the light rail at least two times a week, meaning that there is considerable non-commuting use of it, probably for reaching Portland. Some 22 percent use bus or light rail, compared to 5 percent on average for the region. And 69 percent of residents are using public transit more in Orenco than in their previous place of residence. Another 2.7 percent carpool, bike or always walk for commuting. A resident said: "I am already making walks through the neighborhood a regular part of my routine as well as making regular use of the Orenco MAX station."

Smart developers are embracing and marketing access to transit.

At Riverside Park, a 222-unit rental apartment complex in an old Virginia suburb near Washington, D.C., a Metro subway station can be reached by walking one-half mile or taking a free shuttle bus. Sixty-three percent of residents use Metro to commute to work. There are shops there also, and a shuttle takes residents to a supermarket on Saturdays. Many residents do not have cars.

At King Farm in Maryland there are two free shuttle bus routes that some 700 riders a day use to move around the new community and get to the nearby metro rail station.

Rivermark is in the heart of Santa Clara, California, within Silicon Valley. Reduced car use is easy because it is close to major employment centers, and also to a light rail station and two bus routes. With nearly 1,900 homes of various types and a high density of 18 units per acre it is very successful. A resident said "The New Urbanism of Rivermark means everything I need is nearby. I don't have to drive 15 minutes to drop off my cleaning and another 15 minutes for groceries and so on. I don't have time for that."

Gaslight Commons is a high density 200-unit apartment complex built adjacent to a New Jersey Transit station in South Orange. Sixty-five percent of residents use transit to get to work, and there are only 1.35 cars per unit.

More than a dozen transit locations in the East Bay area of San Francisco are getting transit village developments that will contain some 10,000 new homes.

Transit-oriented development is booming in the greater Dallas, Texas area. Robert Shaw, a developer of New Urbanism apartment buildings said: "More and more people are making a decision based on access to mass transit."

In March 2004 citizens in seven San Francisco area counties voted to increase seven bridge tolls from $2 to $3 to raise money for area transit improvements, even though only 12 percent of area residents use transit. Contrary to what sprawl shills say, people know that everyone benefits from better transit systems, including the business world. A survey of New Economy companies found that access to public transit is very important to 70 percent of them. Companies know that they get higher productivity from workers less stressed by automobile commuting.

Think more about how quality transit could make your life easier.

HEALTHY PLACES RESPECT THE SURROUNDING AREA.

Good design does not level everything for easy construction. The best developers make creative use of structures on the original site, especially ones with historic and architectural significance. They also refrain from using historic land, such as civil war battlefields. David W. Jones was chagrined at what was happening in Virginia: "Tourists, like me, come to your area to visit the fields where our ancestors fought and died, not to see housing developments. If the sprawl continues, many of us will stop coming and take our tourist dollars elsewhere, where intelligent leadership is preserving sacred treasures, not exploiting them for short-term gain." Churches, schools, cemeteries, and other places important in America's history must be respected. It's bad enough that sprawl consumes our present and future, it should not wipe out our historic past.

HEALTHY PLACES should blend harmoniously with the surrounding area, physically and culturally. Designers and planners must carefully consider how the overall motif is linked to the history of the site and surrounding areas, or to the style of the surrounding community in the case of an infill project.

CHECKLIST QUESTION:
10. Does the place have a consistent and distinctive style that blends in with the environmental setting and cultural features of surrounding areas?

Promote distinctive, attractive communities with a strong sense of place, including the rehabilitation and use of historic buildings

Here are some examples of places where developers met these challenges:

Fairview Village in Fairview, Oregon used an architectural style fully consistent with the design and feel of the "old town" of Fairview.

Baldwin Park near Orlando, Florida met the wishes of surrounding residents by not putting any retail on the outside of the new community. There are 28 ways in and out so that traffic to the town center offices and retail will not interfere with pedestrians.

The Village of WestClay, north of Indianapolis, Indiana was designed to reflect "traditional values" by using both architectural styles found in Indiana towns at the turn of the 19th century, and in old Indianapolis neighborhoods.

I'On Village near Charleston, South Carolina borrowed architectural styles of the Carolina Lowcountry and replicated the personality and look of coastal towns like Beaufort, Savannah, and Charleston. The natural environment was preserved and enhanced, including miles of walking and marsh-front paths. Parks were integrated across the neighborhood. Its developer Vince Graham said "We hope people will get out from in front of the TV and use their automobiles less."

The developer of Armory Park del Sol in Tucson, Arizona worked hard for support from surrounding residents. He succeeded. The infill project has 99 homes on only 14 acres and has been immediately successful. Innovative green building design cuts daily energy costs for cooling and heating to less than one dollar. "Universal design" makes homes usable by all, including those with physical and mental limitations.

The Stapleton project master developer focused on making a seamless transition between the surrounding old neighborhoods and the new one.

COMMUNITY DESIGN WITH HONESTY, QUALITY AND TASTE.

In seeking information and using the checklist you will surely examine your own values. When it comes to sprawl development, there is no limit to its lack of conscience and taste.

McMansions are increasingly made to look like castles and other fancy, ornate styles of majestic "old world" architecture. Plastic is used for building intricate decorative walls and other surfaces, the same as ubiquitous Styrofoam disposable coffee cups, only thicker. It can be molded into complex shapes and coated to look like stucco or cement facades of any color. The outside walls feel hollow. A stray golf ball or a woodpecker can easily poke holes in the walls. Water rot of the wood frames behind them have kept lawyers busy. These houses have been called "polystyrene palaces." They are perfect for plastic people who do not need a checklist, just their checkbooks.

Developers and builders of HEALTHY PLACES have a different ethic and mindset. They are more interested in "green building" design and materials that conserve resources, reduce energy use, and cut pollution, and using them in smaller size homes. A "big green house" is an oxymoron. Using "green" to sell sprawl and super-size homes is just another form of sprawl-speak. Village Habitat Design in Atlanta has designed several excellent communities and part of its mission statement is: "We design communities where nature is a part of life everyday, where the residents enjoy community and privacy as they choose, and where places are made for people rather than for cars." To care about real community is also to care about honesty, quality and taste. Decide what you want.

Use the checklist if you want a true alternative to sprawl.

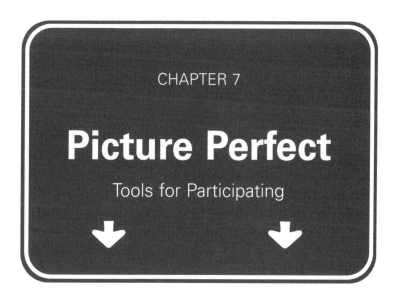

CHAPTER 7

Picture Perfect

Tools for Participating

Sprawl seduces.

"Economic power and political power have been the only two kinds of power at the table. If you want to change the process and change the outcome, you've got to bring this third kind of power – social power – to the table," advised Malcolm Gladwell, author of *The Tipping Point* to an audience of some 1,400 people. They were packed into a room for a visioning activity of the six-county Sacramento Area of Council of Governments on April 30, 2004.

Previously, some 5,000 people had participated in smaller meetings. Computer generated maps and computer-assisted voting helped attendees make choices on how the region would look after adding 1.7 million more people by 2050, on top of the current 1.9 million residents. With a smart growth strategy, transportation capital costs would drop by $1.7 billion, newly developed land would be cut by 60 percent, and a third of future housing would be near transit producing a six-fold increase in transit use. Only one percent voted in favor of continuing sprawl. *The Sacramento Bee* editorialized "A new mix of growth is OK. Growth as usual is not."

You cannot depend on the housing industry and professional planners, designers and architects to give you a community that supports active living, promotes neighborliness, and helps reduce car use. To regain autonomy over your life, you need a chance to shape your built environment to make it healthy and outstanding. This chapter is about implementing the smart growth principle: "Encourage citizen and stakeholder participation in development decisions."

Just as the map is not the territory and the plan is not the place, the place is not the community unless residents make it so. Professionals often think that their plans, designs and buildings make communities. But technical expertise is not enough. People have a right to be more than consumers and residents. They have a right to be collaborators.

Robert Davis, the celebrated founder of the Seaside community in Florida, said:

The default setting for land use politics – the easy answer – is more sprawl. This must change. It is time to abandon developer-driven, project-oriented, reactive planning. Let citizens determine how their community should grow, using a visioning and planning process. When confronted with sprawling subdivisions that consume farms and forests vs. compact, livable communities, most people will make the better choices.

For the built environment, a picture is worth a lot more than a thousand words. Words generate different mental images among people. Pictures clarify concepts and facilitate mutual understanding that helps build consensus about community design. People remember striking images and their impressions. People need visual images to know what characteristics and design features define communities worth living in.

When you see pictures of the many features of an existing place, you understand it better. You cannot fully know sprawl when immersed in it. You must step outside it to see it more objectively. Pictures can be viewed and discussed in some depth and compared to images of other places. This reveals the pluses and minuses of a place, and how it can be changed for the better. Modern technology, like digital photographs and computer simulations, can vividly show how existing locations can be improved (see Figure 7-1). Incredibly accurate pictures and even three-dimensional simulations of possible built environments, even with different changes to the natural landscape, can be created. People can "taste" a new community as the recipe is steadily changed to meet the multiple needs and preferences of many individuals, guided by a master chef called a community designer.

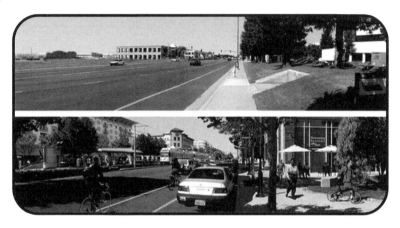

Figure 7-1. Top is photo of actual area; bottom is computer simulation showing additions of mixed-use buildings and pedestrian friendly amenities.

Few people normally get an opportunity to contribute to planning and designing a significant new part of their built environment. For decades, professionals in planning, design and architecture, in combination with developers and government agencies, have dictated the built environment. That combination covered America with sprawl un-places. There was minimal involvement of people who would live in those places or use the highways and shopping centers, or would be greatly impacted by them. You could take it or leave it. You could complain afterwards. This elitist and exclusionary approach made sprawl ubiquitous. What is the key lesson learned? *Ask not what professionals can do for you. Ask what you can do for yourself.*

More people should have an opportunity to participate in "community based planning and design." Those trying to create HEALTHY PLACES are advocates of this new interactive grassroots approach. It has historic importance. It should replace "public participation" and "community involvement" activities that have been required by government for decades. Countless public hearings, open houses, and flip-chart and power point presentations offer sham involvement. The public mostly listens to "talking heads" – the experts – and watches the show. Public officials listen to residents and then, for the most part, do what they want. Sprawl-speak pollutes the air. Participation is perfunctory. Meetings are boring. Coffee is bad and chairs are hard. Consultants get rich. Sometimes citizens can speak, but only for limited times, often just a few minutes. They vent their anger over something they don't want. Confrontation, not collaboration is the norm. Angry opposition is not the best form of civic engagement.

Many government officials and developers resent even token public participation and do things to undermine or avoid it. In June 2003, the *New York City Gotham Gazette* ran a story on ethical problems in government land use decisions. A professional planner in the Brooklyn Office of City Planning had resigned in protest against her agency. In a letter that went public she said: "I was instructed to participate in a process that would specifically avoid community involvement. While participating in meetings with the project developers, their attorneys, and City Planning staff, I witnessed our own staff utilize the zoning code to assist the developers in designing an as-of-right project in order to avoid community engagement." A similar project had previously been rejected by the community. Few planning professionals have the courage to take such a stand.

The planning system derives power from preventing citizen scrutiny, as historian Richard White revealed in his 1995 book *The Organic Machine*:

> Planning is an exercise of power, and in a modern state much real power is suffused with boredom. The agents of planning are usually boring; the planning process is boring; the implementation of plans is always boring. In a democracy boredom works for bureaucracies and corporations as smell works for a skunk. It keeps danger away. ...The audience is asleep.

Boring planning departments and processes produce blandburbs that create bored and boring residents. Community based planning and design makes planning exciting for citizens and shifts power from planning professionals to them.

CONTRIBUTING TO COMMUNITY DESIGN PROTECTS YOUR HEALTH.

"Our sprawling cities and suburbs, linked together by endless ribbons of freeways, match our sprawling waistlines. ...Density is healthier than sprawl. ...Land use policy is public health policy," said Roger Valdez of the Washington State Public Health Association in a 2004 column in *The Seattle Times*.

Americans need and deserve to be in the "driver's seat" for design so that they can literally get out of the driver's seat. At best, Americans have heard something about zoning. But unless a landowner pursues a conflict with local government, zoning is mysterious and unintelligible. Zoning is supposed to protect *public* health, safety and welfare. Traditionally, this has meant making distinctions among residential, commercial and industrial land uses. Polluting smokestack industries were kept away from housing and shopping. But the problem in the 21st century is communities that are not walkable and pedestrian friendly, that lack everyday destinations close to homes. Zoning that supports sprawl over mixed-use communities should be illegal. Health professionals should help reshape zoning. New "form-based" zoning codes focus on community design and architectural quality.

If you are attracted to HEALTHY PLACES you probably value neighborliness, social capital, civic engagement and the opportunity to participate in the planning, design, and governing of *your* community. Residents offer the unique ability to see the wholeness of their community and how all its parts interact. Residents are best able to ensure that the community is greater than the sum of its parts. They can focus on longer term sustainability. They will safeguard their personal health and safety. In HEALTHY PLACES there is vision-based participation and bottom-up decision making, compared to rule-based, top-down decision making in blandburbs.

You should reject developers who eat up endless hours talking about their preconceived design. Ditto for government experts and their consultants who come to communities with plans and designs in hand. If places are to be built for people on a human, not automobile, scale, then residents must help design those places from the get-go. Professionals should guide and inform the process without dominating or manipulating it because they know "what's right."

Ironically, time-poor people find it hard to take on the added responsibility of shaping their own neighborhood and community – their own future. Tired and time-poor consumers are just what sprawl developers want. They are willing to leave everything to professionals. *This accommodates sprawl that is a generic, commodity form of housing.* And so sprawl breeds more sprawl.

Why should consumers work harder in a collaborative process? Here are several reasons:

+ You may get a better housing option in the geographical area where you now reside.
+ You can ensure place personality and uniqueness. You can help keep your community stay on track as it expands, evolves and goes through build-out over a number of years.
+ You can help shape a general, comprehensive or master plan for your area that leads to more HEALTHY PLACES.

CHARRETTES ARE FUN.

Over the past several years, many groups that have been advancing HEALTHY PLACES have had considerable success with an intensive interactive process between professionals and lay people; it is called a charrette. Activities that usually are performed in the offices of professionals are time-compressed, taken to the field and conducted in public. It has been termed "designing by democracy." Full-blown charrettes run for a number of days, depending on the size of the contemplated project. They produce a polished and professional outcome, usually a design of a place. But charrette means different things to different people. And it can be misused. Several warnings are necessary. Anyone who is hearing about a charrette that they may want to become involved with should ask these questions:

1. WHO IS SPONSORING THE CHARRETTE?
Commercial developers, government agencies, and some nonprofit groups sponsor charrettes, or even join together to hold one. Citizens should know where the money is coming from and who the prime driver is, and what their goal is. A developer typically wants to build something on a particular piece of land, and a charrette

process may be a way to get a desired action by government. Centex Homes funded a large effort to help it get Santa Paula, California to increase the number of homes that could be built in Fagan Canyon. Instead of 450, it wanted to build from 1,350 to 2,500 homes. A government agency may just want to help develop a community "vision" for future development and growth in a particular area, from a neighborhood, to a city, to a region. Sometimes a government agency wants to develop some type of master plan or other planning document to steer future growth and development. The word "plan" sometimes means producing a document with words only, but in other cases a plan means actual design and images, even if only at a concept level that shows patterns and locations of specific parts of the built environment and open spaces, but not detailed building or street designs.

2. ARE ALL STAKEHOLDERS ABLE TO FULLY PARTICIPATE IN THE PROCESS? Charrettes must be open to all stakeholders in the public and private sectors, including local officials, businesspeople, and members of advocacy groups. Charrettes for substantial projects may involve hundreds of people, although not all of them may participate in every activity. Anyone who perceives being impacted by the potential project should be given the opportunity to participate. No one should be excluded, even people and organizations that may be viewed as "troublemakers" and "opponents." Ordinary citizens and not just community "leaders" and government officials must be encouraged to participate. Be wary of developers and designers who use not-so-public charrettes, where only specifically invited people can participate.

3. WILL THE CHARRETTE PRODUCE A SPECIFIC WORK PRODUCT OR OUTCOME? A charrette is not just informational or educational; it should produce something that is specific, tangible and useful. A design charrette produces a professional quality design of something that can be built. Everything else that may be obtained, including survey results, a vision for future growth and development, and data about the location are subservient to the prime goal of creating a consensus design. Producing a design means producing images, drawings, models and whatever else communicates the layout and style of a

neighborhood or community, as a whole or some critical part of it.

4. ARE THE PROFESSIONALS LEADING THE PROCESS RESPONSIVE TO CITIZENS
AND NOT FORCING THEIR OWN VALUES AND PREFERENCES ON THEM?
A pioneer of mixed-use development, Ray Gindroz of Urban Design
Associates said: "I always like sharing my ideas with people. My
approach to design is not to go off in a corner and meditate. My
approach is to reach out for as much input as possible. People tell us
about their dreams for the future."

Some powerful, articulate, and strong willed design professionals who
run charrettes have staked out their beliefs in great detail for many years.
They have "rules" they believe in. They have styles they consider the best.
They can talk faster and have more facts at their fingertips than ordinary
people. They know what works. They know what is right. They are famous.
They intimidate. They are highly paid. But they must respect ordinary citizens and avoid "loading" the game to get the outcomes they want. For
example, front porches have considerable merit, but you can have a successful HEALTHY PLACE without slavishly requiring all homes to have
front porches.

Despite being hard work, participants often say that charrettes are fun.
Citizens leave with a strong sense of achievement, because they helped
shape the future – *their future* – where they and perhaps their children will
live. Hardly anyone who has attended a zoning hearing, a government
briefing, or a formal presentation by a developer would describe the experience as fun. Few citizens have any desire to attend such boring conventional meetings if their property is not at stake.

The best advice is to talk to several people who have participated in
previous charrettes headed by the design professional handling the one
you are considering. Was the charrette an honest collaboration between
the professionals and the others participating? Did the professionals avoid
dominating meetings and facilitate active participation by everyone? Did
they make everyone participating feel comfortable and valued? Did they
resist the temptation to please whoever funded the charrette? When the
charrette was over, did they faithfully execute the decisions made by the
larger group?

All these questions should also be asked about a charrette that has
already occurred in your area. If the outcomes of the process are to be val-

ued, then its legitimacy should be confirmed.

VISUAL SURVEYS INFORM.

If you listen to sprawl supporters, nobody wants to live in higher density housing. Au contraire.

To understand why people actually like well designed higher density, this is the key question: How do people reach judgments about the look and feel of different residential densities? Researchers at the University of North Carolina asked themselves: Why do people who are asked questions on an opinion survey prefer single-family detached houses in typical, sprawl developments, but have consistently preferred higher-density living in walkable communities when they are shown "visual surveys" with pictures of high quality, mixed-use and higher density places?

Developers and home builders, who profit from sprawl development, consistently cite opinion survey results to defend sprawl and, sometimes, attack smart growth. What these survey measure are outcomes (what people have already chosen) and not determinants (why they have chosen). Most people chose sprawl because they had no other choice.

Opinion survey results are also misleading because responses depend on individual interpretations of the words used in a written questionnaire or asked by an interviewer. If specific definitions or images are not provided, people freely use their own negative views of the word or concept of "density." What one person imagines for "high" density may be very different than the next person. This makes responses to opinion surveys highly subjective and the results misleading, because so many different interpretations are pooled together. References to alternatives to sprawl can evoke mental images of perceived high density, low quality of life places with inferior homes, like lousy inner cities. Sprawl interests who pay for such surveys want respondents to react in these ways to maintain the sprawl status quo and let them proclaim "we just give consumers what they want."

In contrast, by using visual surveys with pictures, people can make sensible trade-offs for the totality of their community. They are better able to process complex information and evaluate many different features or variables in combination, rather than separately. Unlike opinion surveys and polls, visual surveys inform, not just collect responses. By looking at images of alternative real places, *perceived* density produces a much more accurate understanding of actual density. Through visual surveys and discussions, large numbers of people can more effectively reach a common understanding and a shared preference, the goal of community based planning and design.

If people really value settings that are filled with usable greenspaces, walkable and safe streets, and public meeting spaces, and pictures portray these well designed characteristics, then that's what they choose, despite higher residential densities. *Good design always trumps density!* This is the important lesson from hundreds of visual surveys and recent successful projects. In other words, residential density may serve as a useful statistical measure, but it is not a good defining characteristic of a place. Density is far less important than the totality of place design and personality that determine how people perceive the look and feel of a neighborhood or community. People living in Paris or Manhattan's Upper East Side – and the many examples of HEALTHY PLACES given previously – do not think twice about high density. Great community design and amenities make high density irrelevant.

With visual surveys, sprawl un-places inevitably lose. This fact alone tells us that HEALTHY PLACES will compete successfully against sprawl in a fair housing market. Advice to people stuck on high density: Get over it. Stay focused on design that pleases you. And remember that so much public opposition to higher density housing is a result of decades of the sprawl culture. Americans have been conditioned to treasure low density without understanding its negatives.

IMAGE SURVEYS IDENTIFY WHAT PEOPLE VALUE.

Anton C. Nelessen invented the Visual Preference Survey. Firms and nonprofit organizations nationwide now offer many versions of this, including the Community Image Survey. Image surveys are particularly useful in areas where public involvement has been low and distrust of government and developers is high. Image surveys, however, can be used for different purposes.

An ideal use is as a component of a design charrette. But visual surveys are often used strictly for developing a paper product, either some type of "vision" or an actual "plan" for future growth and development within a specified area, from neighborhood to large multi-county regions. Visions and plans can surely have value. But they should not be confused with creating an actual design for a new addition to or change in the built environment. Vision activities typically produce narratives with statements that describe the future social, economic, and physical development preferred by the community. Whether vision statements or plans lead to actual changes and improvements in the built environment is problematic. Once the political system receives vision statements and plans the sprawl lobby may use its influence to protect the status quo.

When part of a design charrette, an image survey identifies a preferred vision based on the specific design features of the built environment that people value, or would like to preserve. The image survey results identify what people want their community to look and feel like in the future. Many of the photographs can be used as the basis for computer simulations that show incremental changes and improvements using different design approaches. The preferred design features can be used together with general smart growth principles to initiate the design process.

An image survey in Burnsville, Minnesota found that the community preferred streets with outdoor dining and wider sidewalks. An image survey in Spanish Lake, in the St. Louis, Missouri area, found that the community preferred pedestrian scale buildings with no more than two stories, parking areas with landscaped islands and green buffers off of streets, and avoidance of garish color schemes and generic corporate architecture for chain retail places.

The usual practice in image surveys is to take many pictures that are representative of the best and worst features of the natural and built environment in the project's area. However, taking pictures of what many people may deem undesirable places poses a problem. Some members of the community associated with negative places, such as builders, developers and businesspeople, may be cast as "villains." If they do not participate in the charrette, it is a loss. One solution is to take pictures of similar features in other communities. Images from other communities can also illustrate design features or principles not found in the survey area.

How do visual surveys work? Participants score individual photographs, often 100 to 200 images in Visual Preference Surveys and 40 to 60 images in Community Image Surveys. Participants should be assured before the "show" begins that there is no right or wrong answer. Images are shown rapidly to get initial, "gut" reactions to the images. A preference scale is used, usually from –10 for least preferred to +10 for most preferred. Scoring is done on paper ballots, which may be machine read, or electronic voting devices to get faster results. Statistical analysis yields conclusions about community preferences.

Next, pairs of images show how participants have scored contrasting design elements and reveal tradeoffs and compromises. Score differences stimulate group discussion that aids the development of a list of design details and principles for the project. People learn how to weigh the importance of different and conflicting features of their community. Figure 7-2 shows two single-family houses and their scores.

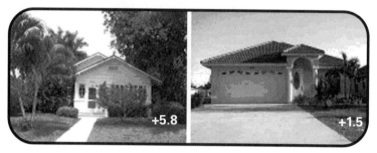

Figure 7-2. Paired images for single-family houses.

As shown on the left, even modestly sized homes are more highly rated when the garage is not the dominant feature of the home. On the right, the dominance of the garage door and wide driveway cause the "snout home" to receive a lower rating. These images are from a Community Image Survey used in conjunction with a design charrette to develop the community character plan for Collier County, Florida, which includes the city of Naples, and has a population of about 200,000. The survey was initially used in the kickoff session and then made available on the county's website. During about a ten-month period 372 people took the survey.

The image on the right is consistent with a much-desired street in a real neighborhood, with wonderful trees and lush landscaping and a sidewalk clearly being used by residents. In contrast, the image on the left is a more typical suburban street without good landscaping; it is clearly oriented almost entirely to the automobile, with a sidewalk too close to traffic, no shade trees, and nothing but fences along the street. For the visioning charrette of Maple Valley, Washington the image survey was taken by about 75 people, including about 20 children between the ages of 5 to 12.

The children did not like fences, dark places, or boring streets.

So much for the process. Ensuring that image survey results are fair, accurate, and representative of the total community is another matter. Figure 7-3 is another example, showing two different residential streets.

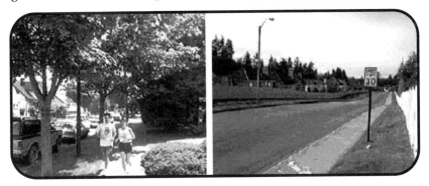

Fgure 7-3. Paired images of residential streets with scores: right, walkable street; left, road lacking safe sidewalk and poor greenspace.

| Adults | -5.3 | Adults | +5.5 |
| Children | +1.0 | Children | +8.0 |

PICTURES SLAUGHTER SPRAWL MYTHS.

A major issue is the number of people taking a visual survey. Is the number truly representative of the broad community? Companies providing visual surveys rarely provide any detailed analysis to demonstrate that the number and characteristics of the participants are a statistically valid, representative sample. Visual survey participants are invariably a tiny fraction of the total population relevant to the project. Unlike phone surveys used to determine public opinions, for image surveys there is no random selection of people with characteristics that reflect broad demographic profiles of the general population. Great effort is needed to increase the number of people participating. *If the group taking the visual survey is not truly representative, then survey results may not help create a design that gets wide public support.*

In Baltimore County, Maryland, with a population over 2 million, about 120 residents took an image survey sponsored by the county. Although a representative sample of county residents was desired, 63 percent of the participants were older, ages 35 to 61, compared to 36 percent for the county population; similarly, the group was more affluent with 46 percent having incomes of $75,000 or higher compared to a county median income of $51,700. These characteristics are not unusual. In San Antonio, Texas, 302 people took a Visual Preference Survey, but the income and education levels were higher than the city's average. Self-selected participants are also more likely to be angry about something in the built environment. The City of Vancouver, British Columbia did not rely on self-selected participants, but found ways to include a number of random respondents. More sponsors of image surveys should do this.

The best practitioners actively pursue creative means of increasing the number of participants and their diversity. They make the visual survey available on one or more Internet sites, on videos that citizens can rent without cost, in printed materials that are widely distributed by community organizations, in kiosks in shopping and office centers, and on local community cable channels so that people can take the survey in the comfort of their own home. Respondents can then email or mail in their scoring sheets.

"Marketing" materials to attract citizens should focus on the positive theme of improving a neighborhood or community, or creating a new one, and not on attacking what some people view negatively. The goal is to capture people's imagination and hopes about *their* future. Here are some examples of image surveys. Note that the numbers of participants are often much less than one percent of the survey area's population.

The town of Weddington, North Carolina, trying to control growth after population doubled in the 1990s to 6,700, conducted an image survey with over 140 images. Over 200 people participated, compared to 1,125 responses to a written survey form from 45 percent of households. Residents clearly preferred features associated with HEALTHY PLACES over ones showing sprawl development and streets.

A Visual Preference Survey with 230 images was used in Milwaukee, Wisconsin, with a population of about 600,000. As part of a Downtown Planning Process over 1,600 people participated over three and one-half months in small and large public meetings and Internet availability. A follow-up workshop where a plan was developed involved 300 people over three days. After that, professionals alone turned the workshop results into a plan that went on for further review and refinement.

In the Hartford, Connecticut region, with a population over 120,000, 573 people completed a Visual Preference Survey in public meetings and in walk-through displays and 170 used the Internet. It was sponsored by the metropolitan planning organization.

In Lockport, Illinois in the Chicago area, with a population over 12,000, nearly 100 people completed a Visual Preference Survey and ranked 180 images. Several local government agencies sponsored the activity as part of a Living with Growth project. Participants ranged from long-active leaders to newcomer families. A follow-up five-hour design workshop had only 35 participants.

The person conducting the survey usually is talking before and during the presentation of the images, these days typically by a power point presentation. Beware of professionals bubbling with passion and enthusiasm who breathlessly exhibit the fervor of a tent revival preacher revealing the Truth. Too much advocacy can diminish honest *community* input. Some professionals may "load" the survey and manipulate the outcomes by controlling the content of photographs and computer simulations. Images can be crafted to turn people on or off. Some things are perceived positively by most people – like flowers, trees, the American flag, and people apparently enjoying themselves, or negatively – like large business road signs, bill boards, and slum-looking areas.

Another problem with images is that they may have so much going on that they do not focus on the intent of the image, typically a specific design feature. When this happens, there is too much idiosyncratic interpretation by participants. This reduces the significance of average rankings, because people are reacting to different parts of the picture.

Beware of verbal statements that bias scoring. Professionals should not try too hard to entertain, nor should they play tricks to ensure they get the results they think are necessary to carry the project *they want* forward. Good development may be referred to as "sensible development" or "smart growth development." Bad development may be called "sprawl development," "unbelievable development," or "cookie-cutter development." Referring to a building as "historic" can produce positive reactions. Calling housing "multi-family" or "high density" can cause negative reactions. Similarly, a grimace, sigh or laugh from the professional running the "show" as an image appears can bias results.

Smart growth and New Urbanism proponents must trust the participants. Hundreds of image surveys have consistently shown a preference for design features associated with HEALTHY PLACES. Pictures can slaughter many sacred cows of the sprawl culture.

Would you like to see an image survey? Go to the Internet. Using a search engine like Google.com, enter phrases like "visual preference survey," "community image survey," or just "image survey." Many places have put there surveys on web sites; sometimes you can look at the results and sometimes you can actually take the survey.

CHARRETTES HELP CONSUMERS MAKE A DIFFERENCE.

Why hold a charrette? It has been shown over some years that a charrette uses time, money and social capital efficiently. When it is done correctly, it can save much money, particularly by eliminating delays and litigation that conventional approaches suffer because of many confrontations over design. An effective charrette streamlines the ordinary design process. Time is saved through a high-intensity effort, as compared to processes that can take many months or even years.

By including stakeholders at the beginning rather than the end of the process, the charrette promotes early negotiation, resolution and consensus. The major parts of design charrettes are presented below. The extent and intensity of each component activity must be adapted to the specific project at hand and the conditions and circumstances of the project location.

PLANNING A CHARRETTE IS A MAJOR EFFORT

Charrette planning includes: decisions about exactly what is to be designed, who participates as professional leaders or consultants and as members of the public, how long the total activity will last, and where the main activities will be held. A usual first step is forming some type of steering or organizing group, committee, or task force. It usually has representatives from the funding source, which typically is a developer or some government agency, and decision makers and opinion shapers in the local community or general geographic area.

A design team is formed. Sometimes a request for proposals from different firms is used to select one or more companies to lead the effort. The team consists of one to three primary community designers with support from professionals in relevant areas, such as the natural environment, traffic engineering, architecture and landscape architecture. A firm that offers image surveys might also be contracted, unless one of the design professionals offers the service. Often one or more professional facilitators are also selected to manage group activities.

Focus groups can be used to obtain opinions and preferences on specific issues and to gauge the likely response of a large group. They can identify the concerns of specific constituencies or interest groups and help the organizing group design the details of the charrette.

An important task is to develop a work plan for inviting all categories of stakeholders to participate in the charrette, either in its entirety or as much of it as they can handle. The planning group must prepare "marketing" materials about the charrette and its purpose, as well as a detailed schedule of specific activities. The most important message to communicate to citizens is that the charrette is an opportunity "to make a difference." One community used the slogan "Together We Decide." Citizens need to know that it will be a citizen-driven design process. The challenge is convincing citizens that the charrette activity is not just another public hearing or conventional public meeting.

Special attention should be given to enticing citizens who are also professionals in various fields that relate to the topics and issues addressed in the charrette, such as local architects, environmental scientists, and health professionals. Another objective should be involving children in the charrette in some realistic way, such as through a special image survey event in a school. Many professionals have not done enough to attract larger numbers of participants, truly representative of all people living in a place. And yet they use the results as if the community has spoken. *Much more effort must be given to attracting the poorest, the least educated, the busiest, the most cynical, and the least concerned citizens to image surveys and charrettes.*

The charrette planning activity can take several months to do well.

A BACKGROUND COMMUNITY ASSESSMENT SUPPLIES IMPORTANT INFORMATION

The goal is to gather baseline information about the natural and built environment of the location for the contemplated project and its surrounding areas. Individuals or small groups can document what exists at the location through photographs taken during walking assessments. Some may be used later for the image survey. Questions that can guide the photographic assessment are:

+ What parts of the natural environment are prized or truly unique?
+ What scenic views are most appealing?
+ Where do people in various age groups like to gather?
+ What parts of the built environment do most people like or find objectionable?
+ What historic buildings exist?
+ What are some of the basic characteristics of nearby communities?

The team of professionals can gather considerable data from Geographical Information Systems (GIS) sources to produce computerized maps showing various environmental and infrastructure data for the site. These are used later to identify possible site locations for specific buildings or open space. Computer generated maps of a region that show land use increases in something like ten year intervals and some projection of what the area will look like in the future with anticipated population growth are very powerful. Aerial photographs taken over time can vividly show land use changes at the site and the surrounding area.

Any existing local or regional plans and zoning requirements that cover the site need to be examined and summarized, with special attention to constraints on development of the site. Some charrettes motivate changes in zoning codes. In most cases, zoning needs to be improved to explicitly allow mixed-use land development.

"Build-out analysis" has been used successfully in Massachusetts to help town residents and public officials learn to manage land development. Several GIS-based maps, along with aerial photographs of the community show the maximum development possible based on existing local policies and regulations. Projections are made for population, households, school enrollment, traffic, and water use, for example. The community's future is shown, first as a baseline, if no changes are made in zoning and other policies, and then as alternative futures through different zoning and policies. Residents are then able to evaluate whether available land is best developed, preserved, or used for other community needs.

KICK-OFF MEETINGS MUST GET PEOPLE ON THE RIGHT TRACK

An introductory evening or weekend social event helps charrette sponsors, members of the design team and citizens become acquainted. Ideas about charrettes are presented. An important message is that charrette participants will get something they want, but no one will get everything they want. Printed materials from the background assessment are provided. The steering group should consider the feasibility of a walking tour of the site just prior to the social event.

A good way of starting things off is through an image survey, because most people will find it exciting and fun. An hour or so is used for introducing and conducting the survey followed by several hours of open and usually intense discussion.

Participants should be introduced to the smart growth principles given in the previous chapter. If stakeholders can agree to these general principles early on, it will enhance the subsequent activities. It is a way to get participants started on a collaboration and consensus process. It also helps citizens raise their concerns about development in general.

Here is an example of a charrette that integrated an image survey: The Downtown Design Charrette in Bakersfield, California, with a population of close to 250,000, involved more than 135 residents and business leaders. They worked with professionals during a three-day charrette to develop implementation tools and general designs for a previously generated vision. During the opening Friday night session a Community Image Survey using 40 slides was given to 95 residents. About 80 people participated in the follow-up discussion of the results in the following morning design workshop. Lists of physical elements and qualities that were deemed positive and negative were drawn up to guide the design. Scores were used to document specific design elements that were favored, such as streets with medians, wide and shaded sidewalks with a planting strip, active storefronts on streets, and mixed-use buildings with retail on the ground floor and housing above.

Design studios and workshops are the crux of the charrette

These comprise the longest and most intense component of the charrette, most likely over three to five days. Energy, passion and commitment provide effective brainstorming and lively discussions, where "people argue with their pencils" and deal with many details. The basic idea is to get everyone to jointly, collaboratively and collegially produce a design. The key message is: What the community wants, the community gets, tempered by the technical facts and constraints given by the professionals. *The most important people in the room are the residents.*

For an effective outcome, all issues are addressed and everyone gets a fair voice. At the beginning, the role of the design professionals is more intense, as they must guide participants in a logical way to address a complex set of design issues.

The design team produces increasingly complex and detailed drawings and models of whatever is being designed, following the preferences determined through the image survey. Discussions or "feedback loops" explore technical, market, finance, political, and social issues. Constraints and opportunities posed by the physical environment are considered. The design team usually works in a temporary office in the site area, and prepares materials for the daily design sessions. Work-in-progress briefings are presented frequently.

Concurrently with the production of the design, the participants must also develop an implementation plan. This must address the relevant political, legal, and financial issues and obstacles that can be anticipated, and how they will be satisfactorily resolved in the shortest time possible. The goal is to make it easy to obtain whatever government approvals are necessary to move from design to actual project execution. Often this means identifying specific constraints of local zoning laws and how they should be removed.

During the course of the design workshops, attention should be given to obtaining local media coverage and inviting citizens to drop in to see the design materials being produced.

Final public presentation must sell the design

A highly professional presentation must be given at a well advertised public meeting. Some charrette participants as well as the design team should contribute to the public presentation. The goal is to get even more citizens involved. The charrette activities are summarized, and the final design presented verbally and visually. Comments from any members of the community are sought. These can cause the design team to make some changes in the design. The public presentation is a critically important opportunity to inform the community and particularly local government officials about changes in zoning that may be needed to move the project forward.

FINAL DOCUMENTATION MUST SUPPORT THE DESIGN

The design team prepares a final report package, after review by the steering group. This report is critically important; it must fully document all charrette activities, findings and accomplishments, and include the final design images.

Listen to these smart words from Marie Kennedy: "A successful transformative planner must carefully listen and respect what people know; help people acknowledge what they already know; and help them back up this 'common sense' and put it in a form that communicates convincingly to others."

COST MATTERS

Cost matters. Many groups cannot afford the $200,000 to $400,000 that the bigger companies usually charge for charrettes lasting from 7 to 10 days. These firms usually have architects and a number of other professionals on the design team. They usually address fairly large projects and extensive designs. They put a lot of emphasis on extensive preparation before the charrette and on high quality production of architectural renderings, images and models afterwards. Trying to cut costs may lead to insufficient time.

Some firms offer smaller scope and shorter charrettes in the $20,000 to $60,000 range. They typically focus on a smaller scope, perhaps the redesign of an old strip mall or a major intersection or street, for example. Mini-charrettes last from 1 to 3 days and may rely more on volunteer professionals for their team.

The higher cost charrettes can usually be handled by developers, but not so easily by small town or city governments and nonprofit groups. For the latter, the issue may come down to a mini-charrette or no charrette. One thing to remember is that providing image surveys and charrettes is a business, not just a noble service by committed professionals. They are also a *marketing tool* used by firms to get business designing and planning projects for developers, and sometimes for government agencies.

DEVELOPERS MUST LEARN TO WORK WITH CITIZENS.

Proponents of community based planning and design should be sensitive to criticism, especially about activities that are too short, too long, too elitist, or too poorly attended. Here are some actual criticisms:

A charrette activity in Williamsburg, Virginia was criticized: "Well-connected 'key players' with the time and patience to sit in meetings, will decide just what the future will look like. The other 12,000 or so residents of Williamsburg have no say in the matter."

A community leader challenged the legitimacy of calling a plan "the community's plan," because the number participating (250) was only .01 percent of the neighborhood population.

A community activist complained that the charrette "did not last more than a day, and so didn't provide time for citizens to come forth with and debate concrete, specific new alternatives for localized design issues."

"Putting the People in Planning," published by the state of Oregon about public participation in land-use planning, said this about charrettes: "It is an effective way of 'getting to yes,' but it requires a big investment of time by participants, and it usually does not represent a cross-section of the community."

While small numbers raise legitimate issues, the greater truth is that in the "normal" approach to planning there is very little participation by anyone other than government officials and the developer.

You may hear that developers resist charrettes because of their time and expense. John Clark, the developer of Haymount in Virginia, has made the case that his front-end spending of $400,000 for several charrettes made economic sense. He compared his cost to a nearby project where the developers only spent $135,000 on planning, but subsequently had to revise their plans several times, which pushed their planning costs up to $8 million. Clark's conclusion was that "clearly they spent more time and money by not using a front-loaded planning process." The lesson for developers: learn how to work with citizens.

Developers may also fear designing in public with a process they cannot control. When developers sponsor charrettes, there is no assurance, of course, that all results will be used. In one case a citizen complained that the developer's "plan is not the plan that the community developed in the design charrette." Ultimately, private investors make decisions that they think make the most business sense and may not follow all the recommendations from a charrette. This happened in Pittsburgh for a downtown project. Some 45 volunteer architects and citizen activists spent a day crafting a new urban plan for a project; they agreed on 18 specific points for the urban revitalization plan. They focused on preservation of buildings, parking, sustainability and other issues. The developer had two representatives there. Several months later the developer rejected more of the charrette's ideas than it accepted. Not all the preservation of buildings recommended survived, for example.

An effective charrette was held in Hercules, California. A seven-member steering committee, comprised of city officials, staff, prominent citizens, and developers' representatives, moved things along. The professional planning and design team spent months gathering information. For a city of only about 20,000 people the cost of $300,000 was stiff, so two developers split the cost with the city. The charrette consisted of a ten-day series of intense, hands-on, problem-solving and sketching sessions held in a local former bank building. An overflow crowd of 400 attended the initial town meeting and 300 residents participated in the various activities thereafter. Citizens wanted: one coherent vision for Central Hercules; a neighborhood center; interconnected living, shopping and employment; to make the most of the area's natural resources; and pedestrian friendly/walkable development. The chairman of the planning commission said: "The questions went from 'Should there be development?' to 'How soon can we get this?' "

In reflecting on the importance of a charrette held to design a revitalizatation plan for the downtown area of South Miami, the vice-mayor said:

> We had literally hundreds of people touching the plan, and that week changed the life of our city. This was a moment when people were really heard, and the energy from that has been sustained for eight years, keeping the plan whole. People still feel ownership; it's their plan, and they forcefully defend and promote it.

A citizen who participated in a charrette in New Bedford, Massachusetts said:

> On Saturday morning, I sat down at a table with 12 strangers, from different backgrounds, and began a discussion which, though a bit stiff in the beginning, became a wonderful organic dialogue, synapses firing, a crescendo of ideas, resulting in a vision that we all could agree upon. We could see ourselves walking down the street, greeting friends on the sidewalk, stopping for coffee on a beautiful spring day, listening to music, and feeling safe and invigorated. ...Everyone should know that this process wants and needs the input of the community through every step of the process.

Something good is going on. We need more of it.

ADVANCING SMART GROWTH WITHOUT REGULATIONS.

Perhaps the best example of outstanding, aggressive, and effective involvement of citizens over several years, and on a large scale, is the work of Envision Utah. This private-public partnership is executing smart growth principles to reshape growth and development in the greater Salt Lake area and other places. It had the support of then Governor Mike Leavitt and business leaders. Thousands of citizens helped build a quality growth strategy for Utah, fine-tuned to meet the special cultural, social and historical circumstances in the state. Scientific surveys and analyses have provided valuable information. Here are some of the impressive activities and results over the years:

In 1999, a growth questionnaire appeared in daily newspapers and weekly ad supplements, and was posted on the group's web site. The headline read "HELP DECIDE THE FUTURE OF THE GREATER WASATCH AREA." People returned 11,214 questionnaires through the mail and 6,277 via the website.

In some 25 public workshops, over 2,000 residents reached these preferences: greater population growth in infill areas rather than greenfield development, minimal development in the main skiing and recreation area, rail as an essential component of the region's growth, the need for walkable developments, and conservation of critical lands.

Two scientific polls were conducted, asking residents if they would support an increase in sales tax for public transportation. The results showed strong support for public transit.

Eight cities hosted site-specific Community Design Workshops to address how Envision Utah growth strategies could be applied to development sites in the communities.

In the spring of 2000, Envision Utah sent teams to visit 89 cities and 10 county commissions in the Greater Wasatch Area to get feedback from local officials on how the group could develop tools and resources to assist communities in their planning efforts. Ultimately, tools were created to assist local municipalities to promote walkable communities, encourage infill and redevelopment, meet housing needs, conserve water resources, promote transit oriented development, and protect sensitive lands.

Note that the population of the greater Salt Lake area is about 1.6 million. Some 25,000 or more people participated in Envision Utah's meetings and submitted questionnaires. Though less than 2 percent of the total population, surely many more family members and friends were educated.

Utah developers have listened and are building HEALTHY PLACES. A mixed-use development that received an award from Envision Utah is The Village at Riverwoods in the Provo area. It is a walkable community for over 500 people in 142 homes, including attached single-family townhouses, single-level residences and urban lofts above neighborhood retail stores to cover a broad price range. Walking is supported by narrow streets that slow traffic, wide sidewalks, bikeways and trails, and plentiful green common areas. Varied earth-toned colors and curved roof forms create a unique identity consistent with the local architecture and incredible natural beauty. It is close to considerable shopping and employment centers. An editorial in Provo's *The Daily Herald* said: "We hope this becomes a model for development, because Utah needs to do something about growth. It's a concept that's worked on the East Coast for years, with people being able to move around major cities without ever owning a car. It's time we heeded the lesson and put it in place here."

An even larger smart growth project is the 4,200-acre Daybreak in South Jordan. Construction started in spring 2004. Over some 30 years, more than 13,000 homes for 40,000 people will be built in several villages that will have town centers with employment, shopping and entertainment. Diverse home options will accommodate a mix of age groups and income levels. There will be access to light rail. About 30 percent of the land will be greenspace. Homes will be close to schools and walking and biking trails. "Water wise" techniques for landscaping and irrigation will mean that residents use 15 percent less water than in sprawl developments.

Politically conservative Utah has shown that smart growth can be achieved through a partnership of citizens, business and government, rather than regulatory approaches. But sprawl shill-meister Wendell Cox defames the Envision Utah effort by calling it "Entangling Utah," claiming it reduces housing affordability, increases traffic congestion and worsens air pollution. Cox ignores market forces and the profit-seeking developers building smart growth projects. Hypocrisy is the hobgoblin of sprawl shills. Cox may have been angry because Salt Lake City chose light rail, a constant target of his. Cox concocts "facts" to deceive people about transit. Renowned transit expert G. B. Arrington examined many of Cox's analyses and concluded: "In every instance, Cox's statements are either inaccurate, distortions or claims not supported by the facts. Cox's technique seems to be to start with a snippet of the truth and stretch it like taffy until it turns into something else that supports his position." University of Cincinnati Professor Haynes Goddard also studied Cox's work and said that he and his colleagues produced "superficial, poorly thought out and misleading arguments;" the work represents "either intellectual laziness, or more seriously, intellectual dishonesty" which results because "all ideologues are blind to reality and to the vacuousness of their arguments." As to Cox's pro-automobile fanaticism, former Milwaukee Mayor John Norquist said: "I think Wendell Cox is one of the biggest advocates of big [government] spending I've ever encountered in my 28-year political career."

PROFESSIONALS GAVE US THE SPRAWL CULTURE.

Community based planning and design befits a true *democracy* – citizen-consumers and professionals working together optimistically to create better communities. It puts into practice what Thomas Jefferson said:

> I know of no safe depository of the ultimate powers of the society but the people themselves; and if we think them not enlightened enough to exercise their control with a wholesome discretion, the remedy is not to take it from them, but to inform their discretion.

For image survey and charrette activities to work effectively there must be a sharing of power. Professionals must be dedicated to the Jeffersonian trust in the "people" and accept that people will sometimes choose sprawl-type development.

Professionals need the right personality. Design professionals must patiently bring people along on a journey of learning new information and seriously questioning conventional wisdom embedded in the nation's sprawl culture. They must lead without dominating. They must speak respectfully to citizens without using professional jargon.

For charrettes, citizens need time and energy; they must accept responsibility, commit to hard work, and be open to new information and principles. They must also overcome biases and all the baggage they have inherited from the sprawl culture and, especially, drop disgust for government and distrust of developers. Residents should see a unique opportunity to be partners in building an ideal community over time. The relatively low numbers of citizens participating in image survey and charrette activities defines an opportunity. If *you* participate in an image survey or charrette, *you* get a disproportionate degree of influence in speaking for the community.

Charrettes sometimes fail. To get a large smart growth infill project approved, a developer hired the "top-gun" to lead a one-week charrette that was well executed in May 2004. There was wide public involvement and the local smart growth advocacy group assisted. At one point, Andres Duany told an audience that smart growth design would "help you stop spoiling this beautiful island the way you've been doing for 50 years." Duany also repeatedly told residents that if they didn't accept smart growth they would get dumb growth. Some 1,000 residents attended the final presentation with just as many shouting at Duany as applauding him, according to one account. Large numbers wanted no development on the 370-acre site of the former Kings Park Psychiatric Center on Long Island. A month later the developer called it quits because of heavy citizen opposition. *The New York Times* used the occasion to editorialize "We like smart growth." and noted: "Long Islanders are not used to hearing developers deplore the barren anonymity of their tract-house lives." Lesson: Don't blame and threaten people living in sprawl, especially on Long Island – the birthplace of sprawl.

The epitome of community based planning and design is "cohousing" – standing for community housing. The goal is to create a close-knit community, like an extended family where neighbors have refrigerator rights. These projects are catching on. In 2004, there were 73 completed cohousing projects and more than a 100 under development. Residents play a decisive role in the original planning and design, and then the management. Besides 15 to 35 separately owned residences, there are shared common areas, such as a community center, workshop, large kitchen, guest unit, hot tub, garden, office space, and playground. Projects are either on greenfield sites or urban infill sites where an old office building or factory is renovated. Cherry Anderson explained her family's choice of the Wild Sage community in Boulder, Colorado: "We chose cohousing because community was lacking in our previous homes… It was important to us that there were other caring adults who could help watch and mentor my child as he grew up." Sheana Bull resides in Hearthstone in the Denver area and confessed: "Not everybody is going to love each other. But there's a respect and openness among everyone in the community. Our relationships are the most important thing." Sounds like the opposite of a gated McMansion un-place.

Some people *can* get picture perfect places, but not everyone who wants one. For more people to get them, the political power of the sprawl industry must be counterbalanced by citizen power to open up the market. The rest of the world that seems so intent on copying American lifestyles should learn from our mistakes, before they lose their authentic neighborhoods and communities. An army of professionals gave us the sprawl culture and social isolation. Now, we need citizens to curb sprawl. Remember this old adage: Amateurs built the ark, professionals built the Titanic.

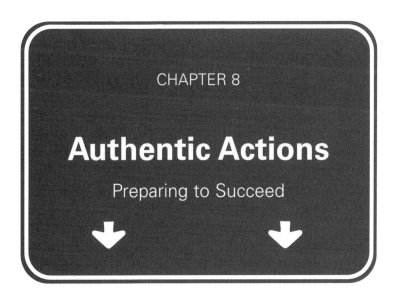

CHAPTER 8

Authentic Actions

Preparing to Succeed

Sprawl succumbs.

So now that you know why sprawl is bad for you and what is good for you, what do *you* do?

An army of sprawl developers, shills, and corrupt politicians have trampled America (see Figure 8-1). *Sprawl has replaced quality with blandness, health with harm, and time with traffic.* Sprawl has sown the seeds of its own destruction by causing a landslide of negative impacts on individuals. Better late than never – sprawl is choking on its own success, as its residents choke on traffic and bad air. Sprawl is not sustainable unless it is propped up by government. Thankfully, sprawl is more vulnerable than ever. Backlash against sprawl mounts as people connect the sprawl dots. Once, only airplane views showed sprawl's land gluttony. Now, people easily see sprawl's blitzkrieg moving in all directions.

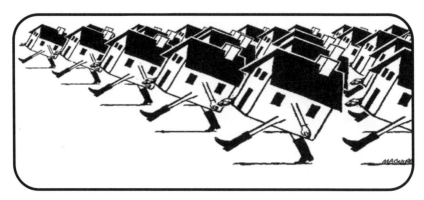

Figure 8-1. The blitzkrieg march of gluttonous sprawl developers.

Everyone experiences the ill effects of sprawl, not just those living in it. The sprawl industry remains arrogant. Why not? For decades it has beat back repeated attacks. But momentum is not destiny. Sprawl's past success must stop propelling future sprawl. New housing decisions must reshape the market. True, consumers must buy what is made available. Homelessness is not an option. But without perceiving an alternative, consumer preference for sprawl means nothing. Sprawl is not so much preferred as it is endured.

Sprawl around small towns and cities has caused the federal government to create a new category called "micropolitan" areas, in contrast to metropolitan ones. More than 28 million people, about one in ten Americans, live in these 565 micros, with at least 10,000 residents (but less than 50,000) in their central cities. Roanoke Rapids, North Carolina has 17,000 city residents in 8 square miles, but its micropolitan area has 76,000 people sprawled across 1,360 square miles in two counties.

Without using the s-word, pro-development author Joel Kotkin said in 2004: "This fundamentally horizontal form of urbanism – based around the car and relatively low density development – has few admirers in planning schools, think tanks or among 'progressive' politicians, but seems to have won overwhelmingly as the first choice of the individuals and businesses who have migrated there." As if Americans had a choice besides sprawl, as if there is no sprawl lobby, as if there is no demand for something else. Kotkin is a sprawl shill.

Say "sprawl" and almost everyone thinks suburbs. It was not always that way. Suburbs started blooming in America in the mid 1800s. For about one hundred years there were three vibrant American lifestyles –

cities, rural areas and suburbs, each with its own unique character. Cities were dominated by manufacturing industries and housing for their workers. Rural areas prospered as Americans worked the land in resource-based industries: farming, ranching, mining and forestry. Now, large land-owning agriculture, timber and mining companies are selling their land for sprawl development or doing it themselves. Suburbs depended on jobs in nearby cities reached mostly by rail or trolley; they were often called "streetcar suburbs." Now, jobs are in suburbs, but people must drive to them. For all three lifestyles, neighborhoods were mixed-use, relatively high density, and walkable. They had a people-focus and social capital was high. There were great public spaces. Housing and population densities were much higher than modern sprawl suburbs. Public transportation was important, and cars did not dominate lives and the landscape. In pre-World War II St. Louis, Missouri, for example, 99 percent of all residents were served directly by streetcars and buses.

Now, suburbs *are* synonymous with sprawl. Some sprawl is super-size single-family houses on enormous lots. Sprawl for lower incomes consists of low quality townhouses crowded together near highways and far from jobs. Rural small towns are mostly under sprawl siege. Progress should mean suburbs with plenty of HEALTHY PLACES.

SPRAWL SHOULD HAVE TO COMPETE.

In his 1957 anti-suburb novel *The Crack in the Picture Window*, John Keats described suburbs as "developments conceived in error, nurtured by greed, corroding everything they touch." That caustic criticism was right in sprawl's early years and even more right today.

The sprawl-for-profit formula is used over and over. Blandburbs have cookie-cutter sprawl housing and chain-dominated shopping. In the "United States of Sameness," from house designs to roadside signs, to restaurant menus, to products in chain stores, consumers find the same choices everywhere and see the same surroundings everywhere. In the sprawl culture *products get branded, places get blanded and — for sprawl residents – minds get stranded.*

Sprawl developers have a perverse sense of pride. They think they got it right. They revel because they have turned nothing – just the natural environment – into something. For them undeveloped land is a waste, a lost money-making opportunity. Where others see sprawl infestation, bland-burb developers see achievement. The Covenant of Sprawl may as well hang on the wall of every sprawl developer and shill.

The Covenant of Sprawl

We build what Americans want
We are blessed with limitless land
We trust zoning that supports sprawl
We provide the American dream
In sprawl we trust

We reject paying impact fees
We reject paying for new roads and schools
We provide housing, shopping and offices
Taxpayers must pay for what government builds
In sprawl we trust

We build bigger homes on bigger lots
We buy rural land
We turn greenspace into profits
We pave over land for progress
In sprawl we trust

We marvel at smart growth theories
Americans love their suburbs and cars
Politicians want growth
Our profits support democracy
In sprawl we trust

We trust the free market
We support American freedom
We sustain economic growth
In sprawl we trust
We made the American dream

The sprawl industry should be as vulnerable to market forces as any other industry. Logically, building HEALTHY PLACES instead of blandburbs means selling a different kind of housing, not less housing. Industries with an obsolete product rarely survive by switching to the competing innovation. For the most part, industries and companies die and are replaced by new ones. If sprawl declines, carpenters and other skilled workers can just as easily build HEALTHY PLACES. The group Good Jobs First found that smart growth policies increase construction jobs and an AFL-CIO resolution in 2001 denounced sprawl.

Suppliers of materials can just as easily provide them for HEALTHY PLACES. Land owners can sell to developers of HEALTHY PLACES. Architects can design HEALTHY PLACES, and real estate agents can sell them. But Brooke Warrick, president of a housing market research firm, got it right in an article published in 2003 by the National Association of Realtors that said its members "are accustomed to selling houses. They are not accustomed to selling community. Most people don't know how to explain community." It is time for them to learn.

With little growth in agriculture and manufacturing many states pursue economic prosperity through sprawl land development. But instead of prosperity governments get stuck with high infrastructure costs. Some politicians fall for this and fail to see smart growth as the solution. In 2004 William Denish, a 30-year resident of Mesa, Arizona, wrote in *The Republic* about his state's dismal economic condition: "During the '90s, the growth-for-the-sake-of-growth mentality continued with abandon by double-dealing politicians, land developers and real estate moguls… With an apathetic public and growth moguls continually bankrolling state and local politicians into office, an economy based on land speculation and a plethora of bottom-feeder jobs are the future for Arizona." The sprawl industry holds government hostage because home building is important to economies. But sprawl-caused problems cause high-tech employers to go elsewhere. Silicon Valley in California, Austin, Texas, and Northern Virginia suburbs of Washington, D.C. have lost competitiveness because of traffic congestion and other sprawl impacts on employees.

As a mature industry producing a commodity product, the sprawl industry benefits relatively little from new knowledge. Nor is there any emphasis on quality house design. Indeed, houses are probably the most costly product purchased by people for which outstanding design is irrelevant. Buy land, build sprawl. Then do it again. The risk is small. Some companies are exporting sprawl. For example, Pulte Homes Inc., one of the largest U.S. home builders, has built sprawl subdivisions in Mexico

and Argentina. Listen to Steven J. Guttman, an industry insider and former chairman of Federal Reality, which built some great mixed-use places
as well as conventional projects. "Most developers, if they only are interested in making money, will build the simplest, most cookie-cutter product they can. The way great fortunes are made in real estate has been to
have a cookie cutter and keep producing it." Sprawl developers keep feeding rural land into the sprawl production machine, and keep feeding
money to politicians to block competition.

Emerging Trends in Real Estate for 2002 told the investment community about the sprawl industry: "Booming populations and wide open
spaces in the Sunbelt's expanding suburban agglomerations can provide
developers and investors with short-term opportunities to cash in on
growth waves – but the returns, on average, have not been competitive."
In its 2003 report, investors were warned about places where "pedestrians
are an endangered species" and "banal commercial strips and gasoline
alleys" dominate. Sadly, the financial sector keeps supporting sprawl
developers.

In theory, the sprawl industry could reinvent itself and change. The
sprawl industry does not have an enormous amount of financial capital
invested in physical facilities that cannot produce HEALTHY PLACES.
They need information, expertise and courage. They must be willing to
change and then find the resources needed to faithfully produce HEALTHY
PLACES. But the sprawl industry focuses on sales, not true marketing. It
wants people to buy what it offers (sprawl) rather than find out what many
customers truly want (HEALTHY PLACES) and then meet that demand.
Why fiddle with success?

Developer Brent E. Herrington has seen the future and believes in
HEALTHY PLACES. In 2004 he said that there is "a massive gap between
what developers and home builders are producing and what today's home
buyers say they want." "Home buyers of the 21st century want to live in
pedestrian-friendly communities that foster casual, spontaneous interaction among neighbors. …Developers take heed! Your customers are ready
for change," he said.

But the sprawl industry uses sprawl-speak to support smart growth at
a broad, nebulous policy level while at the grassroots level they work hard
to stop competition to sprawl. They portray smart growth as the enemy of
the American Dream rather than competition to sprawl. Stephen Snell,
executive director of the Realtors Association of York and Adams Counties

in Pennsylvania, did just this when he accused the local smart growth group of "threatening the ability of working families to own a home." Warren Evans with the Eastern York County Smart Growth Coalition responded: "This is pure nonsense, and he and his Realtor friends should be ashamed to make such unfounded claims." The real issue was the rezoning of agriculture lands so that developers could build sprawl subdivisions with large homes, rather than build in older areas with available land.

The Washington Post ran a front page story in early 2003 "When Business Plans Go Bust." The theme was that the strategies used by major industries "are no longer working." Adrian J. Slywotsky, author of *The Profit Zone*, noted "You can name any number of industries right now in which there needs to be a new business model, but there's no clue what that is." But the housing industry was not analyzed, and it is clear what the new business model and strategy should be — HEALTHY PLACES.

Rather than change its business model, the sprawl industry is consolidating. The top 10 home builders doubled their market share to 23 percent from 1997 to 2003 and are projected to reach 40 percent by 2010. Land consumption is accelerating because of consolidation. Mega-companies with financial strength stockpile land, often for five years of home production. Credit Suisse First Boston found that the 13 largest home builders increased their land purchases by 22 percent between 2002 and 2003 and would boost it by 15 percent in 2004.

Sprawl companies have a successful business model and they want to keep it. Developers manage risk by minimizing delays and uncertainties, most easily done by building sprawl. Home builders expand revenues by increasing house size and selling many options. Proof is that if house prices are adjusted for inflation, houses of the same size and comparable amenities have the same price now as they had in the 1970s. Larger houses bring more revenues, made easy by expanding outward to cheaper land. Just as sprawl fits undemanding consumers, sprawl fits uncreative developers and the companies that finance them. As with all mature industries with major market share, the path of least resistance is the sprawl status quo.

A reinvention or restructuring of the housing and real estate industry should be seen positively as "creative destruction," which keeps capitalism vital and successful, according to the theory of the noted economist E. F. Schumpeter. Old products and industries give way to new ones; to subsidize outmoded ones is the antithesis of capitalism and a market economy. What Harvard Professor Shoshana Zuboff said about business in general applies to the sprawl industry: "There's a century-old pattern here: a business model hits its stride, only to be overtaken by rigidity, resistance to change, and vested interests. Its wealth-creating power and zest for innovation go into decline, and everyone is left to fight over a shrinking pie." And for the embryonic business of building HEALTHY PLACES: "New business models are invented that connect with new people and release the economic value concealed in their unmet needs." The unmet demand for HEALTHY PLACES defines a giant business opportunity.

But the sprawl industry is not grabbing that opportunity, because its leaders either do not perceive HEALTHY PLACES as a business threat, or see their appeal to many consumers but lack the capabilities to produce them. HEALTHY PLACES resemble what existed a few decades ago in the automobile industry. Foreign-made cars seemed to face insurmountable obstacles. Arrogant American automakers did not recognize the unmet needs of consumers. But foreign automakers gave consumers better products, just as developers of HEALTHY PLACES are doing.

Publications by the National Association of Home Builders seemed to show strong support for smart growth. The façade of that support collapsed in January 2003. A prestigious award from Professional Builder magazine to the American Planning Association's Growing Smart initiative was withdrawn shortly before it was to be presented at the annual builders' convention. This was the official explanation: "Our 127,000 home builder subscribers are not supportive of the Growing Smart initiative and were vocal in letting us know their positions." Why? The initiative produced model state planning and zoning statutes, which 14 state legislatures had already used. Home builders cannot stomach reforming state laws that remove preferences for sprawl. As an advocate for replacing "dumb growth" with cluster development by changing Massachusetts state law, Jack Clarke, Chairman of the Gloucester Planning Board, complained in 2004: "Efforts to tame the rules on sprawl are routinely defeated [in the legislature] by wealthy and well-connected special interests within the building and real estate industry." Beware of the slick trick of publicly supporting smart growth without opposing, which does more to keep the sprawl status quo than promote smart growth.

Toronto Star columnist Royson James was upset over a report on stemming unbridled sprawl in Ontario, Canada: "Where revolution is needed, the [politicians promoting smart growth] are proposing slow evolution that barely upsets the status quo. ...But it is too subtle, too soft, too gradual, and too accommodating of the debilitating practices that threaten to cripple southern Ontario to have a significant impact." This applies to many smart growth "initiatives."

A real danger is letting "sprawl" become a cliché. Sprawl is land use, built environment, product, industry, mindset, lifestyle, and culture. We must take its many impacts seriously. Sprawl supporters would like it to be a hollow cliché, but this dishonors all the people who have paid a heavy price for sprawl's rampage. Sprawl should scare. You should care.

HEALTHY PLACE DEVELOPERS WANT MORE THAN PROFITS.

Listen to Stewart Greenebaum, a former sprawl developer and more recently the developer of Maple Lawn in Maryland. He publicly announced his new commitment to HEALTHY PLACES by saying "After a lifetime of sin, I'm now addicted to virtue." He admitted that sprawl developers build "any piece of crap that you want." Referring to conventional sprawl development, he told the Baltimore County Planning Board that "What we're doing is wrong. It's our fault; we forced it." He was right when he said "There will never be enough money or concrete for us to pave our way out of the traffic congestion."

Ex-sprawl developers who feel guilty about their sprawl-building history have at least found redemption through building HEALTHY PLACES. But those developers still committed to sprawl are guilty of all the good they have not done. Perhaps they are destined for sprawl hell, stuck forever in traffic congestion behind an old school bus belching diesel fumes, alone in a small vehicle without air conditioning, a stereo system and a cell phone.

It is good news that for about 20 years a small number of developers, planners, architects and others have been nucleating the HEALTHY PLACE paradigm, with the pace picking up in the past few years. Years after they succeeded in replacing what previously prevailed, paradigm changes or revolutions look like they occurred relatively quickly. They actually take considerable time. The transistor-silicon chip took decades to change the world through computers and electronic communication; it was invented in 1947, as was the wireless cellular phone. In just a few blinks it seemed as if Starbucks popped up on every other street in America. Actually, it took some 20 years for Starbucks to become ubiquitous and for consumers to find it normal to spend several dollars for a coffee drinking *experience*. Sprawl will never be completely replaced. The goal is increasing consumption of HEALTHY PLACES until a "tipping point" is reached and an abrupt increase takes place. Just like waking up one day and realizing that every other person is using a cell phone and driving an SUV, one day nearly everyone should know someone who is thrilled with their life in a HEALTHY PLACE.

Statistics now work against HEALTHY PLACES. Few people have had the opportunity to live in HEALTHY PLACES and spread the word about the benefits they have obtained. Conventional word of mouth and "digital word of mouse" do not work effectively with so few people talking first-hand about HEALTHY PLACES. Nevertheless, once HEALTHY PLACES are built they succeed, and with more success the endangered sprawl industry will fight back with two tactics. They will use more sprawl-speak to hide the negative effects of sprawl and make people afraid of smart growth. And they will spend even more money to keep government protection and block smart growth initiatives.

When sprawl companies compete against HEALTHY PLACES they do so semantically with sprawl-speak, not substantively. Saying in advertisements that consumers can get real neighborhood or small town living is so much easier than building real neighborhoods and town centers. As to house design, nothing is more cynical and sleazy than putting tiny, dysfunctional front porches on widely separated houses on streets without sidewalks. Developers and home builders often use only one or two of the ten smart growth principles, or some New Urbanism features, and falsely claim that their product is not sprawl. As architect Rick New observed, "lots of times builders only use [New Urbanism] as a marketing gimmick by just putting a garage in the back of the house and the porch in front."

The terms of competition against sprawl housing are important. HEALTHY PLACES compete more on the basis of quality of life benefits and outdoor community design and amenities, rather than on home price, size, and indoor amenities. The full market impact of this change has yet to be seen. Success can be reached by stressing quality, service and experience over price for groceries (Whole Foods versus Wal-Mart) or coffee (Starbucks versus Dunkin' Donuts).

Unlike the sprawl business, producing HEALTHY PLACES is much more of a *knowledge industry.* Value-added activity is focused on the front end of the process, where quality design determines the more sophisticated, tailored product and its market success. Creative thinking is used, not formula methods. More technical expertise is needed for commercial buildings, public spaces, and green infrastructure. Community based planning and design is used to create "places of the heart." It sounds sappy but developers of HEALTHY PLACES want something besides profits. They want to be proud of their communities, proud of the legacy they leave to future generations. In many cases, they live in their innovative communities. An advantage is lower unit housing costs from higher residential density and lower marketing costs than for sprawl subdivisions competing against each other.

The developer Jonathan Rose shrewdly made the business case for HEALTHY PLACES:

> We have found that walkable, mixed-use, mixed-income communities designed to have a sense of place are not only healthier for their residents, but they are also healthier for the developer because they appeal to multiple markets and mitigate development risk.

If only more developers learned this lesson.

URBAN REVITALIZATION REQUIRES MIXED-USE NEIGHBORHOODS.

"If your downtown is not a neighborhood, it's not going to work. The number one priority is that a city has to be an attractive place to live. That has to be ahead of an attractive place to visit and an attractive place to do business." Lou Glazer, President of Michigan Future Inc., is absolutely correct.

Where traditional attempts at urban revitalization have failed, smart growth thinking can succeed in making cities more attractive. Not in any coercive way, but by offering consumers what they want. Millions more people could be accommodated in cities, which is significant considering the yearly national increase of some 3 million more people. Vibrant cities are also needed for the suburbs around them to be successful.

Neighborhood-scale HEALTHY PLACES within cities attract singles, childless couples, and aging baby boomers, which now represent a high fraction of households. They seek active street life in walkable, mixed-use neighborhoods with access to public transit. The right kind of urban redevelopment is taking place on a grand scale in New Jersey. The Landings at Harborside in Perth Amboy is a mixed-use project attracting empty nesters fleeing suburbia; it includes 2,100 units in condominium buildings, town houses, duplexes, and triplexes, as well as underground parking, three waterside parks, retail shops, an international market, and restaurants. "It's about a place that encourages people to leave their cars behind and go out on foot to socialize, relax, shop and play," so boasted architect Ted Liebman. An associate said "Most people will not have experienced this kind of lifestyle, this sense of community and security, in any other setting in which they have lived."

In the past, the desire for good schools drove much of the outward migration of households with children to suburban homes, and kept others from moving to cities. A strategy to greatly improve city schools to keep and attract families with children is extremely expensive and unlikely to succeed. Using tax revenues for the other aspects of municipal infrastructure will be better supported by residents without children. School voucher programs make more sense by assisting city families with children to attend private schools.

Spending large sums of money on building sports stadiums is also ill-conceived. Sports and gambling destinations do not help build true 24-7 cities. Streets often become deserted at the end of the business day and when tourist "attractions" empty out. Residents and their local shopping activities are essential for downtown revitalization programs. Infill projects must promote walkable mixed-use neighborhoods convenient to public transit and ensure easy access to green infrastructure. City streets must be made pedestrian friendly. Neighborhoods need smaller parks and plazas. Trails and greenways that connect neighborhoods to commercial areas and cultural attractions should promote walking and bicycling. New York City's Central Park was part of urban renewal and replaced a shantytown. Its stability against incalculable Manhattan land value demonstrates the value of urban greenspace. Without Central Park, Manhattan would not be such a prized location. Cities in the worst condition, like Philadelphia and St. Louis that lose population to the newest outer suburbs have considerable abandoned or underused land perfect for infill mixed-use development.

In addition to greenspace, public transit makes city living pleasurable without the need for vehicles, battling traffic and suffering parking hassles. Just as higher population density is needed for transit, transit is needed for high population density. A successful national trend is the construction of light rail and trolley systems in cities. These are much lower cost than heavy rail or subway systems. In 1975, only seven cities had light rail systems. Now there are over 20 built or under construction and over 40 more are in the planning stage. There is solid evidence that light rail attracts riders who would not use bus systems. The hourly rider capacity of light rail is about double that of buses. City governments must target areas around light rail stations for mixed-use development.

What happens when city population declines? Remaining residents protest high property taxes relative to poor services. Can urban real estate taxes be brought down to earth? Yes, literally down to land. There is a tax strategy that stimulates development in established urban areas and benefits residents. Systems usually tax land and improvements on it equally; they can be replaced with a graded or split tax system that taxes land more heavily than structures on it. Taxing the development value of land motivates landowners to develop it to generate more revenue. Unused or underused urban land becomes more competitive to sprawl development. Say goodbye to large surface parking lots, abandoned factories and warehouses, and rows of rundown houses. Welcome mixed-use development.

A few local governments have successfully used this tax approach, including Pittsburgh where, until recently, land was taxed six times more than buildings; after administrative problems in 2001 the city reverted to an ordinary tax, but has faced fiscal problems, in part because 40 percent of real estate is tax exempt. Fifteen other Pennsylvania cities, 100 irrigation districts in California, and three towns in Delaware also use this approach.

Why care? Residents can benefit because the majority of home owners get lower real estate taxes. This is important if some people are to choose city living over suburban sprawl. Here are examples of the consistent proof for the benefits of the split tax:

> In Fairfax City, Virginia, 88 percent of homeowners would pay less tax while city services would be maintained, and large corporate land owners and commercial interests would pay higher taxes.

In Philadelphia, Pennsylvania taxes would drop for 78 percent of homeowners, and increase for 50 percent of commercial properties, such as parking lots and car dealerships.

In Baltimore, Maryland a split tax would result in reduced taxes on all types of homes, varying from 5 percent less on single family houses to 12 percent less on condominiums, and 10 percent less for owners of apartment buildings.

In Asheville, North Carolina, 70 percent of residential properties would see a tax decrease or no change with a split tax.

In Harrisburg, Pennsylvania the split tax is credited with helping to reduce vacant buildings on abandoned lots from over 4,000 to less than 500 over the past two decades, while businesses increased from 1,900 to 5,600.

Eight Nobel Prize economists have endorsed this approach, including Milton Friedman who said: "Land should be taxed as much as possible, and improvements as little as possible." And a 1980 report by a U.S. House Subcommittee said: "One of the major causes of sprawl is the upside-down incentives of state and local property tax systems which invite land speculation. In the nation's 100 largest cities, nearly one-fourth of all the privately held land is vacant. Taxes on idle (urban) land are typically low, making it profitable to keep parcels unused while land values are rising." In economic downturns, this approach means less impact on residents.

Smart growth needs this smart tax. Why is it hardly used? Think about it. A system that benefits ordinary city home owners, which is most voters, has not caught on. Sprawl companies do not want the competition, and urban land speculators and businesses do not want higher taxes. The main obstacle is political, not technical or administrative; it is the influence of real estate and business interests on politicians and on voters through advertising and misinformation. High property taxes force low to middle income people to leave for lower cost sprawl housing, causing gentrification. The split tax promotes affordable housing.

Something to pay attention to is the use of formerly contaminated sites, so called brownfields, usually in urban areas targeted for revitalization. Using these former industrial sites after effective cleanup makes perfect sense, if the cleanups are truly effective. Second-rate cleanups by agencies or developers can expose future residents to toxic substances. In New Jersey, residents in a multi-unit condo building that had been a General Electric factory producing mercury vapor lamps became ill; testing showed that the building was loaded with mercury, as were its residents. Despite its industrial history, it had not been tested for mercury. It became an EPA Superfund site, and 16 families were evacuated and relocated. In Ohio, the Lexington Manor subdivision became a Superfund cleanup site after lead contamination was found because of the site's previous use, despite testing that said it was clean; many homeowners were bought out and compensated by Ryland Homes

Cities can compete with suburban sprawl growth. Some speak of "comeback cities." Mostly there are comeback *parts* of cities. We need "get real" cities. The most expert mayor on community design is Charleston, South Carolina Mayor Joseph P. Riley, Jr. Here is some of his wisdom:

> The idea is to give citizens pride in their communities by creating places that gives them a sense of ownership, of belonging. That's the true American Dream. …A key component of urban design is a belief in the value of the public realm, which every citizen owns. …If you build beautiful places – whether they are parks, parking garages, or public housing – the land next to these places becomes more successful. …If you make a city special for those who live there, then the tourists will come. …Controlling sprawl does not mean stopping growth. Controlling sprawl means strategically shaping growth. If we don't do that, then we are giving a nation of diminished value to our great grandchildren.

Juxtapose these insights with the right-wing rhetoric of sprawl shill C.C. Kraemer who believes that smart growth advocates "are on the brink of urging local governments to seize private homes through eminent domain so they can be replaced with high-rises." Sheer nonsense. Better to rant about the seizing of small businesses to grab land for big box chain stores like Wal-Mart.

SPRAWL IS A CHRONIC HEALTH THREAT.

Ugliness does not kill people. Like medicine, sprawl housing should do no harm. Through government, society manages home health threats like fires, lead paint, asbestos, radon, carbon monoxide, and more recently mold. Structurally unsafe buildings are condemned. Smoke alarms are ubiquitous. Hazards like natural gas and electricity in homes are well managed. But the ill effects of sprawl living have been ignored. Society's inattention reflects the difference between acute and chronic threats, and also between public *safety* versus public *health*. Americans have higher expectations for public safety than for public health functions of government, except when there is a major health crisis, such as polio or small pox.

Traditionally, consumers are best protected against acute home dangers that produce large short-term consequences, and where measurable quantities allow clear-cut protective standards. This allows testing for unsafe levels of smoke, carbon monoxide, lead paint and radon in homes, for example. More insidious are chronic or longer-term threats that are not easily confirmed through laboratory testing and where the harmful impacts creep up over time. *Sprawl is a chronic health threat.* Getting doses of sprawl living year after year is like accumulating a slow-acting toxin in your body. Public health departments must become involved. This is not social engineering, it is social responsibility.

Nothing is worse than a product with varying health consequences *and* different possible causes for those effects. It's difficult to convince people to protect themselves from such a product. With multiple causes, people believe that they can escape harm. Illusive scientific "proof" is not the sole salvation. Scientific certainty is a myth, one of the greatest. Common sense and personal experience are needed. Being physically inactive, stressed-out, and time-poor does not feel good, connecting them to the sprawl lifestyle can help you feel better.

Susan Muller explained why her family moved from a suburban sprawl location in Massachusetts to a higher density, more urbanized area: "It gave us the opportunity to live in the center of town. And now our children walk to school, we walk to church, and the Acton Arboretum is in our backyard." The Mullers found a HEALTHY PLACE. And so should you.

HAVE INDIVIDUALISM AND CONNECTEDNESS.

Recall the book and movie Pay It Forward, and the old adage "what goes around comes around."

Much of the case for HEALTHY PLACES is about community. Americans cherish individual freedom. No sacrifice of individual freedom is necessary to benefit from belonging to a community. Social interdependence does not negate personal freedom. Communities that work provide opportunities for a wide-ranging set of relationships as well as individual freedom. The individual freely forms relationships that are self-defined as beneficial. You choose privacy when it is desired and which neighbors are close friends.

A crude and extreme interpretation of the American ideal of rugged individualism and personal freedom can lead to social disconnection and isolation. Excessive emphasis on personal freedom displaces civic engagement and fosters anti-social behavior. Recall the Unibomber and his secluded shack in Montana. This is the core paradox of community: Individualism and social connectedness can coexist and support each other. Those cherishing the rugged individualism of early pioneers settling vast stretches of virgin land need to remember that survival meant relying on neighbors, even if they were distant.

The concept of serial reciprocity is helpful. Social connectedness works over time. Equitable benefits are not obtained through a complex chain of relationships among community residents over time. Mary serves Joan in some direct or indirect way. Joan does not repay the service by directly and immediately serving Mary, but by serving Ann next week. Ann serves others and eventually Mary benefits, but she does not see how some of her previous acts helped provide the benefits. One good deed is not bartered for another. The matrix of good deeds pays forward.

Neighborliness is a community's social fabric and quality of life support system. Neighborliness and privacy can be balanced. In blandburbs, residents are in a self-imposed prison of privacy and automobile addiction. In HEALTHY PLACES, the community is greater than the sum of its individuals. Lives are connected, but not with chains that bind. Freedom and privacy are protected by following this hierarchy of common sense "rules":

1. Take care of yourself and family.
2. Take care of your friends and neighbors.
3. Take care of your community.

Residents in real communities feel a connection to a deeper place, something beyond geography. The community is a "place of the heart," so much more than a collection of buildings, streets, and amenities. It is not a temporary place until moving on. You want to stay in a HEALTHY PLACE.

KEEPING THE GROWTH IN SMART GROWTH.

We might as well replace "In God We Trust" on our currency with "In Growth We Trust."

Emily Kueny of Dallas, Texas bemoaned the loss of "a little string of shops" that was "replaced with a Walgreens that is a gigantic concrete cube" and close by "a CVS in the shape of a concrete cube. I'm sure if you asked around, nine out of 10 people would tell you they do not want their neighborhood becoming a boring, faceless neighborhood with no character," she asserted. True local character is squashed by chain retailing prospering from automobile-dependent shopping.

So much money is made from sprawl – directly in land development and housing, and indirectly in road building, fast food, automobiles, petroleum, big box retailing, and pharmaceuticals. Products for overweight and obese people also benefit; almost half the clothes sold over the Home Shopping Network are "plus-size" women's items. From 1985 to 2003 the most popular size for women's sportswear jumped from size 8 to 14. Men's shirts are now sold in size XXXXXXXXXL. WideBodies Furniture sells an eight-legged couch to handle a 500-pound person. Airlines buy 150 to 200 seat-belt extenders a month. *Helping people through accommodation also protects sprawl and sedentary lifestyles.*

In early 2003, when many local government officials and smart growth advocates tried to get the Virginia legislature to enact some badly needed growth management laws, the executive vice president of the Home Builders Association of Virginia bragged: "Had it not been for our industry in the last two years, the state and the nation would likely be in full recession. ...[smart growth] measures would bring the economies of the 25 fastest-growing localities in the state to a complete halt." Builders used semantic terrorism to frighten the public and government. As Glen Brand of the Sierra Club said: "The major characteristic of these folks is intellectual dishonesty and ideological extremism."

Business supports sprawl, because sprawl supports business. Curbing sprawl and its sedentary lifestyle threatens much of corporate America. In 2003, fear of transit caused General Motors Canada to use an advertisement saying that buses are full of "creeps and weirdos" and suggested that riding the bus exposed people to "Hours of Hell" and "Bacterial Stew." Public uproar forced them to stop. Writing in the New York Press, Andrey Slivka made the point that sprawl "is the geographical expression of the contemporary corporate order – it's the physical reality that corporate capitalism constructs for us." Sprawl enables chain business success; virtually all growth of chains depends on more sprawl, which means the stock market counts on more sprawl.

Sprawl kills more than people. In the past decade, 50 percent of independent bookstores closed, the number of independent pharmacies dropped 30 percent, and many pizza restaurants, burger joints, ice cream parlors, and coffee shops disappeared. In the 1950s more than half of grocery stores were mom-and-pop stores, now it is only 17 percent. One chain restaurant promotes itself as a local place but does not belong in a HEALTHY PLACE. Applebee's Neighborhood Grill & Bar says it is "America's Favorite Neighbor" – all 1,600 of them. Who believes that customers really walk down to their "favorite neighbor" and afterwards over to the local mom and pop Wal-Mart and then take a nice stroll back home? Spare the sprawl-speak.

HEALTHY PLACES support "entrepreneurial capitalism" and local economies by favoring locally owned shops and restaurants. Places where art on the wall is from local people rather than art reproduced thousands of times for chains. One study found that local merchants generate three times as much local economic impact than national chain stores. A new option is community owned business like The Mercantile in Powell, Wyoming; residents bought 800 shares at $500 a piece to raise the capital to start the business in 2002. It has competed successfully against a Wal-Mart and a shopping mall. Big-business corporate capitalism uses money and power to manipulate the public psyche to shape mass consumer demand. Entrepreneurial capitalism finds a genuine need and fills it, often in the most innovative ways. Sprawl underpins corporate capitalism; the financial sector needs to imagine a consumer economy that is not dependent on roads and cars, like so much business in cities worldwide.

More Americans can and should rediscover the joys and benefits of unique neighborhood businesses. Self-service means no service. Driving some distance to save money costs time *and* money. Value means more than low price. There is product quality, style and uniqueness as well as personalized service, pleasurable experience, and near-home convenience. Some local governments with public support are restricting the size of new retail stores to address the impacts of big box stores. In some places fast food chains and other "formula" stores are being rejected. San Francisco passed a citywide ordinance to regulate formula retail, defined as chains of 12 or more stores. As one community leader said: "We don't want San Francisco to look like Trenton, New Jersey, or Topeka, Kansas." Coronado, California has a limit of 10 chain restaurants. In the excellent Village of WestClay in Indiana there will be no Starbucks, because the booming town center is reserved for entrepreneurs, and instead of a Safeway there is Broccoli Bill's Vintage Market.

Nothing symbolizes the sprawl and corporate culture more than the success of Wal-Mart, a business that never had any urban roots. No single company has benefited more from mushrooming sprawl than Wal-Mart, often called "Sprawl-Mart" by its many opponents. Wal-Mart is part of the sprawl industry. Every month Wal-Mart approves more than $1 billion of land purchases for new stores. Huge parking lots surround cheap cinder-block buildings that used to be 100,000 square feet and now are often 200,000 square feet on 25 to 50 acres. More land is used for nearby roads, and for gas stations and fast food stores located to profit from heavy traffic. Big box stores attract others and soon a large area is nothing but nothing, just mindless asphaltism run amok. In West Sadsbury, Pennsylvania a Wal-Mart Supercenter spurred a 67-acre shopping center. Local residents complain because blazing lights – "Wal-Mart sunshine" – block seeing the stars for miles around the site.

Without public spending on roads, Wal-Mart would not prosper. A report by Good Jobs First found that Wal-Mart has collected well over $1 billion in state and local government subsidies, despite negative impacts on local communities and small businesses. When a new supercenter opens two local grocery stores are likely to close. That is how Wal-Mart became the biggest seller of groceries in the nation. Professor Floyd J. McKay created this apt image: "Wal-Mart is like a neutron bomb, sucking life out of small towns, leaving buildings without the essence of civic life."

On a human scale, Wal-Mart creates a large number of dead-end, low-wage jobs. That smiling face of a Wal-Mart greeter is not the whole story. Half the Wal-Mart workforce qualifies for food stamps. No wonder every year half the workforce turns over, some 600,000 workers. And a little known fact is that half the states allow chains like Wal-Mart to avoid paying state income taxes because local profits can be transferred to tax free states like Delaware. Desperate local governments often exempt the chains from local taxes for years. All this shifts tax burdens to the public. The final economic insult is that almost everything sold is manufactured in foreign countries with cheap labor, causing loss of good jobs in the United States. Along with Wal-Mart workers themselves, the unemployed increase the burden on remaining taxpayers for public health care and welfare services. Low prices are indirectly subsidized, a kind of hidden welfare program funded through higher taxes. In 2003 the average American spent $761 in Wal-Mart stores because of lower prices, but that means a savings of perhaps $85, assuming an average 10 percent savings (actually Wal-Mart claims only a 4.4 percent saving). That savings comes with considerable costs to Americans taxpayers.

The "Wal-Martization" of our economy offers low priced goods to low wage earners, the unemployed, and sprawl residents spending too much money on driving in sprawlspace. Margaret Kimberley saw the absurdity: "The Wal-Martization of America provides us with the lower cost goods we will all need when our wages are lowered by the Wal-Marts of the world." Wal-Mart is the booby prize for those winning the race to the *bottom* of the economic ladder. In fact, Wal-Mart targets households with less than $35,000 income.

Americans now have a love-hate relationship with Wal-Mart – love the prices, hate the company. Fighting new Wal-Mart stores is one thing, threatening the whole economy is quite another. For smart growth and HEALTHY PLACES to succeed, national economic growth must not be threatened. Growth is a national mandate, unassailable dogma. *Like it or not, American economic prosperity depends on GROWTH.* The American economy is like a giant Ponzi scheme; without certain future growth the economy would plummet. But the Gross National Product measures economic activity, not quality of life. Smart growth must emphasize both smart and *growth* to succeed. If the anti-sprawl movement is equated with no-growth, it will be opposed by government officials, unions, financial institutions, the business community, and much of the public. Advocates of no growth who label themselves as smart growth adherents help smart growth's opponents. Slow growth and building moratorium proponents usually want time to figure out what current residents want for their future and to promote smart growth. But the sprawl industry thinks no growth, slow growth, controlling growth, and smart growth are all bad for business. Smart growth is really a middle ground between total capitulation to developers and unproductive attempts to stop all new land development. Baltimore developer Bill Struever got it right: "Rather than being anti-growth, Smart Growth is all about promoting growth in targeted areas." The style and character of growth matter. Growth by choice beats growth by chance.

Though the smart growth movement must acquiesce to growth and the need for more housing to succeed, as a consumer you have choices. You can support independent, locally owned businesses rather than chains. You can practice "political consumerism." Shop outside the box and your money will do more than buy things; it will work for your community.

SPRAWL SUPPORTS CONSUMPTION AND CONSUMPTION SUPPORTS SPRAWL.

"This is the paradox. Here we are, living at the pinnacle of human possibility, awash in material abundance. We get what we say we want, only to discover that it doesn't satisfy us," so observed psychologist Barry Schwartz about the overabundance of choice.

On a 20-mile stretch of highway in Arizona there are six Wal-Marts, and 14 more nearby. Sprawl supports consumption and consumption supports sprawl. Mall after strip mall after mini-mall after big box store after fast food store after convenience store after gas station, and over again - this is the commercial sprawlscape — built to snatch your dollars. Americans are united not by interpersonal relationships but by similar patterns of consumption, buying and eating the same products in the same chains. A society of segregated strangers connected by what they consume rather than by involvement in their shared community. Writing in the *Los Angeles Times*, author Patrick Moore caught the essence of the sprawl culture and economy when he identified "a creeping blandness in American life, fueled by the culture's endless packaging and sale of all that is unique." We have "a culture consisting mainly of marketing messages," he said. But there are no big companies marketing HEALTHY PLACES.

American consumerism is a paradox. Yes, the United States is home to pluralism and diversity. But large market share defines product success.

Less successful products disappear, or survive by serving niche rather than mass markets. Retail chains foster consistency. The American culture of consumption is also the culture of conformity. Like some commercial cancer, the genius of American marketing replicates success everywhere. Sprawlspace is brand-rich: Burger King or McDonald's or Subway, Circuit City or Best Buy, Wal-Mart or K-Mart or Target, CVS or Walgreens or Rite-Aid, Red Lobster or Outback Steakhouse or Olive Garden or Applebee's, Staples or Office Depot. And when you travel you can choose among chains in hotel-strips, from which you cannot walk to anything. These chains bind you to the consumer economy…and bore you. Stores and restaurants may appear to be local businesses but are not. You can get Mexican food at Chipotle where workers are mostly Hispanic; the chain is owned by McDonald's.

Once inside stores you face the illusion of choice, daunting arrays of products, like 20 kinds of toothpaste, 50 kinds of television sets, dozens of jeans, etc. Competition among companies is largely superficial however, because products in a specific category are more alike than dissimilar. For time-poor Americans, trivial choice masks blandness, eats up time and adds to stress from "choice congestion." Corporate America knows that consumers relish choice, but it is out of control. Often one company will make many variations of essentially the same product, like six or more kinds of orange juice or toothpaste under the same brand. Worse yet, what appear as different brands and companies are often just parts of the same corporate conglomerate. Giving us more meaningless choices manipulates us to buy more meaningless products.

Competition among products and companies is less than meets the eye. The best product does not necessarily succeed. Marketing trumps performance. As market share swells competition becomes more difficult. So IBM-style personal computers conquer Apple computers, and Microsoft Word beats WordPerfect software. Cars replace trolleys, railroads and buses. Chain big box stores wipe out neighborhood mom-and-pop shops. Blandburbs preempt HEALTHY PLACES. In the sprawl economy, market share success is the mother of blandness.

Most Americans feel neither pleasure nor disgust driving through repetitive commercial tastelessness. These surroundings hide in plain sight, because people are blinded by their blandness. People periodically seek surroundings that make them feel better. They escape to vacation spots that have place personality, environmental beauty, and walkable streets. But most of the time Americans keep driving to buy more stuff for their cocoons. In blandburbs, consumption is compulsive and conspicuous. Sedentary, automobile addicted sprawl residents are compliant consumers. When Wal-Mart became and stayed number one on the Fortune 500 list of the biggest U.S. companies, America's economy unmistakably became the sprawl economy. Battles against Wal-Mart are part of the war against sprawl and its bland conformity.

The consumer economy got a shot of adrenalin in the 1970s. Bigger and more costly housing, higher vehicle costs and – most importantly – suburban loneliness and blandness prompted many married women to become wage earners outside the home. They were surely repulsed by the subservient suburban housewives in 1975's *The Stepford Wives*. The exodus from suburbia to jobs signaled the change from suburban dream to nightmare. Ironically, victims of sprawl made sprawl worse by increasing vehicle use and traffic. Working women became time-poor, stuck in traffic, and sedentary. Eating habits worsened as home cooking disappeared from daily routines. The Centers for Disease Control and Prevention found that, for the 1980s and 1990s, baby boomer women in their mid-thirties and early forties had a 32 percent increase in deaths from heart attacks. Women sought freedom and self-fulfillment, but sloth, gluttony, traffic congestion and stress found them.

So called "bleeding-heart liberals", environmental activists and social responsibility advocates have bemoaned intense American consumerism, claiming it threatens the global environment, uses unfair amounts of natural resources, and drives pollution. "Conservative" thinkers believe that technology comes to the rescue to prevent resource depletion and pollution from causing calamities. When some supporters of smart growth condemn and belittle consumers they sound anti-American and set up smart growth for attack by sprawl shills. Of course, each of us is both consumer and citizen. Americans should embrace "political consumerism" that supports preferred values. A home purchase makes a big statement. Choosing a HEALTHY PLACE is a vote in favor of the public realm and civic engagement, and a vote against sprawl.

Political consumerism empowers individuals and reduces dependence on government action; it is individualized collective action that can transform the housing market. Choosing a HEALTHY PLACE is like rejecting products associated with foreign child labor, environmental pollution, poor labor practices, and destruction of rain forests. And it is also like buying low carbohydrate, low fat or organic foods that you believe provide a health benefit. Our society needs a "buycott" of sprawl because it is a "bad" product, bad for individuals and bad for society.

Being a consumer is inevitable, but not being an obsessive consumer. The American lifestyle trap is working long hours to afford voracious consumption. It has been termed "affluenza," an epidemic of over-consumption, an unappeasable hunger for goods and services, and a craving for choice. Shop till you drop has new meaning. While great for corporate America, compulsive consumption is not working for individuals. Happiness and self-fulfillment have not risen with rising incomes and materialism. Intense consumption makes people time-poor and sedentary. People spend more time buying things, using them, taking care of them, and updating them. More stuff requires more home space. The Worldwatch Institute's State of the World 2004 said: "Higher levels of obesity and personal debt, chronic time shortages, and a degraded environment are all signs that excessive consumption is diminishing the quality of life for many people."

A vacuum of meaning afflicts Americans. The Bland American Dream implodes one person at a time. Bored and stressed residents become sedentary and fat amidst their plentiful possessions. In the past 30 years of rising affluence, retailing and sprawl, the fraction of women and men saying they are happy has declined and more and more of them and their children are clinically depressed. In "How not to buy happiness" in *Daedalus*, Cornell University Professor Robert H. Frank offered this explanation: "Considerable evidence suggests that if we use an increase in our incomes, as many of us do, simply to buy bigger houses and more expensive cares, then we do not end up any happier than before. …The less we spend on conspicuous consumption goods, the better we can afford to alleviate [traffic] congestion; and the more time we can devote to family and friends, to exercise, sleep, travel and other restorative activities." Individuals could better spend time and money on civic engagement to offset the political influence of the sprawl lobby. A reallocation of time and money strategy would "result in healthier, longer – and happier lives," said Frank. This fits perfectly with pursuing life in a HEALTHY PLACE, even if it means a smaller but not cheaper house, especially if it cuts car use and promotes active living.

What is blocking Americans from waking up to their pseudo-reality and switching strategies? Americans have been brainwashed by corporate capitalism to consume as if enough is never enough. Personal compulsive consumption is like a military arms race. Armed with credit cards consumers feel compelled to join cancerous consumption patterns defined as American "success," even if it means working harder and having less time to be healthy and happy. It is spending for the sake of GNP and Wall Street, not personal well-being. A society that steers its citizens to seek possessions and unhappiness is surely a social phantasy system.

Answer these questions: If Americans prized more of what is *outside* their homes, would there be less consumption? If homes were not cocoons to luxuriate in, would there be less consumption? If homes had not become bigger and bigger, would people buy less stuff to put in them? If people spent more time being physically active, would they buy less stuff? If Americans drove less through the commercial sprawlscape, would they buy less? If you answered affirmatively to these questions, then you agree that excessive consumption of goods and food goes hand in hand with excessive land consumption. If so, sprawl surely supports consumption and consumption surely supports sprawl.

Patriotism does not require compulsive consumption. True enough, if a great many Americans suddenly consumed less, the economy would tank. Entrepreneurial capitalism, political consumerism and "smart business" must replace quantity with quality and discounts with service and convenience. Two examples of "smart business" are Starbucks and Whole Foods Market. Both serve the mass market profitably by selling higher priced quality products, offering a pleasing shopping experience, and providing a "neighborhood" store atmosphere.

Nicholas von Hoffman asked in *The Nation*, "isn't one of the traits of conservatism to give us more of what we already have too much of and to withhold what we have too little of?" Yes, and that helps explain why shills work for sprawl and against HEALTHY PLACES.

BABY BOOMERS AND GEN XERS WANT A CHOICE.

Imagine what might have happened if, in The Graduate (1967), Dustin Hoffman had been told to get into sprawl land development rather than "plastics." Back then popular culture had not yet embraced anti-sprawl sentiments, and "plastics" was a good metaphor for mainstream American culture that so many young people were rebelling against. Now, anti-sprawl sentiment is part of contemporary culture.

The greatest contribution to American society by the coming tsunami of baby boomers may be as the market force that breaks the back of sprawl. Like a counter-culture echo from the 1960s, the boomers finally change America by recognizing how sprawl's social and geographical separateness corrodes quality of life by promoting isolation, indolence, technology dependence and indulgent consumption. They apply E. F. Schumaker's ideas in Small Is Beautiful – A Study of Economics as if People Mattered and help demolish sprawl's bigger-is-better-mentality.

Demographically, many of the 77 million aging baby boomers will seek alternatives to sterile sprawl living, especially the 30 percent who are not inclined to stay in their current homes as they age. They will seek a HEALTHY PLACE, because they want a more urban place, but not necessarily a city center. They will be very health oriented and dissatisfied with the same suburban schlock found everywhere. They will want to walk more and drive less, a lot less. A survey by the developer Del Webb found that walking is the favorite form of exercise of nearly 90 percent of baby boomers. The boomers do not want to waste their precious time in cars and painful traffic. For the last decades of their lives, they will want a real community with place personality. Pam Vaughn has studied boomer homebuyers and said: "They are not looking at this stage in life to mow the lawn and rake the leaves. Cookie cutter neighborhoods where all the homes look alike turn them off. They don't see themselves as old now or ever getting old. Living in an active adult community carries a stigma."

While the baby boomers are likely to seek HEALTHY PLACES in their later years, about 20 million post-boomer Generation Xers are ready right now to embrace HEALTHY PLACES. J. Walker Smith, the head of Yankelovich, Inc., said that the Gen Xers want "planned communities that foster togetherness and neighborhood life." They value public gathering places, sidewalks, porches, and inclusive neighborhoods, which reflect their priority for human values over property values. "Expect to continue to find Xers in mixed-use communities filled with an eclectic mix of office facilities and retailers within walking distance of their homes," said Smith. Developer Brent E. Herrington has studied Gen Xers and said: "The friends and neighbors who are coming over have refrigerator privileges." They "view a great neighborhood as an extension of great parenting," he said. Moreover, Harrington found that they "find suburbia homogeneous and uninteresting," and have "extreme disillusionment with the bland, vanilla suburbs."

At least one-third of consumers want an alternative to sprawl, according to a 2001 report produced for the National Governors Association, "New Community Design to the Rescue – Fulfilling Another American Dream." This will surely rise to 50 percent with better information. The Congress for the New Urbanism talks about home buyers willing to pay a 25 to 40 percent premium for property in walkable communities where they can reduce their car use. Its report "The Coming Demand" noted: "The American housing market is constrained by policies that promote sprawl and the natural inertia of an interdependent, multi-billion dollar industry. ...Whereas a third of housing consumers in many markets say they would prefer to live in a walkable neighborhood with small lots, the number of such units actually developed is negligible against the vast scale of the American real estate industry."

Have no uncertainty about this consumer demand. Here is ample evidence of it; take a mind walk through this field of statistics.

Robert Charles Lesser & Company, a real estate advisor to developers, studied Atlanta, Phoenix, Denver, Provo, Albuquerque, Boise, and Chattanooga; a consistent 25 to 33 percent of residents would seriously consider buying a HEALTHY PLACE.

A 2002 survey of California adults by the Public Policy Institute of California found that, other things being equal: 49 percent would choose to live in a small house with a small backyard, if it meant having a short commute to work; 47 percent would choose to live in a mixed-use neighborhood where they can walk to stores, schools, and services; 31 percent would choose to live in a high-density neighborhood where it was convenient to use public transit when traveling locally.

The 1998 Vermonters Attitudes on Sprawl Survey found that 48 percent of people preferred communities with houses, stores, and services within walking distance of one another.

National surveys show that consumers prefer smaller lots and/or clustered housing: 37 percent in the 1998 Professional Builder survey, and 57 percent in the 1996 National Association of Home

Builders survey.

A 2002 survey for the National Association of Realtors found that in choosing a community the following were very important to quality of life: parks and open spaces, 92 percent of people; streets with sidewalks, 70 percent; shorter commute, 64 percent; access to shops and restaurants, 52 percent. The conclusion was that one-fourth to one-third of Americans "is willing to consider the Smart Growth option."

A 2004 survey of Sacramento area residents found that 73 percent prefer single family housing close to work, versus 48 percent who preferred suburban single family housing even with a long commute; 43 percent want to live close to parks.

In late 1998 the state of Maine surveyed 602 recent homebuyers and found that 37 to 45 percent of homebuyers could be consumers of HEALTHY PLACES. But homebuilders were skeptical that consumers wanted alternatives to sprawl.

The Detroit Area Study of the multi-county metro area found that 30 percent of people favored a HEALTHY PLACE alternative over sprawl; over 50 percent supported smart growth initiatives and less than 10 percent opposed them.

A 1999 survey by American LIVES of home-buyers in five states found that 72 percent favored clustered housing around a town center with a village green surrounded by shops, civic buildings, churches, and similar facilities; 78 percent favored homes with garages hidden behind them, front porches to encourage neighborly interactions, and streets with shade trees; 64 percent preferred a place with less automobile dependency.

A survey found that 84 percent of people felt that homes, stores, and services within walking distance of each other in their community was extremely or somewhat desirable. Another survey found that 76 percent of people felt that it was very or somewhat important to have neighborhood shops.

A survey found that 74 percent of people strongly agreed that they wanted a town with a rich texture of housing styles and a variety of people and lifestyles.

The city of Tucson surveyed 300 residents and found that 80 percent would be willing to pay a $5,000 to $10,000 premium to live in a place designed with "resource conservation and community features."

Minnesota's Metropolitan Council found that 88 percent of people agreed that their neighborhood should have a mix of homes, shops, offices, schools and parks, so people can more easily meet their everyday needs.

A survey found that 46 percent of people agree that businesses and homes should be built closer together to shorten commutes and limit traffic.

For some 16 years Los Angeles has had the honor of being the number one traffic congested urban area in the nation. Because of car pain people want to reduce their car use, especially by living closer to work. An October 2003 article in the Los Angeles Times concluded: "Choosing a house based on commuting arguably marks the most dramatic shift in home-buying attitudes among Southern Californians since the post-World War II march to the suburbs began." Research at the University of Southern California found that the fraction of consumers who prefer denser, walkable communities will comprise one-third to one-half of new homebuyers by 2010, double that in previous decades.

A 2002 survey of AAA members in Arizona, 98 percent of whom depend on motor vehicles for daily transportation, found that 36 percent would choose a community where they could walk or take public transit to work, shopping, and restaurants but had less private space, as compared to a conventional car-dependent sprawl un-place. Interestingly, the preference for the sprawl-alternative rose with decreasing household income, reaching 64 percent for annual incomes under $25,000. The survey also found stronger support for public transit than building new roads.

And the Funders' Network for Smart Growth and Livable Communities, representing philanthropic foundations supporting smart growth, concluded that conventional consumer preference data, such as that widely circulated by the National Association of Home Builders, is biased. Survey data overstate demand for detached homes on large suburban lots and seriously underestimate demand for HEALTHY PLACES. The core problem is that most residents only know sprawl. In fact, usually over 80 percent of respondents own detached sprawl houses; one survey found that 32 percent of people do not think that alternatives to sprawl even exist.

In turning latent demand into actual home buying decisions, is there self-selection of customers of HEALTHY PLACES? Are people choosing places that fit them? Or are people from sprawl un-places changing their behavior? It does not matter. But logically, if latent demand for HEALTHY PLACES is at least one-third of housing consumers, then most of those people are living in blandburbs. Do physically inactive automobile addicts want to live in HEALTHY PLACES? We have a direct answer.

Professor Larry Frank and colleagues at the Georgia Institute of Technology questioned large numbers of people living in the Atlanta metropolitan area. People living in sprawl un-places were given a number of tough choices and trade-offs about communities with contrasting features. They consistently chose the HEALTHY PLACES option: 37 percent prefer smaller homes that allow them to walk, bike or use public transit more, over larger homes that require driving for all trips; 70 percent prefer a community with more space for walking and biking and less space for cars over a place designed for cars but lacking walkability; and 33 percent prefer a home on a smaller lot within a community that would be 3 to 4 miles to everyday destinations like work, school and shopping over a home on a larger lot, but where they would have to drive 15 to 18 miles to everyday destinations. Remember, these are people already living in automobile dependent blandburbs who would rather live in HEALTHY PLACES, even though few have seen such places or fully understand all the health and other benefits of them.

Despite all this evidence on demand, the housing industry produces far less than one percent of HEALTHY PLACES. What will it take to supply this demand? Action by unhappy consumers, which should be easy because: "The only people in the suburbs who like what's happening are the developers, who are getting rich, and the city councils, which are mostly in the developers' pockets," according to urban analyst Myron Orfield

New York Times columnist David Brooks is a sprawl shill hiding behind witty ramblings about things that don't actually exist. In his 2004 article, "Our Sprawling, Supersize Utopia," he talked about the "unsatisfactory present" being overcome by the "Paradise Spell: the tendency to see the present from the vantage point of the future." "Suburban America…is also a transcendent place infused with everyday utopianism." Brooks sees people having "more choice over which sort of neighborhood to live in" and "congregate with people who are basically like yourself." Imagine, the absence of diversity in blandburbs is good. Brooks justifies self-delusion to avoid the pain of the "unsatisfactory present" failing to deliver yesterday's fantasy about the future. Sprawl does not deliver dreams, but Brooks is happy that people keep chasing them. By seeing sprawl as historic inevitability and failing to grasp that most Americans have no choice but sprawl, Brooks earned his sprawl shill status. Practical utopia seekers seek HEALTHY PLACES.

HEALTHY PLACES ARE A BUSINESS SUCCESS.

In 1998 sprawl shill Peter Gordon, supposedly a believer in markets, said this about New Urbanism: "If there were a grain of truth in their view, we would soon see people demanding it, and developers would strive to provide it." Well, that's exactly what's going on.

Annual surveys by New Urban News have documented a steady rise in the number of HEALTHY PLACES completed or in some stage of construction. In 2003 there were 369 such projects, compared to 272 in 2002, 213 in 2001, 155 in 2000, and 124 in 1999. About half the projects are on greenfield sites, meaning totally new communities, and the other half are various types of infill projects in areas with existing infrastructure. But only projects 15 acres or above are counted, which means that many smaller urban infill projects are not counted. Not all these projects may do well when evaluated with the checklist given in Chapter 6.

These constructed and planned HEALTHY PLACES are in 37 states; the top ten states are Florida, California, North Carolina, Maryland, Virginia, Texas, Colorado, Georgia, South Carolina, and Pennsylvania. Wherever you want to live there is a good chance that a HEALTHY PLACE already exists or is being planned, but more of them are needed to satisfy demand.

Contrary to disinformation from sprawl shills, there is proof of the financial success of HEALTHY PLACES, which could only happen if consumers wanted them:

The developer of Carpenter Village in North Carolina said that "After we got 3 or 4 phases done, people could visualize the entire project, and sales went through the roof."

The River Ranch in Lafayette, Louisiana developer has received two to four times the land prices in sprawl subdivisions in the area. Build-out will drop from eight years to six.

The developer of Newpoint, near Beaufort, South Carolina, had revenue per net acre 84 percent higher than a conventional adjacent property.

At Highlands Garden Village in Denver, houses have sold as high as $400,000 higher than original projections. Homes sold before they or the retail center were built. Prices increased 25 percent yearly from 1999 to 2002, compared to 10 percent in the surrounding area. Though the apartment vacancy rate was 12 percent in the Denver metropolitan area, the rate in the Village was only 1 percent.

At Village Homes in Davis, California, units sell in less than one-third the normal listing time, if they have not already been snapped up by word of mouth before listing; homes fetch about $10 to $25 per square foot above normal market value.

Eighty-four percent of residents in HEALTHY PLACES in Maryland, Tennessee, Florida and California said they paid a premium price to live in those communities.

In Kentlands, Maryland, a study of 1,850 sales found that buyers paid a premium of 12 to 13 percent, or $24,000 to $30,000, which was directly attributable to smart growth or new urbanism advantges.

The developer-builder of Doe Mill Neighborhood in Chico, California is receiving a 20 percent premium over conventional housing, even with smaller homes on smaller lots and explained it thusly: "Our home buyers understand the benefits of the neighborhood beyond their own house and yard."

Washington's Landing in Pittsburgh is a mixed-use community built on a former brownfields site; $140,000 townhomes bought in 1996 have more than doubled in value.

Charles Lockwood found that pedestrian-oriented, mixed-use town centers have higher office and retail lease rates, higher prices for apartments and townhouses, and higher retail sales and sales tax revenues than conventional single land use, suburban developments. They also produce a "halo effect" of higher property values in surrounding areas.

OFTEN, SALES HAPPEN QUICKLY.

In Lakelands in Maryland all homes will be sold a year ahead of projections.

In Fall Creek Place in Indianapolis, Indiana, the first year goal of selling 40 homes was exceeded by the sale of 200 homes, with a waiting list for others.

In Baldwin Park, near Orlando, Florida, one builder had sold 35 of its 144 lots in the first week; another builder got deposits on 60 of its 146 lots in the first three weeks.

Instead of taking 15 to 20 years for build-out, only 5 or 6 years will bring Wyndhurst in Lynchburg, Virginia to completion; all the land was sold out in 3 years.

At Metropolis at Dadeland, part of a new mixed-use urban center in Kendall, Florida, 95 percent of the 397 condo units were pre-sold before ground was broken and almost two years from completion.

In the initial phase of Cherry Hill Village in Canton, Michigan, buyer interest was so high that a lottery was used.

With fast sales, build-out for King Farm in Maryland will drop from 10 to 8 years.

At Serenbe, outside Atlanta, Georgia, 32 of the first 40 lots were sold when they were first made available.

The last 45 lots in Middleton Hills near Madison, Wisconsin sold out in 15 minutes.

While the land was still being graded, 350 homes were sold in New Town at St. Charles in the St. Louis, Missouri metro area.

At Maple Lawn in Maryland, because hundreds of customers showed up for just nine townhouses, a lottery was used.

There you have it. Yet, sprawl shills ignore market success. They should listen to professionals in the business. Developer Bill Struever said: "Smart Growth developers and builders like me are booming… From a business perspective, Smart Growth is really about leveling the economic playing field by eliminating the disincentives for reinvestment in older communities and reducing the incentives for sprawl." Community designer Ray Gindroz said: "What's happening nationally is that developments built to New Urbanist principles sell faster, and at higher prices." In the academic world, University of South Florida Professor Trent Green said innovative developers of HEALTHY PLACES "can realize a premium by developing in this manner. The financial benefits are making themselves more and more evident as each new project comes online."

CHILDLESS HOUSEHOLDS ARE THE NEW MARKET FORCE.

General demand is one thing, but exactly what kinds of people are drawn to HEALTHY PLACES? Look at the data below. A 2001 marketing study for a proposed suburban HEALTHY PLACE in the Kansas City area found families with children were more attracted than other households. The opposite trend was found in a study for an urban infill project in Lexington, Kentucky, which shows how high fractions of younger professionals, aging baby boomers, and older retirees drive demand for HEALTHY PLACES.

HOUSEHOLD TYPE	SUBURBAN	URBAN
Families with children	**44 percent**	10 percent
Empty nesters and retirees	31 percent	23 percent
Younger singles and couples without children	25 percent	**67 percent**

Childless households are a steadily increasing fraction of home seekers. In the 1950s when sprawl was exploding married-couple households dominated the housing market at nearly 80 percent. In 2001 they were down to 67 percent, only half with kids. One-third of home buyers were single adults, and only about one-third of these had children. With less than 10 percent of households nationally having two parents and two children under age 18, suburbia should change. In many places, households with singles exceed those with married couples with children. Clearly, schools are not an issue for many home buyers. Households without children can more easily tradeoff home floor space for community, the public realm, street life, and walking access to shopping and other amenities. Sprawl has grown old and ill-fitting for current demographics.

A genuine HEALTHY PLACE should serve the needs of children and the elderly and be pedestrian friendly, walkable, and safe for residents at both ends of the age spectrum. This way, everyone in between will also be well served. Sprawl is just the opposite. It does not serve the needs of the young and old. When baby boomers leave full-time work they will shift from being time-poor to time-rich, and HEALTHY PLACES will provide them with more opportunities for using their new time-wealth, especially for physical activity.

TRAFFIC-SUFFERERS HAVE A PERSONAL SOLUTION.

This is the ugly truth. All the negative consequences of sprawl on the quality of life of so many people cannot be easily fixed by government, especially eliminating traffic congestion. It cannot happen. It is technically impossible.

Build more roads or widen existing ones, and you simply attract more traffic. This "induced demand" – the "build it and they will come" phenomenon – results from people in the area shifting their routes or modes of travel to use the new capacity. The important study, "Analysis of Metropolitan Highway Capacity and the Growth in Vehicle Miles of Travel" found that data for 70 urbanized areas showed from 15 to 45 percent of traffic is caused just by expanding road networks; this means that traffic congestion would have grown less rapidly if no new or wider highways were built at all. A 2002 study in Transportation Research said available research shows "strong evidence that new transportation capacity induces increased travel, both due to short run effects and long run changes in land use development patterns."

New suburban road capacity triggers new development. In the Tampa, Florida area the 2001 opening of the Suncoast Parkway, a state toll road going nearly 60 miles north and costing about $5 one-way, opened up sprawl development in once rural counties. Developers have exploited land along Interstate 85 where four of the five most sprawling metro areas in the nation are exploding in North Carolina, South Carolina and Georgia. Montgomery County, Maryland received $200 million to expand Interstate 270 up to 12 lanes, the "rolling parking lot" that connects Maryland sprawl residents to jobs in Washington, D.C. and Virginia. In the 5 years before widening, 1,745 new homes were approved in the 12 miles north of Rockville, the older suburb on the route. In the following 5 years, 13,642 new homes were approved, and the road stayed congested, despite the expensive widening.

Live with traffic congestion, or react to it with a personal solution. There is no big picture cure for traffic congestion, not road building or wider use of congestion-priced toll roads, nor public transit. Population growth makes more congestion a certainty. The sprawl industry – from home builders to Wal-Mart – benefits from unchecked population growth, much of it from illegal immigrants and their offspring. Suffer in pedestrian sprawl or be a pedestrian and walk away from traffic crawl.

The Wall Street Journal ran an article "Developers building luxury homes in undesirable spots" in 2004. Because of land scarcity in popular areas and because of "people who don't want frustratingly long commutes," developers are selling homes for $500,000 to $1 million or more that are built close to garbage collection centers, airports, noisy highways, train repair yards, low-income housing and cemeteries. That's how strong the desire to minimize car use is.

Likewise, do not expect government to willingly replace zoning laws that promote sprawl with ones that give developers the right to build HEALTHY PLACES. A 2003 survey of city and county governments in the metro Atlanta area, after many years of runaway sprawl, found that only 10 out of 26 had specific mixed-use zoning codes. Government can and should change zoning, but it will take too long, if ever. Elected officials rarely lead efforts to change longstanding behavior, because they are followers of current public tastes and receive support from status quo interests.

Consider changing your home location or your job to reduce your dependence on cars. Don't wait for the "system" to help. Find a HEALTHY PLACE.

THE HUBRIS OF THE SPRAWL INDUSTRY WILL BE ITS DOWNFALL.

Considering sprawl's bad karma it should lose market share. We face two possible future scenarios, success or failure for HEALTHY PLACES. Success means an American Dream Community available to all who want it. Failure means continuing dominance of blandburbs and the sprawl culture. As Bob Ewegen of *The Denver Post* opined: "The legacy of dumb growth will be with us until the next ice age, when the glaciers scrape off the sprawl and allow our descendents to start all over." Unless we restrain sprawl now.

For individuals, just living in HEALTHY PLACES constitutes success. But true market success means giving many Americans that opportunity. Increasing market share will also help ease prices. We need a 100 time's greater level of annual housing units in new HEALTHY PLACES to start the national shift from sprawl. Three things are needed.

First, we need loud voices and consistent votes of citizen-consumers. As the noted economist Henry George said "We cannot safely leave politics to politicians. ...The people themselves must think, because the people alone can act." Practicing political consumerism, Americans must pressure the housing industry – or at least parts of it – to "see the light" and change their business model from sprawl to smart growth. Anger and frustration over traffic congestion and other ill effects of sprawl, especially health impacts, need to become loud demands for more HEALTHY PLACES.

Voter-power surfaces when it comes to paying for open space preservation. In the 2002 off-year election, 85 percent of ballot land preservation measures passed. From 1998 to 2002 ballot measures nationwide generated over $23 billion for land preservation, according to the Trust for Public Land. It is even more important to support elected officials with uncompromising commitment to smart growth. Ironically, civic engagement is less likely for time-poor sprawl residents. Data from some 30,000 interviews and census data showed that people living in neighborhoods built after 1950 are less likely to belong to political organizations, belong to a local reform organization, attend a partisan political event, attend a march or demonstration, vote in a national election or attend a public meeting. Americans who feel the pain of sprawl must act to protect their quality of life and health.

But outspoken citizens and grassroots groups risk "SLAPP suits," standing for Strategic Lawsuits Against Public Participation. Their goal is intimidation, to force activists to back down by making them spend time and money defending themselves, typically against suits accusing them of slander, libel, and defamation. Only 21 states have laws against SLAPP suits aimed at stifling civic engagement. In May 2002 the Colorado Association of Home Builders took credit for defeating anti-SLAPP legislation in the state senate. In September 2003 a SLAPP action was brought against a citizen opposing a development in Loudoun County, Virginia. The developer accused the citizen of stirring up "opposition among the neighbors in a deliberate, willful and malicious effort" to stop the project. The action was described as intimidation by local government officials. In New Jersey, Helen Henderson was sued by a strip mall developer. As a volunteer for the state Department of Environmental Protection she had reported wetlands on the developer's property. The state verified her finding and agreed to pay for her defense. Attempts in New Jersey to pass anti-SLAPP legislation have failed for about seven years.

Why stop at lawsuits? After his rezoning request to develop farmland was denied by Oconee County, Georgia, the sprawl developer got even with local residents who fought his project. Besides suing the county, he dumped tons of fresh poultry manure on his property. Neighbors could spend little time outdoors because of the incredible stench and swarms of flies. They also saw his ad in the local paper for a hog farmer to lease his 34 acres for just $1 per acre. Sprawl happens.

Secondly, we need public support for developers of HEALTHY PLACES so they obtain government and citizen approvals. Public interest, environmental, consumer, religious and social equity organizations should use the checklist presented in Chapter 6 and similar tools, and support genuine HEALTHY PLACES. Some groups are doing this. The Greenbelt Alliance in the San Francisco area has a Livable Communities Endorsement Program; it provides an endorsement letter to a developer, which can be used before government bodies. The group also directly intervenes when appropriate to support a project and get news media coverage for it. The 1000 Friends of Minnesota group has a Smart Growth Design Awards program for constructed projects. The Vermont Smart Growth Collaborative has a Housing Endorsement Program based on smart growth criteria. Such efforts need public health officials to publicize the health advantages of alternatives to sprawl development.

Thirdly, resist blaming NIMBY-citizens for opposing higher density smart growth projects. Remember that the sprawl lobby, sprawl shills, and corrupt elected officials have ensured that local comprehensive plans and zoning rules usually do not directly support smart growth. If they don't, why should citizens have confidence in smart growth? Why should people be "sacrificial lambs" because a region needs new housing? Smart growth developers and their supporters must use community based planning and design, presented in Chapter 7, to address citizen concerns about traffic congestion, crowded schools and other issues. Traffic increases can be mitigated through mixed-use design that cuts car use, and school crowding can be prevented through mixed-income and diverse housing that attracts households without children, and assisted living facilities and senior housing. A superb new town center can offer many amenities for surrounding sprawl residents and help keep local taxes down. The goal should be to tempt some current area residents to move into the new project.

Deafened by decades of success, the hubris of the sprawl industry will be its downfall. With so many smart growth advocates and so many Americans fed up with sprawl, the tipping point for massive societal change is within sight. This is a real fight of good against bad, of people against corruption, of truth against lies. "Kill sprawl before sprawl kills you" – now there's a call to battle to rattle sprawl. Sprawl is a formidable enemy. Sprawl shills practice "intellectual terrorism" to make Americans fearful of smart growth. The sprawl lobby spends whatever it takes and uses trickier tactics to navigate through anti-sprawl storms.

New Jersey Governor James E. McGreevey's anti-sprawl rhetoric was striking, but in July 2004 without the usual fanfare, he signed into law the Permit Streamlining in Smart Growth Areas bill. Environmental and smart growth groups had begged the governor to veto the bill and threatened court action. They correctly viewed the bill as payback to the sprawl industry, because of the passage a month earlier of a bill to preserve 120,000 acres in the Highlands area. The second bill was concealed until its rushed passage in three days with no floor debate, causing The New York Times to comment that it was "a stunning display of the construction lobby's political muscle." The sprawl industry would get access to 43 percent of the state's developable land. State permits would have to be granted if applications were not finalized in 90 days. Developers and builders could overwhelm government agencies with applications and then automatically get permits after 90 days. Environmentalists screamed about scarce time for public reviews. The governor asserted that if development was prevented in the "wrong" places, it must be allowed in the "right" places, particularly for urban revitalization. True enough. But the second law did not exclude suburban sprawl development. Groups that had supported the first law had been hoodwinked by the backroom deals for the second law. They should have recalled that McGreevey had received more than $1.5 million from developers and builders to win the governorship; the head of the New Jersey Builders Association had said: "If we're public enemy number one, why does the governor keep taking our money?" Lesson: Follow the money.

A day before McGreevey's bill signing, Florida Governor and ex-developer Jeb Bush surprised many Floridians by vetoing a bill that critics had called the "Sprawl Forever Act." It would have cut local governments' ability to manage land use, eased rezoning of agricultural land for development, and gutted water regulations. It had been pushed through the legislature by the Florida Farm Bureau and other agriculture interests. Perhaps they forgot a 2001 statewide poll that found 60 percent of voters believed sprawl, uncontrolled growth and overdevelopment were out of control and needed to be regulated. As in New Jersey, many environmental and smart growth groups loudly urged the governor to veto the bill. In this case, local government groups, the state land management agency, and many newspapers, supported a veto. Why no support for the bill by Florida's powerful sprawl industry? The logical answer is a concern about higher prices for farmland and anticipation of a public backlash because of the strong, broad opposition to the bill, especially by local governments. Lesson: With a broad coalition, smart growth can win, especially if the sprawl lobby is not in the fight.

This tale of two governors showed that legislators in Florida and New Jersey easily passed bills that did not serve smart growth values or the public interest; they served sprawl business interests and sources of campaign contributions.

SPRAWL BENEFITED FROM THE ENVIRONMENTAL ETHOS.

Smart growth's most fanatic opponents see environmentalism as anti-sprawl; they are obsessed with property rights and see "enviro-communists trying to get control of your land." They see no need for land preservation. As sprawl shill Doug Kendall said: "When over 95 percent of the surface area of this country is still undeveloped…there is no crisis." That dangerous land-lie does not stop sprawl shill-meister Randal O'Toole being against wind farms and solar power alternatives to fossil fuels because they require so much land. To review right-wing thinking: We have plenty of land for more sprawl and so much that we do not need any land conservation, but not enough for wind and solar renewable energy. Got that?

If there is a *Guinness Book of Records* category for great paradoxes, here is a winner. The environmental movement inadvertently promoted sprawl. Through books, crusades, disasters, crises, laws and regulations, Earth Day celebrations, ecology topics in school curricula, and pop culture "stars" promoting environmental causes, most Americans became environmentally conscious. But when millions of "environmentalists" bought into sprawl they individually and collectively destroyed the natural world they valued. This mass ironic behavior was the Great Sprawl Paradox. Developers found it easy to sell "greener, cleaner and safer" suburban housing in contrast to "dirty, unsafe" cities. If "nature" was worth protecting and saving, then why not move into it and live the good life? People idealized a greener, rural setting but with urban salaries to afford a consumer lifestyle. But large homes on large lots in "the country" do not protect and preserve the natural environment in its highest quality, biologically diverse state. Nor should use of green building methods calm the conscience of those building and buying super-size houses. Large house size offsets the environmental benefits of green building and is as hypocritical as seeking "fuel-efficient" SUVs.

On the Delmarva Peninsula between the Chesapeake Bay and the Atlantic Ocean, six Maryland towns with an "everyone-knows-everyone" culture are facing a 170 percent increase in population as sprawl subdivisions and strip malls quickly suck up farmland. Retirees and baby boomers escaping Baltimore, Washington, D.C., and Philadelphia smother the beaches, rivers, wildlife, and forests that attract them. Chestertown Mayor Margo G. Bailey said she "was absolutely flabbergasted at the uniform monotony" of new "soulless" sprawl homes. "It's absolutely dreadful. It has nothing to do with this place." So much for Maryland smart growth.

Too few Americans understand the "tragedy of the commons" that results when many people do what would be inconsequential if just a few people did it. You walk in a park and see an area of beautiful flowers and pluck just one. One less flower will not matter. But if countless others also pluck a flower the scene is destroyed. When hordes of people move to rural areas, boondocks become blandburbs. When everyone gets everywhere by car, roads become hell. As *Washington Post* columnist E. J. Dionne Jr. said in 1999: "When so many people make the same decision, the suburban dream gives way to those choked roads, crowded schools and the loss of the very green spaces that inspired the journey beyond city limits." Americans seem to be time-blind to patterns and consequences of mass behavior until they personally suffer and hope that government will come to the rescue.

When environmentalists woke up to the sprawl blitzkrieg they latched onto land preservation to limit sprawl development and urban revitalization to lure people back to cities. They also helped create the smart growth movement because "back to nature" had turned into "buy sprawl." Smart growth was also a backdoor way to address population growth, especially for the Sierra Club. On the political left, liberals must understand that even with smart growth the nation cannot tolerate continued high population growth through illegal immigration. Conservatives have a bigger problem; they want to control illegal immigration but not continued sprawl. The sane strategy is to better control both land use and illegal immigration.

It would help if all professed environmentalists rejected sprawl. Joining environmental organizations, giving money to environmental causes, buying green products, and supporting land preservation may do good and feel good. But the higher moral and social responsibility is to oppose sprawl, automobile addiction, and gluttonous land consumption by one's choice of housing.

The Great Sprawl Paradox II is that the smart growth movement cannot succeed if it overemphasizes urban revitalization and open space preservation. Urban revitalization cannot save the country from continued sprawl, because so many people need homes, and want them in a suburban location. And too much new housing in cities is for the affluent. Land preservation by itself is no cure-all. There is not enough money in the universe to buy enough land to curb sprawl, nor can conservation easements do the job. Moreover, developers have learned to co-opt farmland preservation programs. The Pittsburgh Tribune-Review revealed in July 2004 how two Pennsylvania laws designed to stop sprawl and preserve farmland had become tools for developers to legally escape millions of dollars in property taxes. Fewer than 6 percent of Allegheny County land labeled as farm or forest was actually owned by farmers. One developer was saving $48,054 in annual property taxes. Penn State farm economist Stamford Lembeck summed it up: "Purely and simply, what we're seeing here is a subsidy for developers."

Environmental conscience does not curb sprawl. Need proof? The past 25 years or more of a strong environmental ethic did not put a dent in sprawl. The primary marketing of smart growth should be about better homes and communities. Ninety percent of Americans believe that economic growth and protecting the environment are fully compatible. But most people "drive the jive" rather than "walk the talk." They need to admit that economic growth driven by car-centric sprawl is bad for the environment.

SOME CONSERVATIVES OPPOSE SPRAWL.

Hardly heard in the national squealing about sprawl and smart growth are Republicans and conservatives who see sprawl negatively. Too few people know about the REP America group, the national grassroots organization of Republicans for Environmental Protection, faithful believers in the conservation legacy of Teddy Roosevelt. Martha Marks, its President, made the case against sprawl in 2002. She said "people who consider themselves conservatives should fight sprawl whenever and wherever it raises its ugly head…because sprawl is harming our country. …Sprawl has been slowly, quietly and mercilessly undermining our families, our communities and the very character of our country." No left-wing liberal could say it better.

Marks' anti-sprawl position was based on: concern for future generations; belief that "individual freedom is bound at the hip with responsibility" and limits land use; prudence to not ruin natural resources and not build in the path of natural hazards; and "piety towards nature" that supports land and natural habitat conservation. Marks acknowledged that "it's up to us conservatives – who say we care about family life and communities – to insist that government stop doing the things that are having such a negative impact on our country." She also made the case that "sprawl is not the result of market forces, but of poorly thought out" government policies that have "led to a sprawl-prone society" and "the often-dysfunctional society we know today. …I believe that ending sprawl is worth the doing. It would be a sign of how mature our society has become if we could say, 'Enough already!' … and really mean it."

Colorado REP America member John Hereford wrote in 2004 that the Republican Party "has shifted from its conservation and environmental roots." The GOP's opposition to "sensible land-use planning" was noted, even though a growing number of self-described conservatives "worry greatly about the impact of sprawl and bad planning on our community, our values and spiritual integrity." "Moderates are not voicing their opinions on these issues in sufficient strength or at sufficient volume to neutralize the more vocal and significantly better-organized ideological wing of the party," he said. Exactly the problem – right-wing sprawl shills do not represent all conservatives, yet the news media use them out to balance the views of smart growth advocates.

Also in 2004, columnist Froma Harrop wrote about sprawl in Southern states and how "Southerners are paralyzed by their conservative ideology. …When alarmed citizens bring up land-use planning, developers speak darkly of government bureaucrats stomping on property rights." She correctly observed that "developers want matters of land-use planning sent down, down, down to the lowest level of government. Real-estate interests know they can have their way with weak local officials." They get their way with money.

A bi-partisan smart growth movement must help moderate, environmentally responsible conservatives get more visibility to show the nuttiness of extremist conservatives and dampen their influence. In 2004, Tom DeWeese of the American Policy Center said that it was not enough to fight smart growth: "If you want to keep your guns, your property, your children and your God...if you love liberty... Then Sustainable Development is your enemy!" Such people have no interest in saving land, water, natural habitats, forests and other resources for future generations, which is what sustainable development and smart growth aim for.

A REVOLUTION IN THE HOUSING MARKET IS OVERDUE.

On a road trip across the country not so long ago the celebrated writer William Gibson, creator of the term cyberspace, looked out the car window at the passing scene and remarked "We're in something here and it's out of control." More Americans need to see sprawl truth.

Fighting sprawl is one thing, but the extremist Earth Liberation Front is a domestic eco-terrorist effort that uses vandalism and arson against suburban development that destroys wetlands, scenic areas, and just greenspace. According to the FBI, there were 46 such attacks in 2000, and 59 in 2003. The group said "urban sprawl has become a central issue in the struggle to protect the earth." It targets McMansions and SUVs. Alas, the group does not seem to differentiate between sprawl and smart growth.

Sprawl shills and supporters pay attention. People can be – and I am – anti-sprawl and pro-growth, pro-development, and pro-housing. I do not claim that HEALTHY PLACES are utopias or panaceas for all of society's ills or for all personal problems. Not all developers and home builders are sprawl hacks. Not all suburbanites are sedentary and socially isolated. Nor do I claim that all people go through the three stages of unhealthy sprawl life presented in Chapter 4: Suburban Blandness Syndrome, Sprawl Stress Syndrome and Sedentary Death Syndrome. Nor do I claim that all people hate sprawl and want an alternative to it.

I do claim this. Building and seeking HEALTHY PLACES are noble and moral endeavors in this 21st century. No national crisis has stimulated a revolt against sprawl, nor is one likely. Smart growth needs market forces to turn the tide against sprawl. Tragically, in the sprawl culture people become accustomed to quality of life losses. "Busy-bee" lifestyles block awareness that prosperity might have been achieved without replacing quality with quantity, experience with stuff, conversation with communication, and scenic greenspace with development. In our sprawl culture people work like dogs, drive addictively, buy compulsively and don't connect blandburbs to lives becoming emptier and bodies growing fatter. Americans don't think about what might have been, might have been, without 50 years of sprawl. We need 50 years of increases in HEALTHY PLACES to improve our culture.

Thinking that suburban sprawl is a "necessary evil" in American society is half right. Evil? Yes. Necessary? No. And the same goes for automobile addiction and its flip-side sedentariness. Only a society obsessed with market success and consumption accepts such necessary evils.

There is cause for optimism. As more Americans benefit from living in HEALTHY PLACES, others will learn about those benefits and lead the "revolution" to replace new sprawl with HEALTHY PLACES. The sprawl glass may still look full, but if it is upset a little, it will quickly empty because of the unseen hole in the bottom. When more Americans become aware of sprawl's penalties, acceptance of sprawl will dissipate. A market equalizer will be born.

The *Sprawl Kills* "idea virus" must spread like wildfire so that consumers "catch" the bug and reject blandburbs and condemn sprawl politics. Then the HEALTHY PLACES idea virus must spread as the solution to sprawl. There are many sprawl haters to spread the first virus, but few residents of HEALTHY PLACES to spread the second. Twenty-first century pioneers will seek the American Dream Community and demand the end to sprawl politics. Three segments of the population have a natural preference for HEALTHY PLACES. They have been defined mostly through values, lifestyle, and consumption.

In *The Cultural Creatives: How 50 Million People Are Changing the World*, a sub-culture was identified whose values and preferred lifestyles mesh very well the themes of *Sprawl Kills*. "They want to stay far away from tract houses in treeless suburbs," said the authors. About a quarter of adults were identified as cultural creatives who feel alienated from the dominant culture – the sprawl culture – which measures success by money, possessions and power. They care about rebuilding their neighborhoods and communities, want to be involved in creating a new and better way of life in our country, want access to walking and biking paths, and are deeply concerned about destroying our natural environment. Rather than being individualistic and self-concerned they are community centered. Subsequently, marketing research identified cultural creatives as people with Lifestyles of Health and Sustainability; they were estimated at about 30 percent of adults, or over 60 million consumers.

In contrast to the isolationist "cocooning" in blandburbs, is the notion of "hiving." Hiving refers to a desire for more engagement with community and neighbors, consistent with HEALTHY PLACES. Yankelvich Inc. announced in August 2003 that 64 percent of people preferred hiving, compared to 33 percent preferring the isolation of a cocoon. The president of the company said that "people see more value in community." "Hivers" need HEALTHY PLACES.

Some people drive trends, shape public opinion, spread idea viruses, and determine tipping points. According to The Influentials, about 10 percent of the population has remarkable influence. They have values and preferences that should make them supporters of HEALTHY PLACES. Seventy-four percent believe that their community is an important part of "who I am," and 84 percent believe that they have responsibilities to their neighbors and community beyond what is required by law. They value more family time, take advantage of social capital and practice civic engagement, and are receptive to active living, shopping in their local community and in smaller stores. Among serious problems for their children and grandchildren, congestion of cities and highways was the third highest at 83 percent.

So, besides the direct evidence presented earlier that at least one-third of Americans want HEALTHY PLACES, many of the cultural creatives, hivers, and influentials are potential consumers of HEALTHY PLACES, but may not know it yet. Just beyond the intersection of housing, culture and consumption lies the tipping point for the smart growth movement.

A plethora of organizations passionately push their agendas. More of them should support smart growth. It's useful to recognize how HEALTHY PLACES connect to other issues of personal and social importance. You probably care about some of the following: family values, fighting crime, clean air and water, better schools, fighting government corruption, fighting corporate welfare, biodiversity, energy conservation, children's health, saving rural towns and culture, pedestrian safety, reducing overweight and obesity, fighting diabetes and heart disease, green buildings, excessive materialistic consumption, global warming, illegal immigration, fighting junk foods, civic engagement, entrepreneurial capitalism, pollution prevention, preventive health care, social equity, environmental justice, more local sports fields, preventing natural disasters, wetlands preservation, and fair competitive markets. Smart growth can help these and many other efforts. Past attempts to curb sprawl have failed because of too little mass support. Issue-linkage can attract countless people new to smart growth.

The fight against sprawl and for smart growth can unite Americans. As Ann Arbor Mayor John Hieftje observed: "Sprawl harms the business community as much as it does environmentalists, Republicans as much as Democrats, city folk as much as township residents. It is an issue that actually brings people together."

What must not be ignored is the undeniable consumer demand for something better and healthier than blandburbs. Now you know what that something is. The innovative developer Chris Leinberger proclaimed: "You don't mess with Mother Nature and you don't mess with Mother Market. The market is eventually going to get what it wants." It wants HEALTHY PLACES.

I look forward to writing about the fall of sprawl. The Greeks said "the peak is the moment of descent." Reversal of fortune becomes clear when success has ended. The sprawl industry will know that it has peaked when smart growth reaches the tipping point, when it is common knowledge that sprawl kills, and common for Americans to seek HEALTHY PLACEs.

More people must wake from their sprawl stupor and realize that they have been sedated by the sprawl culture and harmed by the sprawl industry and its shills. More people must become outraged about sprawl and the culture of consumption it drives. A war rages in the United States, the people against the tyranny of relentless, runaway suburban sprawl. Silence supports sprawl. You are needed. Feel the sprawl rage. Just say no to sprawl. Don't sprawl yourself short.

Seek a HEALTHY PLACE. Do not be time blind. As land runs out, so does time. See sprawl's inevitable consequences. Be smart. Be demanding. Most of all, be healthier.

Do your part. Spread the word. Sprawl kills.

BIBLIOGRAPHY

Most people in today's world find it much more convenient to get information and publications on the Internet rather than in libraries. In the Internet age, providing exhaustive footnotes and references is no longer effective, especially for a general audience. My goal is to inform and assist readers, not to look scholarly. Nearly all of the source materials for the information provided can be found on the Internet. I urge readers to use the Google.com search engine to find sources and additional materials on any topic covered in this book. It is time to recognize the universal use of the Internet for research and information collection.

There are also Internet sites for nearly all the HEALTHY PLACES mentioned. Just use the name of the development in a search engine and you can locate the home page as well as many other materials on the community.

To help readers pursue topics presented in this book, I provide the following list of Internet sites, along with a comment on the particular usefulness of the site. The numbers given in parentheses refer to the chapters that used the Internet site as a source of information. The subsequent section provides a list of recommended books that also served as general sources.

INTERNET SITES

A

http://www.aarp.org/health-active/walking; this AARP site offers good materials on walking (4)

http://www.abag.ca.gov/planning/smartgrowth; the site of the Association of Bay Area Governments offers some excellent materials on smart growth (2, 3, 6)

http://www.aboutplanning.org/; a treasure of materials on planning (1-8)

http://www.activeliving.org/; the Active Living Network site offers information on the health and active living aspect of communities (4)

http://www.activelivingbydesign.org/; the Active Living by Design program site provides excellent information, especially web links and access to publications (4)

http://www.alpes.ws/; good information on the health and physical activity connection (4)

http://www.americantrails.org; the best site on trails, including their health benefits (4)

http://www.americawalks.org/; the America Walks site promotes walkable communities (4, 6)

http://www.atlreg.com/qualitygrowth/qualitygrowth.html; the Atlanta Regional Commission has various materials on quality (smart) growth topics (2, 6)

B

http://www.bettertogether.org/; to get information on social capital use this site (2- 4)

http://www.bikefed.org/; the National Center for Bicycling and Walking site is a first rate source of information on many aspects of active living (4)

http://www.biodiversitypartners.org/; information on the impact of sprawl on biodiversity is available (2, 4)

http://www.brook.edu/es/urban/urban.htm; the Brookings Institute Center for Urban and Metropolitan Policy offers many first rate reports on growth management issues (2, 3, 6, 8)

C

http://www.calthorpe.com; Calthorpe Associates is a leading company doing mixed-use community design; the site has useful materials, some on projects (2, 3, 6)

http://www.carfree.com/; good source of information about alternatives to cars (2-4)

http://www.cdc.gov/healthyplaces/default.htm; this CDC offers excellent materials on the design and benefits of HEALTHY PLACES (2-4)

http://www.cdc.gov/nccdphp/dnpa/physicalactivity.htm; this CDC site is a good way to access this agency's materials on the benefits of physical activity (4)

http://www.charrettecenter.com/; if you are interested in community based planning and design, this site is useful (7)

http://www.charretteinstitute.org; the National Charrette Institute site is essential for learning more about this process (7)

http://www.citistates.com; the Citistates Group site offers good access to growth management information (1, 2, 3)

http://www.cnu.org/; the Congress for the New Urbanism site is very useful (2, 3, 8)

http://www.commpres.env.state.ma.us; the community preservation site of the state of Massachusetts contains many excellent materials (2, 3, 6, 7)

http://www.communityrights.org; the site of Community Rights Counsel, a public interest law firm, addresses property rights issues raised by critics of smart growth (1)

http://www.communityschools.org/; the site of the Coalition for Community Schools offers useful information (3)

http://www.culturalcreatives.org; the key site for learning about cultural creatives (8)

http://www.cultural-creatives.net; a site for becoming active in the cultural creatives subculture (8)

http://www.cyburbia.org; this is a must use site for all kinds of information related to this book (1-8)

D

http://www.davidsuzuki.org/Climate_Change/Sprawl.asp; The Driven to Action – Stopping Sprawl in Your Community materials are aimed at the anti-sprawl effort in Canada, but others will find the materials useful. (8)

http://www.designadvisor.org/home.html; the focus is on affordable housing, and there is good information and images on mixed use and other community design features (3, 6)

http://www.designcollective.com/; one of the premier design companies offers information on many of their projects (3, 6)

http://www.design.ncsu.edu:1820/cud/; an excellent source of information about universal design (6)

http://www.dot.ca.gov/hq/MassTrans/tod.htm; this site offers a number of fine reports on transit oriented development (3, 6)

http://www.doverkohl.com; the Dover, Kohl & Partners company is a leading company doing mixed-use community design; the site has considerable useful information, including some projects (2, 3, 6)

http://www.dpz.com; the Duany Plater-Zyberk & Company is probably the leading firm doing true sprawl alternative community design; it has much useful information, some on specific projects (2, 3, 6)

E

http://www.envisionutah.org/; the Envision Utah public private partnership is excel-

lent, and many useful materials are provided (2, 3, 5, 7)
http://www.epa.gov/livability/; this is EPA's smart growth page and is a great resource (2-6, 8)

F

http://www.farmland.org; the site of American Farmland Trust has excellent materials on sprawl's impact on farmland (1, 2)
http://www.fitness.gov; the President's Council on Physical Fitness and Sports site has many useful documents on the benefits of active living (4)
http://www.fundersnetwork.org/; the Funders' Network for Smart Growth and Livable Communities site provides excellent documents on many aspects of smart growth (2-7, 8)

G

http://www.ggw.org/RochesterEnvironment/urban.htm; the Dumb-Growth Cycle is available on this site (2-4)
http://www.growingsensibly.org/; the Campaign for Sensible Growth provides great materials on what is going on in the Chicago metropolitan area (2, 3, 6)

H

http://www.hadd.com; the site of Homeowners Against Deficient Dwellings provides consumer protection information on corruption and sleazy practices by developers and builders (1)
http://www.harmonyinstitute.org/; this unusual group focuses on better integration of environmental and community values (3, 4, 6)
http://www.hbns.org/; the site of the Health Behavior News Service designed primarily for health journalists offers some excellent materials (4)
http://www.herl.uiuc.edu/; the site for the Human-Environment Research Laboratory has considerable information on the benefits of green infrastructure (4)
http://www.housingzone.com/pb/; not an easy site to use, but it offers good material on the home building and sprawl industry and access to Professional Builder magazine contents (1)

F

http://i4sd.org; the site of the Florida House Institute for Sustainable Development has materials on community based planning and design (7)
http://www.impactfees.com; good information on impact fees (1, 5, 8)

J

http://www.jointventure.org/resources/photosims/sim_index.html; provides great computer simulations on community design, including those given in this book (7)

L

http://www.lesstraffic.com/; very good source of information on traffic calming (6)
http://www.lohasjournal.com; a site to access information on people with Lifestyles of Health and Sustainability (8)

M

http://www.metrocouncil.org; Minnesota's Metropolitan Council is arguably the best regional planning organization in the nation and this site has many useful materials, but it takes some searching (6)
http://www.mlui.org/index.asp; the Michigan Land Use Institute site offers very useful materials (1, 2, 3, 6,)
http://www.mhc.gov/papers.html; has a number of reports on connections between housing and sprawl and smart growth (2, 4, 6)

N

http://www.nasites.com/collier_character/image_survey_results.asp; the Collier County Image Survey is available here (7)

http://www.nationalgeographic.com/earthpulse/sprawl/us.html; this high-tech site provides an interactive opportunity to learn the basics about community design (7)

http://www.nationaltrust.org/; the National Trust for Historic Preservation site has very good materials on smart growth and saving smaller schools (3, 6)

http://www.ncppa.org/; the National Coalition for Promoting Physical Activity site provides access to many useful materials on the health and active living benefit (4)

http://www.newdream.org; the Center for a New American Dream site offers many useful writings (5)

http://www.newurbanism.org/pages/416429/index.htm; access to many materials on topics in this book (1-8)

http://www.newurbannews.com/; this is an invaluable site for materials and links (1-8)

http://www.nga.org; the National Governors Association site offers a number of reports on growth management and new community design and many other useful materials, many conceived and written by this author (1-8)

http://www.nrdc.org/cities/smartGrowth/default.asp; the smart growth page of the Natural Resources Defense Council's site offers some very useful materials (2, 3, 6)

http://www.nsbn.org/; site of the New Schools Better Neighborhoods organization offers good materials on the benefits of small schools (3, 5)

P

http://www.pedbikeimages.org; the Image Library provides over 2,500 categorized photographs illustrating community design features associated with smart growth (3, 6, 7)

http://www.pedestrians.org/; this is a great site for information on perils for pedestrians (4)

http://www.picturesmartgrowth.org; this is a remarkable site for seeing photographs of almost all aspects of smart growth and HEALTHY PLACES   (2, 3, 6)

http://www.placematters.com; an important site for materials on community based planning and design (7)

http://www.planetizen.com/; if you want to follow smart growth and related topics this site is worth looking at on a daily basis; it provides access to articles and reports published nationwide (1-8)

http://www.planneronline.homestead.com/NewPlanningMeridian.html; the Planner Online site offers a diverse range of materials on many topics covered in this book, including contrarian viewpoints (1-8)

http://www.plannersnetwork.org; the Planners Network represents a more socially conscious model for planning and this site has some excellent materials (1, 7)

http://www.plannersweb.com/sprawl/home.html; this is an incredibly useful site for tracking down many kinds of resources on sprawl and smart growth (1-8)

http://www.planning.org/index.html; the American Planning Association site is necessary to follow the national smart growth movement (1-8)

http://www.pps.org/; the Project for Public Spaces site is the best site for information on any aspect of public places in community design (3, 6)

http://www.preservenet.com/politics/NewUrb.html; this site provides many useful Internet links (1-8)

http://www.progress.org/sprawl/; the Sprawl Information Center provides good materials (1-6)

http://www.publichealthadvocacy.org;   the California Center for Public Health

Advocacy has good materials on health impacts of inactivity (4)

http://www.qualityplaces.marc.org/; this is a very useful site for pursuing resources on specific topics (2, 3, 6)

R

http://www.rep.org; this group represents moderate, environmentally conscious conservatives

S

http://www.saveourlandsaveourtowns.org; Tom Hylton's site offers writings on the sprawl issue and entices people to read his book (2, 3)

http://www.sflcv.org; this excellent site provides an interactive way of seeing the characteristics of different residential densities in San Francisco, and also a series of computer simulations of converting actual places into smart growth type areas (3, 5, 7)

http://www.sierraclub.org/sprawl/; the Sierra Club site on sprawl offers many useful materials (1, 3-6)

http://www.smallschoolsproject; a useful site for information on the benefits of small schools (5)

http://www.smartgrowth.org/; the site of the Smart Growth Network is first rate for current news (1-8)

http://www.smartgrowthamerica.com/; this is an essential site with first rate materials (1-8)

http://www.smartgrowthgateway.org; although conceived for New Jersey residents, it offers many useful materials on smart growth (2-8)

http://www.sprawlaction.org/; the Colorado Sprawl Action Center site provides a wealth of information, including excellent aerial photos of sprawl (3, 4, 6)

http://www.sprawl-busters.com/; this is the premier site on the anti-big box store movement (3)

http://www.sprawlcity.org/index.html; this site focuses on land consumption and the link to population growth (1, 2)

http://www.sprawlkills.com; my site offers my latest writings and opinions (1-8)

http://www.sprawlwatch.org/; the Sprawl Watch Clearinghouse provides many useful materials on sprawl and smart growth (1-8)

http://www.state.ri.us/dem/programs/bpoladm/suswshed/desmanul/toc.htm; this site of the Rhode Island Department of Environmental Management gives access to the South County Design Manual, one of the best reports done on alternatives to sprawl (3, 6)

http://www.sustainable.doe.gov/; the site of the Smart Communities Network offers good materials, especially the toolkit section that includes excellent materials on community based planning and design (7)

http://www.sustainable.org/; the Sustainable Communities Network site offers many materials on all aspects of community and smart growth (1-8)

http://www.sustainableloudoun.org/; although designed for northern Virginia citizens, it has many excellent documents (1, 2, 6)

T

http://www.tcrponline.org; the Transit Cooperative Research Program site offers many publications related to transit (3, 6)

http://www.terrain.org/unsprawl; the UnSprawl case studies offer details on some HEALTHY PLACES (2, 3, 6)

http://thecommunityguide.org/pa; excellent materials on the health benefits of physical activity are on this site (4)

http://www.tndhomes.com; provides excellent information on community design (2, 3, 6)
http://www.tndtownpaper.com/; this excellent site, among many useful materials, provides a list of HEALTHY PLACES with links to their Internet sites (2, 3, 8)
http://www.tpl.org/; the Trust for Public Land site is very good for information on the green and land conservation aspects of smart growth (3, 5, 8)
http://www.transact.org/; the Surface Transportation Policy Project site is the premier site for information on transportation issues relating to mobility choices and community design (2-6)
http://www.transittown.org; offers information on transit oriented design (3, 6)
http://www.transitvillages.org/pages/448644/index.htm; this is useful site for information on transit-friendly communities (3, 6)
http://www.trb.org/; the Transportation Research Board site is complex and difficult to use, but by using its search engine some excellent reports can be found (3, 4, 6)

U

http://www.urban-advantage.com/index.html; this is a wonderful site for photographs, computer simulations showing smart growth improvements, and links (3, 6, 7)
http://www.urbandesignassociates.com/index.html; this is one of the best community design companies and information on a number of places is provided (3, 6)

V

http://www.vtpi.org/; the Victoria Transport Policy Institute site provides a wealth of resources on all aspects of transportation (3-6)

W

http://www.walkable.org/; this is the premier site on walkable communities (3-6)
http://www.walkinginfo.org/; if you want information on walking and walkability, this site is great (3, 4, 6)

Z

http://www.zva.cc; site of Zimmerman/Volk Associates has materials on estimating the market for smart growth places (8)

BOOKS

A

Affluenza: The All-Consuming Epidemic, John De Graaf et al, 2001, Berrett-Koehler
A Better Place to Live: Reshaping the American Suburb, Philip Langdon, 1994,
    University of Massachusetts Press
*Asphalt Nation: How the Automobile Took Over America, and How We Can Take It
    Back,* Jane Holtz Kay, 1998, University of California Press

B

Better Not Bigger, Eben Fodor, 1999, New Society Publishers
Better than Well – American Medicine Meets the American Dream, Carl Elliott, 2003,
    W.W. Norton & Company
Bowling Alone: The Collapse and Renewal of American Community, Robert D.
    Putnam, 2001, Touchstone Books

C

Community and the Politics of Place, Daniel Kemmis, 1990, University of Oklahoma
    Press
Crabgrass Frontier – The Suburbanization of the United States, Kenneth T. Jackson,
    1985, Oxford University Press

The Complete Guide to Walking for Health, Weight Loss, and Fitness, Mark Fenton, 2001, The Lyons Press

The Cultural Creatives: How 50 Million People Are Changing the World, Paul H. Ray and Sherry Ruth Anderson, 2000, Harmony

F

Fast Food Nation: The Dark Side of the All-American Meal, Eric Schlosser, 2002, HarperCollins

Fortress America: Gated Communities in the United States, Edward J. Blakely, Mary Gail Snyder, 1997, Brookings Institute Press

G

The Geography of Nowhere, James Howard Kunstler, 1994, Touchstone Books

H

High and Mighty: SUVs – The World's Most Dangerous Vehicles and How They Got That Way, Keith Bradsher, 2002, PublicAffairs

Home from Nowhere, James Howard Kunstler, 1998, Touchstone Books

How Cities Work – Suburbs, Sprawl, and the Roads Not Taken, Alex Marshall, 2000, Univ. of Texas Press

I

The Influentials, Ed Keller and Jon Berry, 2003, The Free Press

L

The Last Landscape, William H. Whyte, 1968, Doubleday

Luxury Fever: Why Money Fails to Satisfy In an Era of Excess, Robert H. Frank, 1999, Free Press

N

The Next American Metropolis: Ecology, Community, and the American Dream, Peter Calthorpe, 1993, Princeton Architectural Press

P

The Paradox of Choice: Why More Is Less, Barry Schwartz, 2004, Ecco

Picture Windows – How the Suburbs Happened, Rosalyn Baxandall and Elizabeth Ewen, 2000, Basic Books

R

Refrigerator Rights: Creating Connections and Restoring Relationships, Will Miller and Glenn Sparks, 2002, Perigee

S

Save Our Land, Save Out Towns, Thomas Hylton, 2000, RB Books

Solving Sprawl: Models of Smart Growth in Communities Across America, F. Kaid Benfield et al, 2001, Natural Resources Defense Council

Suburban Nation: the Rise of Sprawl and the Decline of the American Dream, Andres Duany, Elizabeth Plater-Zyberk, Jeff Speck, 2000, North Point Press

T

The Tipping Point: How Little Things Can Make A Big Difference, Malcolm Gladwell, 2000, Little Brown and Company

W

Wanderlust – A History of Walking, Rebecca Solnit, 2000, Penguin Books

INDEX

New Urbanism 49, 66, 73, 85, 108, 298-299, 318, 342, 360, 364-365, 384